Medical Informatics and Data Analysis

Medical Informatics and Data Analysis

Editor

Pentti Nieminen

MDPI • Basel • Beijing • Wuhan • Barcelona • Belgrade • Manchester • Tokyo • Cluj • Tianjin

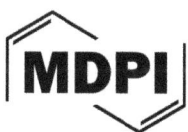

Editor
Pentti Nieminen
University of Oulu
Finland

Editorial Office
MDPI
St. Alban-Anlage 66
4052 Basel, Switzerland

This is a reprint of articles from the Special Issue published online in the open access journal *Applied Sciences* (ISSN 2076-3417) (available at: https://www.mdpi.com/journal/applsci/special_issues/Medical_Informatics_Data_Analysis).

For citation purposes, cite each article independently as indicated on the article page online and as indicated below:

LastName, A.A.; LastName, B.B.; LastName, C.C. Article Title. *Journal Name* **Year**, *Volume Number*, Page Range.

ISBN 978-3-0365-0098-0 (Hbk)
ISBN 978-3-0365-0099-7 (PDF)

Cover image courtesy of Pentti Nieminen.

© 2021 by the authors. Articles in this book are Open Access and distributed under the Creative Commons Attribution (CC BY) license, which allows users to download, copy and build upon published articles, as long as the author and publisher are properly credited, which ensures maximum dissemination and a wider impact of our publications.

The book as a whole is distributed by MDPI under the terms and conditions of the Creative Commons license CC BY-NC-ND.

Contents

About the Editor vii

Pentti Nieminen
Applications of Medical Informatics and Data Analysis Methods
Reprinted from: *Appl. Sci.* **2020**, *10*, 7359, doi:10.3390/app10207359 1

Hanan M. Hammouri, Roy T. Sabo, Rasha Alsaadawi and Khalid A. Kheirallah
Handling Skewed Data: A Comparison of Two Popular Methods
Reprinted from: *Appl. Sci.* **2020**, *10*, 6247, doi:10.3390/app10186247 7

Pentti Nieminen
Ten Points for High-Quality Statistical Reporting and Data Presentation
Reprinted from: *Appl. Sci.* **2020**, *10*, 3885, doi:10.3390/app10113885 21

Byung Mook Weon
Stretched Exponential Survival Analysis for South Korean Females
Reprinted from: *Appl. Sci.* **2019**, *9*, 4230, doi:10.3390/app9204230 39

Shun-Hsing Chen, Fan-Yun Pai and Tsu-Ming Yeh
Using the Importance–Satisfaction Model and Service Quality Performance Matrix to Improve
Long-Term Care Service Quality in Taiwan
Reprinted from: *Appl. Sci.* **2020**, *10*, 85, doi:10.3390/app10010085 49

Zhengdong Lei, Laura Fasanella, Lisa Martignetti, Nicole Yee-Key Li-Jessen and Luc Mongeau
Investigation of Vocal Fatigue Using a Dose-Based Vocal Loading Task
Reprinted from: *Appl. Sci.* **2020**, *10*, 1192, doi:10.3390/app10031192 67

Piotr Wąż, Agnieszka Bielińska and Dorota Bielińska-Wąż
Classification Maps in Studies on the Retirement Threshold
Reprinted from: *Appl. Sci.* **2020**, *10*, 1282, doi:10.3390/app10041282 83

Jihwan Park, Mi Jung Rho, Hyong Woo Moon and Ji Youl Lee
Castration-Resistant Prostate Cancer Outcome Prediction Using Phased Long Short-Term
Memory with Irregularly Sampled Serial Data
Reprinted from: *Appl. Sci.* **2020**, *10*, 2000, doi:10.3390/app10062000 99

Elias Moons, Aditya Khanna, Abbas Akkasi and Marie-Francine Moens
A Comparison of Deep Learning Methods for ICD Coding of Clinical Records
Reprinted from: *Appl. Sci.* **2020**, *10*, 5262, doi:10.3390/app10155262 111

Juan de la Torre, Javier Marin, Sergio Ilarri and Jose J. Marin
Applying Machine Learning for Healthcare: A Case Study on Cervical Pain Assessment with
Motion Capture
Reprinted from: *Appl. Sci.* **2020**, *10*, 5942, doi:10.3390/app10175942 131

Afnan M. Alhassan and Wan Mohd Nazmee Wan Zainon
Taylor Bird Swarm Algorithm Based on Deep Belief Network for Heart Disease Diagnosis
Reprinted from: *Appl. Sci.* **2020**, *10*, 6626, doi:10.3390/app10186626 159

Daniel Clavel, Cristian Mahulea, Jorge Albareda, and Manuel Silva
A Decision Support System for Elective Surgery Scheduling under Uncertain Durations
Reprinted from: *Appl. Sci.* **2020**, *10*, 1937, doi:10.3390/app10061937 . . . . **179**

Christian Mata, Joaquín Rodríguez, Gilberto Ochoa-Ruiz
A Prostate MRI Segmentation Tool Based on Active Contour Models Using a Gradient
Vector Flow
Reprinted from: *Appl. Sci.* **2020**, *10*, 6163, doi:10.3390/app10186163 . . . . **201**

Martín Hernández-Ordoñez, Marco Aurelio Nuño-Maganda, Carlos Adrián Calles-Arriaga, Abelardo Rodríguez-León, Guillermo Efren Ovando-Chacon, Rolando Salazar-Hernández, Omar Montaño-Rivas and José Margarito Canseco-Cortinas
Medical Assistant Mobile Application for Diabetes Control by Simulating a Compartmental Model
Reprinted from: *Appl. Sci.* **2020**, *10*, 6846, doi:10.3390/app10196846 . . . . **223**

About the Editor

Pentti Nieminen is a senior scientist at the University of Oulu. He completed his Ph.D. degree in 1996 and is employed as professor emeritus in medical informatics and data analysis at the University of Oulu. He has worked over 40 years as an academic teacher in knowledge management and data analysis. Much of his teaching and research work has been conducted within the following fields: biostatistics, data analysis methods in health care and medicine, data informatics, statistics in scientific journals, statistical modeling, publications, bibliometrics, information retrieval, and educational practices in teaching scientific research and communication. To date, he has published over 240 scientific articles. His current research projects include studies of statistical intensity, statistical reporting, and quality of data presentation in medical articles. His goal is to improve the quality of published research papers and thus to contribute to societal welfare and human well-being through his experience in data analysis. Outside of professional interests, he enjoys orienteering, hiking, and traveling.

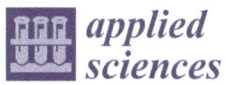

Editorial

Applications of Medical Informatics and Data Analysis Methods

Pentti Nieminen

Medical Informatics and Data Analysis Research Group, University of Oulu, 90014 Oulu, Finland; pentti.nieminen@oulu.fi

Received: 14 October 2020; Accepted: 16 October 2020; Published: 21 October 2020

1. Introduction

The science of statistics contributes to the development and application of tools for the design, analysis, and interpretation of empirical medical studies. The development of new statistical tools for medical applications depends on the innovative use of statistical inference theory, good understanding of clinical and epidemiological research questions, and an understanding of the importance of statistical software. First, statisticians develop a method in response to a need felt in a particular field of the health sciences, after which the new method is disseminated in the form of presentations, reports, and publications. It is also necessary to develop tools for implementing the method: software and manuals. From this point onwards, the extent to which the procedure is adopted will depend on its usefulness. The broader introduction and acceptance of a new analysis method (as useful as the method might be) into medical and health care publications seems to require the method being incorporated into the standard statistical packages generally used by researchers. In addition, if readers do not understand the mathematics or reporting style, or if the conclusions have been drawn on the basis of advanced mathematics or computationally complex procedures not visible in the data (tables or graphs) presented, then clinicians may not be convinced of the results. The lead time from the description of a new technique to its entering into the practice of medical investigators is long [1].

Unsustainable promises and unfulfillable expectations should be avoided in the context of data mining and machine learning [2]. The broader introduction and expansion of a new analysis method to medical publication seems to require that the method helps to solve a data analysis problem, where basic statistical methods have not been useful or applicable. Simpler classical approaches can often provide elegant and sufficient answers to important questions.

This Special Issue on *Medical Informatics and Data Analysis* was an opportunity for the scientific community to present research on the application and complexity of data analytical methods, and to give insight into new challenges in biostatistics, epidemiology health sciences, dentistry, and clinical medicine. The 13 contributed articles belong to four broad groups: (i) basic statistical methods, (ii) data-oriented practical approaches, (iii) complex machine learning and deep learning predictive algorithms, (iv) medical informatics.

2. Basic Statistical Methods

All basic data analysis methods and multivariable techniques depend on assumptions about the characteristics of the data [3]. If an analysis is performed without satisfying these assumptions, incorrect conclusions may be made on the basis of erroneous results. A normal distribution of main outcome variables is a strong requirement in several statistical techniques and should be verified and reported. In their work, Hanan M. Hammouri and coworkers [4] compare the use of a *t*-test on log-transformed data and the use of a generalized linear model (GLM) on untransformed skewed data. Scientists in biomedical and psychosocial research need to deal with non-normal skewed data all the time. Hammouri et al. [4] present three examples with real-life data. Their findings show that the *t*-test with log transformation has superior performance over the GLM method for any data that are not normal and follow beta or gamma distributions. Alternatively, for exponentially distributed data, the GLM method has superior performance over the *t*-test with log transformation.

Several findings have demonstrated that too many medical articles do not provide a sufficiently clear, accurate, or complete account of what was done and what was found. In his article, *Ten Points for High-Quality Statistical Reporting and Data Presentation* [5], Pentti Nieminen proposes an applicable checklist for quickly testing the statistical reporting quality of manuscripts and published research papers. The developed instrument is applicable for a wide variety of medical and health care research forums, including both clinical and basic sciences. Editors and reviewers could use the short quality test proposed in this paper for deciding when the presentation in a manuscript is clearly inadequate. If the reviewer cannot find the basic information and description related to the data analysis, the reviewer does not need to read the whole article. After checking tables and figures and reading through the statistical analysis subsection in the methods section, the reviewer can reject the manuscript on good grounds. When the proposed simple quality test shows that the statistical reporting and data presentation are appropriate, the whole article needs to be read and further reviewed [5].

3. Data-Oriented Practical Approaches

Advances in health information technology are enabling a transformation in health research that could facilitate studies that were not feasible in the past, and thus, lead to new insights regarding health and disease. The extent to which new procedures are adopted will depend on their usefulness. It is important that new methods are applied on real data that arise in medical research. Special attention should be given to the practical aspects of analysis and the presentation of the results.

Byung Mook Weon [6] contributes to the Special Issue with applications of modelling life expectancy and population dynamics. The title of this nice piece of work is *Stretched Exponential Survival Analysis for South Korean Females*. The paper focuses on studying current trends of lifespan among South Korean females using modified survival curves. The study shows the quantitative and comparative evidence for a remarkable rapid increase in female lifespan in South Korea during three recent decades, from 1987 to 2016.

Long-term care (LTC) involves a variety of services designed to meet people's health or personal care needs during a short or long period of time. A paper authored by Shun-Hsing Chen, Fan-Yun Pa, and Tsu-Ming Yeh [7] includes an interesting review of different models and methods to examine long-term care service demands and satisfaction improvement. Using data from the older adult population in Taiwan ($n = 292$), this study demonstrates how two methods can be integrated to serve as a basis for decision makers to adjust LTC service quality design and improve care for older adults. The reproducibility of the proposed integration is easy.

Vocal fatigue may be experienced by any individuals during their lifetime, but it is more frequently encountered by professional voice users in occupational settings. Vocal fatigue increases vocal effort and decreases speaking stamina. Zhengdong Lei and co-authors [8] give in their contribution an extensive examination of the effect of vocal loading on a large number of voice measures and ratings in a small group of vocally normal young women. The novel aspect of the work is the use of vocal dosing as a criterion for performance. Their paper is rich with data, which provides relevant evidence about the acoustic and perceptual manifestations of vocal fatigue.

The paper *Classification Maps in Studies on the Retirement Threshold* by Agnieszka Bielinska and collaborators [9] is an example of a study about retirement age in Poland. The aim of this work is to present new classification maps in health research and to show that they are useful in data analysis. Groups of individuals and their answers to questions of expectations and worries related to the retirement threshold are analyzed. A statistical method, correspondence analysis, is applied for obtaining these maps. With the classification maps, it is possible to find subgroups of these individuals who answer in a similar way to the specific questions. In addition, the authors compare structures of the maps searching for factors such as gender, marital status, kind of work, and economic situation, which are essential at the retirement threshold.

4. Complex Machine Learning and Deep Learning Predictive Algorithms

During the recent decades, mathematical statisticians have introduced new data analysis methods marked by the rapid expansion of computing efficiency and the advancement in storage capabilities. Examples of these are machine learning and deep learning networks. Many computational methods lie at the nexus of mathematical, statistical, and computational disciplines. Statistical methods often employ approaches that glean predictive capability from diverse and enormous databases of information. Emerging complex computational methods can provide impressive prediction models. However, it is unclear how widely these methods are applied in different medical domains [10,11]. This Special Issue includes four articles that focus on these predictive methods.

It is difficult to predict a patient's outcome with serial data that is collected irregularly, including medications, treatments, and laboratory tests. Typical deep learning methods can be used to analyze serial data. However, they must be improved to handle irregularly sampled serial datasets. In their study, Park and colleagues [12] investigate the accuracy of the phased long-term short-term memory (phased-LSTM) deep learning method in the prediction of patients with prostate cancer who might have castration-resistant prostate cancer (CRPC). The authors found that the phased-LSTM model was able to predict the CRPC outcome with 91.6% and 96.9% using 120 and 360 days of data, respectively.

The paper *A Comparison of Deep Learning Methods for ICD Coding of Clinical Records* authored by Moons and colleagues [13] presents a survey of various deep learning methods for text classification in a hierarchical framework for the domain of medical documents. Methods based on exploiting the taxonomy structure and also flat methods are discussed. These methods are evaluated on publicly available datasets corresponding to ICD-9 and ICD-10 coding, respectively.

In their contribution, de la Torre and co-authors [14] demonstrate the particularities of applying machine learning techniques in the field of healthcare. They focus on cervical assessment, where the goal is to predict the potential presence of cervical pain in patients affected with whiplash diseases. Using a sample of 302 patients, they compared several predictive models, including logistic regression, support vector machines, k-nearest neighbors, gradient boosting, decision trees, random forest, and neural network algorithms.

Afnan M. Alhassan and Wan Mohd Nazmee Wan Zainon [15] present in their article *Taylor Bird Swarm Algorithm Based on Deep Belief Network for Heart Disease Diagnosis* an approach to classify medical data for medical decision making. The method uses a feature selection step, where a sparse Fuzzy-c-mean (FCM) approach is used to select the significant features. Then, the selected features are passed into a deep belief network, which is trained using the Taylor-based bird swarm algorithm. The result of the analysis shows that the method is a promising approach.

5. Medical Informatics

Medical informatics focuses on the information technology that enables the effective collection of data using technology tools to develop medical knowledge and to facilitate the delivery of patient medical care [16]. The goal of medical informatics is to ensure access to critical patient medical information at the precise time and place it is needed to make medical decisions. Medical informatics also focuses on the management of medical data for research and education. Three papers in this Special Issue present applications for clinical decision making.

Daniel Clavel and his co-authors [17] present a decision support system to organize and order possible surgeries. Their study has the potential to reduce the workload of the healthcare system in scheduling—which is very labor-intensive work. A heuristic algorithm is proposed and included in the decision support system. Different features are implemented in a software tool with a friendly user interface. A simulation comparison of the scheduling obtained using the approach presented in this paper and other similar approaches is shown and analyzed. In addition, the impact of the software tool on the efficiency and quality of surgical services is studied in one hospital setting.

In their paper, *A Prostate MRI Segmentation Tool Based on Active Contour Models Using a Gradient Vector Flow* [18], Joaquín Rodríguez, Gilberto Ochoa-Ruiz, and Christian Mata describe in a fully and detailed way a new GUI tool based on a semi-automated prostate segmentation. The purpose is to facilitate the time-consuming segmentation process used for annotating images in clinical practice. To support the efficiency of their method, the authors describe an experimental case.

The paper entitled *Medical Assistant Mobile Application for Diabetes Control by Simulating a Compartmental Model* authored by Hernandez-Ordonez and his coworkers [19] is very interesting and innovative. The authors present an application for mobile phones to assistant patients with type 1 diabetes. The proposed application is based on four mathematical models that describe glucose–insulin–glucagon dynamics using a compartmental model, with additional equations to reproduce aerobic exercise, gastric glucose absorption by the gut, and subcutaneous insulin absorption. Such developments are always welcome since diabetes became a civilization disease that affects a number of people every year.

Funding: This research received no external funding.

Acknowledgments: This issue would not be possible without the contributions of various talented authors, hardworking and professional reviewers, and the dedicated editorial team of *Applied Sciences*. Congratulations to all authors. I would like to take this opportunity to express my sincere gratefulness to all reviewers. The feedback, comments, and suggestions from the reviewers helped the authors to improve their papers. Finally, I thank the editorial team of *Applied Sciences*.

Conflicts of Interest: The author declares no conflict of interest.

References

1. Nieminen, P.; Miettunen, J.; Koponen, H.; Isohanni, M. Statistical methodologies in psychopharmacology: A review. *Hum. Psychopharmacol. Exp.* **2006**, *21*, 195–203. [CrossRef]
2. Caliebe, A.; Leverkus, F.; Antes, G.; Krawczak, M. Does big data require a methodological change in medical research? *BMC Med. Res. Methodol.* **2019**, *19*, 125. [CrossRef]
3. Indrayan, A. Reporting of Basic Statistical Methods in Biomedical Journals: Improved SAMPL Guidelines. *Indian Pediatr.* **2020**, *57*, 43–48. [CrossRef]
4. Hammouri, H.M.; Sabo, R.T.; Alsaadawi, R.; Kheirallah, K.A. Handling Skewed Data: A Comparison of Two Popular Methods. *Appl. Sci.* **2020**, *10*, 6247. [CrossRef]
5. Nieminen, P. Ten points for high-quality statistical reporting and data presentation. *Appl. Sci.* **2020**, *10*, 3885. [CrossRef]
6. Weon, B.M. Stretched exponential survival analysis for South Korean females. *Appl. Sci.* **2019**, *9*, 4230. [CrossRef]
7. Chen, S.H.; Pai, F.Y.; Yeh, T.M. Using the importance-satisfaction model and service quality performance matrix to improve long-term care service quality in Taiwan. *Appl. Sci.* **2020**, *10*, 85. [CrossRef]
8. Lei, Z.; Fasanella, L.; Martignetti, L.; Li-Jessen, N.Y.K.; Mongeau, L. Investigation of vocal fatigue using a dose-based vocal loading task. *Appl. Sci.* **2020**, *10*, 1192. [CrossRef] [PubMed]
9. Bielińska, A.; Bielińska-Waz, D.; Waz, P. Classification maps in studies on the retirement threshold. *Appl. Sci.* **2020**, *10*, 1282. [CrossRef]
10. Nieminen, P.; Kaur, J. Reporting of data analysis methods in psychiatric journals: Trends from 1996 to 2018. *Int. J. Methods Psychiatr. Res.* **2019**, *28*, e1784. [CrossRef] [PubMed]
11. Nieminen, P.; Vähänikkilä, H. Use of data analysis methods in dental publications: Is there evidence of a methodological change? *Publications* **2020**, *8*, 9. [CrossRef]
12. Park, J.; Rho, M.J.; Moon, H.W.; Lee, J.Y. Castration-resistant prostate cancer outcome prediction using phased long short-term memory with irregularly sampled serial data. *Appl. Sci.* **2020**, *10*, 2000. [CrossRef]
13. Moons, E.; Khanna, A.; Akkasi, A.; Moens, M.F. Article a comparison of deep learning methods for ICD coding of clinical records. *Appl. Sci.* **2020**, *10*, 5262. [CrossRef]

14. De la Torre, J.; Marin, J.; Ilarri, S.; Marin, J.J. Applying machine learning for healthcare: A case study on cervical pain assessment with motion capture. *Appl. Sci.* **2020**, *10*, 5942. [CrossRef]
15. Alhassan, A.M.; Wan Zainon, W.M.N. Taylor Bird Swarm Algorithm Based on Deep Belief Network for Heart Disease Diagnosis. *Appl. Sci.* **2020**, *10*, 6626. [CrossRef]
16. Melton, B.L. Systematic Review of Medical Informatics–Supported Medication Decision Making. *Biomed. Inform. Insights* **2017**, *9*, 117822261769797. [CrossRef] [PubMed]
17. Clavel, D.; Mahulea, C.; Albareda, J.; Silva, M. A decision support system for elective surgery scheduling under uncertain durations. *Appl. Sci.* **2020**, *10*, 1937. [CrossRef]
18. Rodríguez, J.; Ochoa-Ruiz, G.; Mata, C. A Prostate MRI Segmentation Tool Based on Active Contour Models Using a Gradient Vector Flow. *Appl. Sci.* **2020**, *10*, 6163. [CrossRef]
19. Hernández-Ordoñez, M.; Nuño-Maganda, M.A.; Calles-Arriaga, C.A.; Rodríguez-Leon, A.; Ovando-Chacon, G.E.; Salazar-Hernández, R.; Montaño-Rivas, O.; Canseco-Cortinas, J.M. Medical Assistant Mobile Application for Diabetes Control by Simulating a Compartmental Model. *Appl. Sci.* **2020**, *10*, 6846. [CrossRef]

Publisher's Note: MDPI stays neutral with regard to jurisdictional claims in published maps and institutional affiliations.

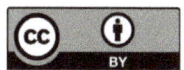

© 2020 by the author. Licensee MDPI, Basel, Switzerland. This article is an open access article distributed under the terms and conditions of the Creative Commons Attribution (CC BY) license (http://creativecommons.org/licenses/by/4.0/).

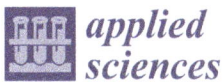

Article

Handling Skewed Data: A Comparison of Two Popular Methods

Hanan M. Hammouri [1,*], Roy T. Sabo [2], Rasha Alsaadawi [1] and Khalid A. Kheirallah [3]

1. Department of Mathematics and Statistics, Faculty of Arts and Science, Jordan University of Science and Technology, Irbid 22110, Jordan; alsaadawir@vcu.edu
2. Department of Biostatistics, School of Medicine, Virginia Commonwealth University, Richmond, VA 23298, USA; roy.sabo@vcuhealth.org
3. Department of Public Health, Faculty of Medicine, Jordan University of Science and Technology, Irbid 22110, Jordan; kakheirallah@just.edu.jo
* Correspondence: hmhammouri@just.edu.jo

Received: 26 July 2020; Accepted: 4 September 2020; Published: 9 September 2020

Abstract: Scientists in biomedical and psychosocial research need to deal with skewed data all the time. In the case of comparing means from two groups, the log transformation is commonly used as a traditional technique to normalize skewed data before utilizing the two-group t-test. An alternative method that does not assume normality is the generalized linear model (GLM) combined with an appropriate link function. In this work, the two techniques are compared using Monte Carlo simulations; each consists of many iterations that simulate two groups of skewed data for three different sampling distributions: gamma, exponential, and beta. Afterward, both methods are compared regarding Type I error rates, power rates and the estimates of the mean differences. We conclude that the t-test with log transformation had superior performance over the GLM method for any data that are not normal and follow beta or gamma distributions. Alternatively, for exponentially distributed data, the GLM method had superior performance over the t-test with log transformation.

Keywords: biostatistics; GLM; skewed data; t-test; Type I error; power simulation; Monte Carlo

---

1. Introduction

In the biosciences, with the escalating numbers of studies involving many variables and subjects, there is a belief between non-biostatistician scientists that the amount of data will simply reveal all there is to understand from it. Unfortunately, this is not always true. Data analysis can be significantly simplified when the variable of interest has a symmetric distribution (preferably normal distribution) across subjects, but usually, this is not the case. The need for this desirable property can be avoided by using very complex modeling that might give results that are harder to interpret and inconvenient for generalizing—so the need for a high level of expertise in data analysis is a necessity.

As biostatisticians with the main responsibility for collaborative research in many biosciences' fields, we are commonly asked the question of whether skewed data should be dealt with using transformation and parametric tests or using nonparametric tests. In this paper, the Monte Carlo simulation is used to investigate this matter in the case of comparing means from two groups.

Monte Carlo simulation is a systematic method of doing what-if analysis that is used to measure the reliability of different analyses' results to draw perceptive inferences regarding the relationship between the variation in conclusion criteria values and the conclusion results [1]. Monte Carlo simulation, which is a handy statistical tool for analyzing uncertain scenarios by providing evaluations of multiple different scenarios in-depth, was first used by Jon von Neumann and Ulam in the 1940s. Nowadays, Monte Carlo simulation describes any simulation that includes repeated random generation of samples and studying the performance of statistical methods' overpopulation samples [2]. Information obtained from random samples is used to estimate the distributions and obtain statistical properties for different situations. Moreover, simulation studies, in general, are computer experiments that are associated with creating data by pseudo-random sampling. An essential asset of simulation studies is the capability to understand and study the performance of statistical methods because parameters of distributions are known in advance from the process of generating the data [3]. In this paper, the Monte Carlo simulation approach is applied to find the Type I error and power for both statistical methods that we are comparing.

Now, it is necessary to explain the aspects of the problem we are investigating. First, the normal distribution holds a central place in statistics, with many classical statistical tests and methods requiring normally or approximately normally distributed measurements, such as t-test, ANOVA, and linear regression. As such, before applying these methods or tests, the measurement normality should be assessed using visual tools like the Q–Q plot, P–P plot, histogram, boxplot, or statistical tests like the Shapiro–Wilk, Kolmogrov–Smirnov, or Anderson–Darling tests. Some work has been done to compare between formal statistical tests and a Q–Q plot for visualization using simulations [4,5].

When testing the difference between two population means with a two-sample t-test, normality of the data is assumed. Therefore, actions improve the normality of such data that must occur before utilizing the t-test. One suggested method for right-skewed measurements is the logarithmic transformation [6]. For example, measurements in biomedical and psychosocial research can often be modelled with log-normal distributions, meaning the values are normally distributed after log transformation. Such log transformations can help to meet the normality assumptions of parametric statistical tests, which can also improve graphical presentation and interpretability (Figure 1a,b). The log transformation is simple to implement, requires minimal expertise to perform, and is available in basic statistical software [6].

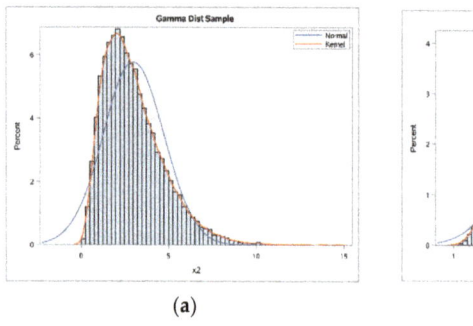
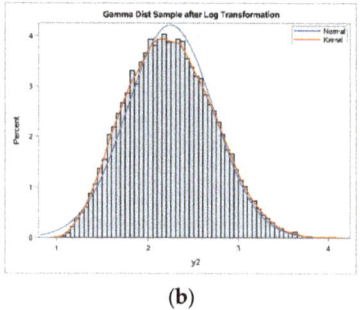

(a)   (b)

Figure 1. Simulated data from gamma distribution before and after log transformation. (a) The histogram of the sample before the application of log transformation with fitted normal and kernel curves; (b) The histogram of the sample after the application of log transformation with fitted normal and kernel curves.

However, while the log transformation can decrease skewness, log-transformed data are not guaranteed to satisfy the normality assumption [7]. Thus, the normality of the data should also be checked after transformation. In addition, the use of log transformations can lead to mathematical errors and misinterpretation of results [6,8].

Similarly, the attitudes of regulatory authorities profoundly influence the trials performed by pharmaceutical companies; Food and Drug Administration (FDA) guidelines state that unnecessary data transformation should be avoided, raising doubts about using transformations. If data transformation is performed, a justification for the optimal data transformation, aside from the interpretation of the estimates of treatment effects based on transformed data, should be given. An industry statistician should not analyze the data using several transformations and choose the transformation that yields the most satisfactory results. Unfortunately, the guideline includes the log transformation with all other kinds of transformation and gives it no special status [9].

An alternative approach is the generalized linear model (GLM), which does not require the normality of data to test for differences between two populations. The GLM is a wide range of models first promoted by Nelder and Wedderburn in 1972 and then by McCullagh and Nelder in 1989 [10,11]. The GLM was presented as a general framework for dealing with a variety of standard statistical models for both normal and non-normal data, like ANOVA, logistic regression, multiple linear regression, log-linear models, and Poisson regression. The GLM can be considered as a flexible generalization of ordinary linear regression, which extends the linear modeling framework to response variables that have non-normal error distributions [12]. It generalizes linear regression by connecting the linear model to the response variable via a link function, and by permitting the magnitude of the variance of each measurement to be a function of its expected value [10].

The GLM consists of:

i   A linear predictor
$$\eta_i = \beta_0 + \beta_1 x_{1i} + \cdots + \beta_p x_{pi} = X\beta, \tag{1}$$
where η_i, $i = 1, 2, \ldots, N$, is a set of independent random variables called response variables, where each η_i is a linear function of explanatory variables x_j, $j = 1, \ldots, p$.

ii A link function that defines how $E(y_i) = \mu_i$ which is the mean or expected value of the outcome y_i, depends on the linear predictor, $g(\mu_i) = \eta_i$, where g is a monotone, differentiable function. The mean μ is thus made a smooth and invertible function of the linear predictor:
$$\mu_i = g^{-1}(\eta_i), \tag{2}$$

iii A variance function that defines how the variance, $Var(y_i)$, depends on the mean $Var(y_i) = \phi V(\mu_i)$, where the dispersion parameter ϕ is a constant. Replacing the μ_i in $V(\mu_i)$ with $g^{-1}(\eta_i)$ also makes the variance a function of the linear predictor.

In the GLM, the form of $E(y_i)$ and $Var(y_i)$ are determined by the distribution of the dependent variable y_i and the link function g. Furthermore, no normality assumption is required [13,14]. All the major statistical software platforms such as STATA, SAS, R and SPSS include facilities for fitting GLMs to data [15].

Because finding appropriate transformations that simultaneously provide constant variance and approximate normality can be challenging, the GLM becomes a more convenient choice, since the choice of the link function and the random component (which specifies the probability distribution for response variable (Y) are separated. If a link function is convenient in the sense that the inverse-linked linear model of explanatory variables adheres to the support for the expected value for that outcome, it does not further need to stabilize variance or produce normality; this is because the fitting process maximizes the likelihood for the choice of the probability distribution for Y, and that choice is not limited to normality [16]. Alternatively, the transformations used on data are often undefined on the boundary of the sample space, like the log transformation with a zero-valued count or a proportion. Generalized linear models are now pervasive in much of applied statistics and are valuable in environmetrics, where we meet non-normal data frequently, as counts or skewed frequency distributions [17].

Lastly, it is worth mentioning that the two methods discussed here are not the only methods available to handle skewed data. Many nonparametric tests can be used, though their use requires the researcher to re-parameterize or reformat the null and alternative hypotheses. For example, The Wilcoxon–Mann–Whitney (WMW) test is an alternative to a *t*-test. Yet, the two have quite different hypotheses; whereas *t*-test compares population means under the assumption of normality, the WMW test compares medians, regardless of the underlying distribution of the outcome; the WMW test can also be thought of as comparing distributions transformed to the rank-order scale [18]. Although the WMW and other tests are valid alternatives to the two-sample *t*-test, we will not consider them further here.

In this work, the two-group *t*-test on log-transformed measures and the generalized linear model (GLM) on the un-transformed measures are compared. Through simulation, we study skewed data from three different sampling distributions to test the difference between two-group means.

2. Materials and Methods

Using Monte Carlo simulations, we simulated continuous skewed data for two groups. We then tested for differences between group means using two methods: a two-group *t*-test for the log-transformed data and a GLM model for the untransformed skewed data. All skewed data were simulated from three different continuous distributions: gamma, exponential, or beta distributions. For each simulated data set, we tested the null hypothesis (H_0) of no difference between the two groups means against the alternative hypothesis (H_a) that there was a difference between the two groups means. The significance level was fixed at $\alpha = 0.05$. Three sample sizes ($N = 25, 50, 100$) were considered. The Shapiro–Wilk test was used to test the normality of the simulated data before and after the application of the log transformation. We applied two conditions (filters) on the data: it was only accepted if it was not normal in the beginning, and then it became normal after log transformation. The only considered scenarios were the ones with more than 10,000 data sets after applying the two conditions and the number of accepted simulated samples = T. We chose T to be greater than 10,000 to overcome minor variations attributable changing the random seed in the SAS code.

Afterward, a *t*-test was applied to transformed data, while a GLM model was fitted to untransformed skewed data. We used the logit link function when the data were simulated from a beta distribution, and we used the log link function when the data were simulated from the exponential distribution or gamma distributions. In each case, a binary indicator of group membership was included as the only covariate.

The two methods were compared regarding Type I error, power rates, and bias. To assess the Type I error rate, which is the probability of rejecting H_0 when H_0 is true, we simulated the two samples from the same distribution with the same parameters. The same parameters guaranteed statistically equal variances between groups, and thus we used the equal-variance two-sample *t*-test. In addition, the GLM method with an appropriate link function was used. If the *p*-value was less than the two-sided 5% significance level, then H_0 was rejected and a Type I error was committed (since H_0 was true). The Type I error rate is then the number of times H_0 was rejected (K for *t*-test and K_{GLM} for GLM) divided by the total number of accepted simulated samples (K/T or K_{GLM}/T).

To assess the power rate, which is the probability of rejecting H_0 when H_a is true and it is the complement of the Type II error rate, we assumed different mean values for the two groups by simulating the two groups from distributions with different parameters. In this case, since the variances are functions of the mean parameter as well, the unequal variance two-sample *t*-test was used. In these situations, if the *p*-value was less than the 5% significance level, then we rejected H_0 knowing that H_a is true. If the *p*-value was larger than the significance level, we failed to reject H_0 and concluded that a Type II error was committed (because H_a was true). Then, the power rate is the number of times H_0 was rejected (K for *t*-test and K_{GLM} for GLM) divided by the total number of accepted simulated samples (K/T or K_{GLM}/T). Each case (sample size, distribution, mean relationship) was repeated five million times (denoted as T_0). The diagram of testing the Type I error algorithm is shown in Figure 2.

Regarding the difference estimates, other methods work on the response differently. The log transformation changes each response value, while the GLM transforms only the mean response through the link function. Researchers tend to transform back estimates after using a *t*-test with transformed data or after using GLM. We wanted to test which method gives a closer estimate to the actual difference estimates. So, while testing Type I error, we transformed back the estimates of the mean difference of the log-transformed data and the GLM-fitted data. Then we compared it with the means difference of the original untransformed data (which should be close to zero under (H_0)) to see which of the two methods gave mean difference estimates that are not significantly different from the estimates of the actual mean difference. We also compared the estimates of the difference of the standard deviations between the log-transformed and the original data under the assumption that H_0 is true (while testing Type I error), so we could use pooled standard deviation.

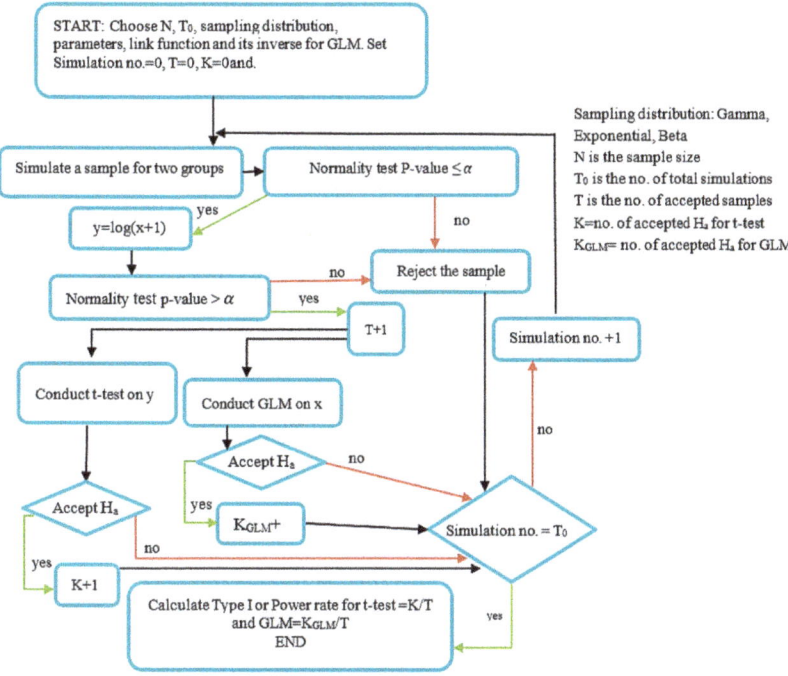

Figure 2. Simulation and Hypothesis Testing algorithm (for Type I error, we simulated data from distributions with the same means, and for power, we simulated data from distributions with different means).

In three applications to real-life data, we applied the two methods to determine whether the methods give consistent or contradicting results. By using visual inspection for this simulation study, Q–Q plots were used to test the normality of the data before and after the application of the log transformation to make sure that targeted variables were not normal before transformation and then became normal after transformation. After that, we used the t-test. Then, we used the bias-corrected Akaike information criterion (AICc) after fitting different continuous distributions to determine which distribution and link function to use with the GLM model [19,20]. Finally, we compared the results from both models. We generated all simulated data and performed all procedures using SAS codes. Moreover, the data that support the findings in the real-life applications of this study are openly available from the JMP software.

3. Results

3.1. Comparisons between the Two Methods

Comparisons were made between log-transformed t-tested data and original GLM-fitted data regarding the following aspects.

3.1.1. Comparison Regarding Type I Error Rates

Table 1 shows the parameters and the results of the alpha values for testing gamma-distributed data using the *t*-test and GLM, where α_1 represents the Type I error rate for the simulated data that was log-transformed and then tested using a two-group *t*-test assuming equal variances. Furthermore, α_2 represents the Type I error rate for the same groups of simulated data tested using GLM for gamma distribution with the log link function. Note that the Type I error rates for both methods are close to alpha = 0.05, but the *t*-test method is closer (0.0499 to 0.0503 in *t*-test data and 0.049 to 0.0577 in GLM data). In about 86% of the simulations, the *t*-test gave lower alpha values than the ones in the GLM. For the other 14% where the GLM gave lower Type I error, though, the *t*-test gave Type I error rates that were close to 0.05.

Table 1. Alpha values for gamma-distributed data tested using *t*-test and GLM.

Example	Sample Size	Parameters (Shape, Scale) [1]	*t*-Test Alpha (α1)	GLM Alpha (α2)	Diff. = α1 − α2
1	25	2, 1	0.0501	0.0490	0.0011
2	50	2, 1	0.0502	0.0499	0.0003
3	100	2, 1	0.0502	0.0499	0.0003
4	25	3, 2	0.0501	0.0526	−0.0024
5	50	3, 2	0.0502	0.0512	−0.0010
6	100	3, 2	0.0500	0.0507	−0.0007
7	25	5, 1	0.0501	0.0555	−0.0054
8	50	5, 1	0.0499	0.0526	−0.0027
9	100	5, 1	0.0500	0.0517	−0.0018
10	25	4, 0.25	0.0503	0.0549	−0.0046
11	50	4, 0.25	0.0503	0.0536	−0.0033
12	100	4, 0.25	0.0502	0.0516	−0.0014
13	25	6, 3	0.0501	0.0562	−0.0062
14	50	6, 3	0.0501	0.0533	−0.0031
15	100	6, 3	0.0500	0.0517	−0.0017
16	25	9, 0.5	0.0502	0.0577	−0.0075
17	50	9, 0.5	0.0500	0.0535	−0.0035
18	100	9, 0.5	0.0500	0.0516	−0.0016
19	25	3, 0.5	0.0501	0.0529	−0.0029
20	50	3, 0.5	0.0501	0.0514	−0.0012
21	100	3, 0.5	0.0501	0.0511	−0.0010

[1] The two simulated groups have the same parameters.

Table 2 contains summary information for the Type I error results for the gamma, exponential and beta distributed data. For the exponentially distributed data examples, the Type I error rates for the GLM across all parameter values were lower than the *t*-test rates in all of the settings, though the *t*-test Type I error rates did not exceed 0.0504 (0.0497 to 0.0504 for the *t*-test; 0.0367 to 0.0477 for the GLM). The *t*-test Type I error rates for beta distributed outcomes were lower than those from the GLM in all settings (0.0497 to 0.0511 for the *t*-test; 0.0518 to 0.0589 for the GLM). Figure 3 shows the Type I error for both methods, which are compared to 0.05 for the three distributions.

Table 2. Summary of Type I error rates for gamma, exponential and beta distributed data tested using the *t*-test and GLM.

Dist.	*t*-Test			GLM		
	Average α	Min α	Max α	Average α	Min α	Max α
Gamma	0.0501	0.0499	0.0503	0.0525	0.0490	0.0577
Exponential	0.0502	0.0497	0.0504	0.0432	0.0367	0.0477
Beta	0.0503	0.0497	0.0511	0.0544	0.0518	0.0589

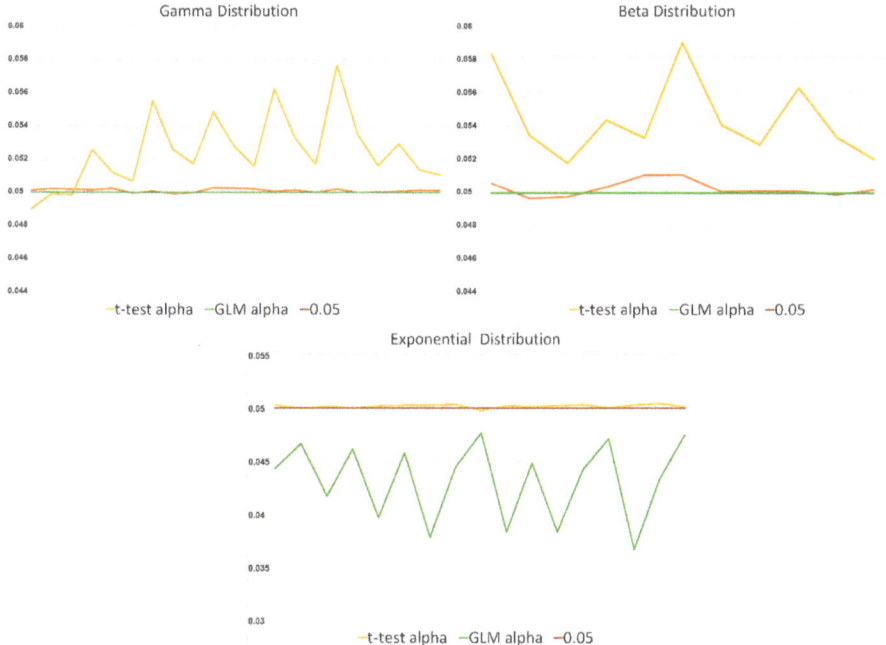

Figure 3. Type I error rates for the *t*-test and GLM compared to 0.05 for the three distributions.

3.1.2. Comparison Regarding Power

Table 3 presents the parameters and power results for the beta-distributed data. P_0 is the power values calculated for the two-group *t*-test using the information provided by knowing the two distributions and their parameters that are used in the simulation process, P_1 is the empirical power of the two-group *t*-test conducted on the log-transformed groups, and P_2 is the empirical power of the GLM-fitted data. Here we note that the GLM power rates were higher than those for the *t*-test with log transformation in 68% of the settings with absolute values of differences ranging from 0 to 0.0884. In 74% of the settings, the GLM power rates exceeded or equalled the calculated power, while the *t*-test power rates exceeded the calculated power in only 58% of the settings. Although the percentage of GLM power rates that exceeded or equalled the computed power was higher than the percentage of *t*-test power rates, the estimated power rates produced by the *t*-test were not that different to those that were produced by the GLM, with a difference of less than 0.1.

Table 4 contains summary information for the power results of gamma, exponential and beta distributed data tested using both methods. In about 86% of the exponentially distributed data examples, the power for the GLM was higher than that for the *t*-test, with absolute values of differences ranging from 0.001 to 0.108. Moreover, in 41% of the settings, GLM power rates exceeded or equalled the calculated power. Then again, in just 10% of the settings, *t*-test power rates exceeded the calculated power, while in the gamma-distributed data examples, the power for the GLM was higher in about 85% of the settings, with absolute values of differences ranging from 0.000 to 0.363. In addition, in 41% of the settings, GLM power rates exceeded or equalled the calculated power. Still, in just 15% of the settings, *t*-test power rates exceeded the calculated power. Figure 4 shows powers for both methods compared to the computed power rates for three distributions.

Table 3. Power values for beta distributed data tested using the *t*-test and GLM: P_0 is the power value of the two-group *t*-test calculated prior to the simulations, P_1 is the empirical power of the two-group *t*-test conducted on the log-transformed groups, and P_2 is the empirical power of the GLM-fitted data.

Example	Sample Size	Group1 Shape Parameters (α, β)	Group2 Shape Parameters (α, β)	Original *t*-Test Power (P_0)	*t*-Test Power (P_1)	GLM Power (P_2)	Power Diff. = $P_1 - P_2$
1	25	5, 3	5, 5	0.792	0.8217 [2]	0.8531 [2]	−0.0314
2	50	5, 3	5, 5	0.977	0.9815 [2]	0.9858 [2]	−0.0043
3	100	5, 3	5, 5	>0.999	0.9998 [2]	0.9999 [2]	−0.0001
4	25	2, 3	0.5, 0.5	0.224	0.1158	0.2042	−0.0884
5	25	2, 3	1, 3	0.75	0.7633 [2]	0.7532	0.0101
6	50	2, 3	1, 3	0.965	0.9552	0.9456	0.0095
7	25	2, 5	1, 3	0.108	0.1262 [2]	0.1142 [2]	0.0120
8	50	2, 5	1, 3	0.17	0.2071 [2]	0.1718 [2]	0.0352
9	25	2, 2	2, 5	0.967	0.9637	0.9739[2]	−0.0102
10	50	2, 2	2, 5	>0.999	0.9995 [2]	0.9997 [2]	−0.0002
11	100	2, 2	2, 5	>0.999	1.0000 [2]	1.0000 [2]	0.0000
12	25	2, 3	2, 2	0.371	0.3909 [2]	0.4318 [2]	−0.0409
13	50	2, 3	2, 2	0.645	0.6374	0.6723 [2]	−0.0350
14	100	2, 3	2, 2	0.912	0.8824	0.9021	−0.0197
15	25	2, 3	2, 5	0.586	0.5948 [2]	0.6321 [2]	−0.0373
16	50	2, 3	2, 5	0.876	0.8599	0.8788 [2]	−0.0189
17	100	2, 3	2, 5	0.993	0.9874	0.9903	−0.0029
18	25	1, 3	2, 2	0.985	0.9822	0.9828	−0.0005
19	50	1, 3	2, 2	>0.999	0.9998 [2]	0.9998 [2]	0.0000

[2] Power exceeds the original *t*-test expected power P_0.

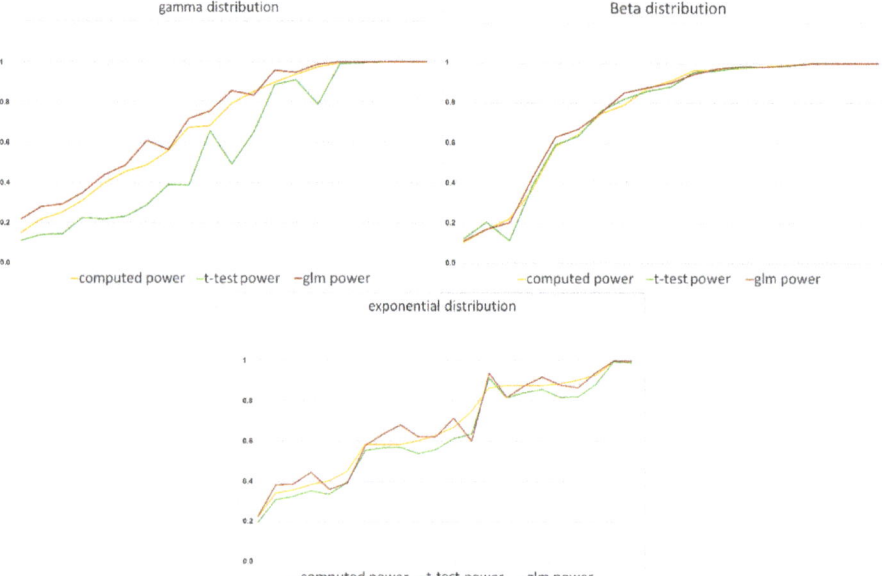

Figure 4. Power rates for the *t*-test and GLM compared to the computed power rates for the three distributions.

Table 4. Summary of power values for exponential and gamma-distributed data tested using the t-test and GLM: P_0 is the power value of the two-group t-test calculated prior to the simulations, P_1 is the empirical power of the two-group t-test conducted on the log-transformed groups, and P_2 is the empirical power of the GLM-fitted data.

Dist.	Difference between t-Test Power and Calculated Power			% ≥ P_0	Difference between GLM Power and Calculated Power			% ≥ P_0	Difference between GLM Power and t-Test Power		
	Average	Min	Max		Average	Min	Max		Average	Min	Max
Gamma	−0.106	−0.299	0.000	15%	0.033	−0.017	0.119	95%	0.138	0.000	0.363
Exponential	−0.040	−0.113	0.049	1%	0.005	−0.148	0.095	59%	0.044	−0.035	0.108
Beta	−0.003	−0.108	0.037	53%	0.009	−0.020	0.061	74%	0.012	−0.035	0.088

3.1.3. Comparison Regarding Estimates of Mean Differences and Standard Deviations

Next, we compared the estimates of the mean difference between the log-transformed data, the GLM-fitted data and the original untransformed data under testing Type I error, simulating every two groups from the same distribution to ensure the mean difference will be close to zero. For all the tested sampling distributions, we transformed back the estimates of the transformed mean differences and they were not significantly different from the actual mean differences according to p-values. On the contrary, we transformed back the estimates of the mean differences in the GLM according to the link function in each scenario and all were significantly different from zero. Table 5 presents the parameters and the back-transformed estimates' values of mean differences of log-transformed and GLM-fitted exponentially distributed data.

Table 5. Mean differences estimates' values for original, log-transformed and GLM-fitted exponential distributed data.

Example	Sample Size	Scale Parameter	Actual Difference	Back Transformed Trans. Mean Diff.	p-Value	Back Transformed GLM Mean Diff.	p-Value
1	25	1	0.0001	0.0131	1	1.0306	<0.0001
2	50	1	0.0011	0.0066	1	1.0135	<0.0001
3	25	1.5	0.0000	0.0202	1	1.0331	<0.0001
4	50	1.5	0.0004	0.0095	1	1.0149	<0.0001
5	25	2	−0.0003	0.0263	1	1.0363	<0.0001
6	50	2	−0.0002	0.0123	1	1.0162	<0.0001
7	25	3	−0.0004	0.0364	1	1.0396	<0.0001
8	50	3	0.0009	0.0086	1	1.0188	<0.0001
9	100	3	0.0002	0.0037	1	1.0084	<0.0001
10	25	2.5	−0.0004	0.0151	1	1.0381	<0.0001
11	50	2.5	0.0003	0.0073	1	1.0178	<0.0001
13	25	3.5	−0.0004	0.0151	1	1.0381	<0.0001
14	50	3.5	0.0006	0.0095	1	1.0195	<0.0001
15	100	3.5	−0.0023	0.0040	1	1.0083	<0.0001
16	25	6	−0.0002	0.0267	1	1.0425	<0.0001
17	50	6	0.0002	0.0131	1	1.0206	<0.0001
18	100	6	−0.0007	0.0130	1	1.0084	<0.0001

Finally, we compared the estimates of the standard deviation between the log-transformed data and the original skewed data. According to the resulting p-values, the estimates of the pooled standard deviation of the log-transformed data were significantly smaller than the estimates of the pooled standard deviation of the original skewed data in all the tested examples, as expected. Table 6 presents the parameters and the estimates values of standard deviation for the original and log-transformed gamma-distributed data. This component, however, was not provided by the GLM procedure.

Table 6. Standard deviation estimates for the original and log-transformed gamma-distributed data.

Example	Sample Size	Parameters (Shape, Scale)	Two-Group t-Test between SD(x_1) and SD(y_1)	
			Trans. Mean	Actual Mean
1	25	2, 1	0.8839	1.4017
2	50	2, 1	0.8767	1.3931
3	100	2, 1	0.87	1.3878
4	25	3, 2	1.0554	3.518
5	50	3, 2	1.0456	3.4678
6	100	3, 2	1.045	3.4814
7	25	5, 1	0.72	2.313
8	50	5, 1	0.7135	2.2487
9	100	5, 1	0.7116	2.2406
10	25	4, 0.25	0.4167	0.5086
11	50	4, 0.25	0.4088	0.4941
12	100	4, 0.25	0.4062	0.4898
13	25	6, 3	0.7747	7.6397
14	50	6, 3	0.7695	7.4241
15	100	6, 3	0.7657	7.4052
16	25	9, 0.5	0.487	1.567
17	50	9, 0.5	0.484	1.5254
18	100	9, 0.5	0.482	1.5037
19	25	3, 0.5	0.6107	0.8733
20	50	3, 0.5	0.6023	0.8558
21	100	3, 0.5	0.6003	0.8534

3.2. Application to Real-Life Data

In this section, we present three examples of real-life data that we imported from JMP software and tested using both of our studied methods.

3.2.1. The Lipid Data

We have real data from 95 subjects at a California hospital and are interested in whether triglyceride levels differ between patients considering their gender. The data were observed to be skewed and fitted to gamma distribution according to AICc values. The Q–Q plot and the frequency histogram of the untransformed and log-transformed lipid data are presented in Figure 5. Using the t-test after log transformation, we got a t-value of $t_{58.47} = 2.56$ with a p-value $= 0.0065$, indicating a significant difference between the two gender means, with the male triglyceride average larger than the average for females. An application of the GLM to the original data with gamma distribution and log link function yielded a p-value $= 0.006$. For this data, the results from the t-test of log-transformed data and the GLM both indicated evidence of a difference in triglyceride means between males and females.

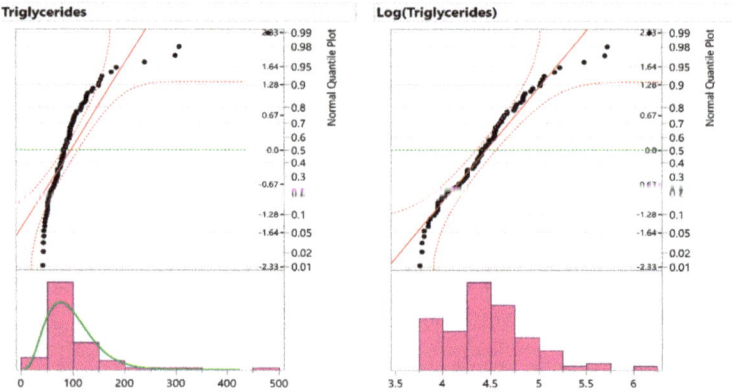

Figure 5. The normal Q–Q plots (up) for the Triglycerides variable before and after transformation and the frequency histogram of the Triglycerides variable on the left (down) is fitted with a gamma distribution (green).

3.2.2. The Catheters Data

We have real data from a sample of 592 children who received multiple attempts to start peripheral IV catheters in the inpatient setting. The data were obtained from a study conducted at two southeastern US hospitals from October 2007 through October 2008 [21]. We are interested in checking the difference in children's weight between children who lost IV vs. those who did not. The weight variable was skewed and fitted to a gamma distribution according to AICc values. The Q–Q plot and the histogram of the untransformed and log-transformed weight variable are given in Figure 6.

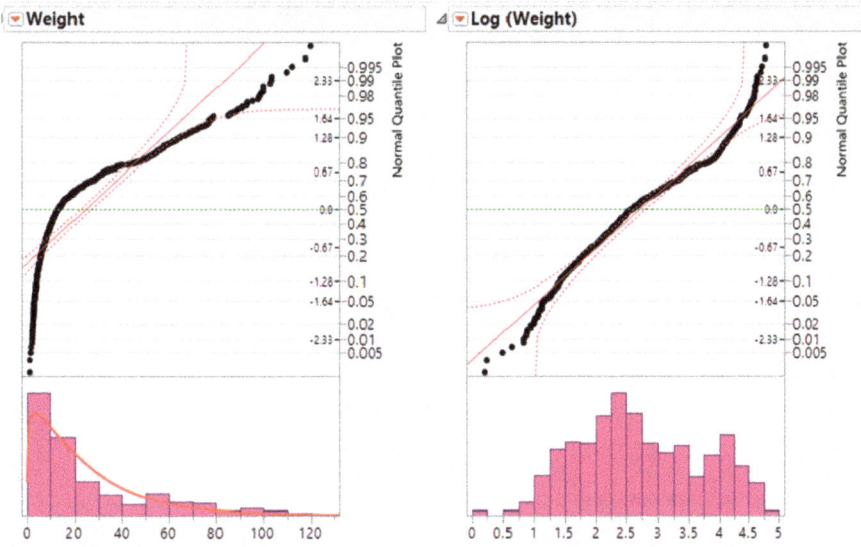

Figure 6. The normal Q–Q plots (up) for the weight variable before and after transformation and the frequency histogram of the weight variable on the left (down) fitted to a gamma distribution (red).

Then, the t-test after log transformation was used; we got $t_{394.29} = -3.39$ with a p-value $= 0.0004$, indicating a significant difference between the two groups; the average for the children who lost the IV weight was lower than that of the other group, who did not lose the IV. An application of the GLM to the original data with gamma distribution and log link function returned a p-value $= 0.0042$. For this data, the results from the t-test with log-transformed data and the GLM indicated evidence of a difference in mean for the weight variable.

3.2.3. The Pharmaceutical and Computer Companies Data

We have a data table of 32 registered companies and some information like the sales, profits, assets, and number of employees in each company. There are two types of companies, computer companies and pharmaceutical companies. We wanted to check if the assets variable is significantly different between the two types. So, we tested the mean difference between the computer and pharmaceutical groups regarding the assets variable. The data was found to be skewed and fitted to an exponential distribution according to AICc values. The Q–Q plot and the frequency histogram of the companies' untransformed and log-transformed data are presented in Figure 7.

We tested the data using both methods. The resulted t-value is $t_{29.99} = 1.97$ with p-value $= 0.0292$, which indicates that there is a significant difference between the two groups' means and that the pharmaceutical companies have a significantly higher assets mean than the computer companies. For the second method, we applied GLM to the original data with a log link function. The resulting *p*-value = 0.4908 indicates that there is no significant difference between the assets' means of the two types of companies. So, the two methods gave contradicting results and this issue puts us on a crossroads. We need to decide which result to adopt.

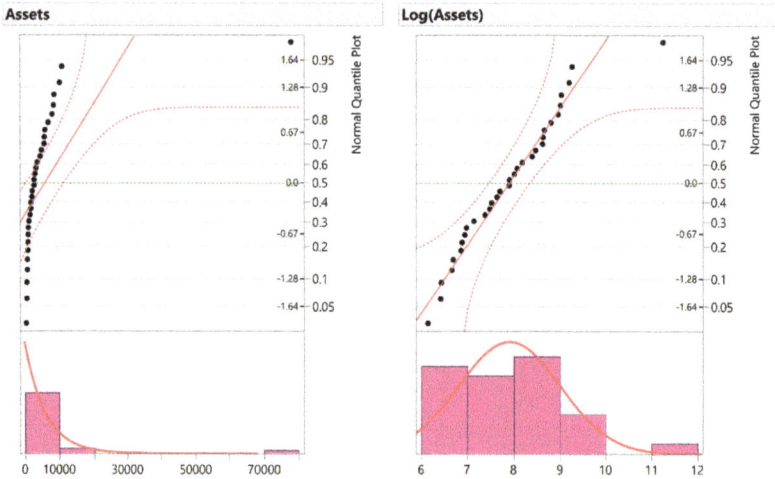

Figure 7. The normal Q–Q plots (up) for the Assets variable before and after transformation and the frequency histogram of the Assets on the left (down) fitted to an exponential distribution (red).

4. Discussion

In this work, we compared the use of a *t*-test on log-transformed data and the use of GLM on untransformed skewed data. The log transformation was studied because it is one of the most common transformations used in biosciences research. If such an approach is used, the scientist must be careful about its limitations; especially when interpreting the significance of the analysis of transformed data for the hypothesis of interest about the original data. Moreover, a researcher who uses log transformation should know how to facilitate log-transformed data to give inferences concerning the original data. Furthermore, log transformation does not always help make data less variable or more normal and may, in some situations, make data more variable and more skewed. For that, the variability and normality should always be examined after applying the log transformation.

On the other hand, GLM was used because other nonparametric tests' inferences concern medians and not means. In addition, GLM models deal differently with response variables depending on their population distributions, which provides the scientist with flexibility in modeling; GLM allows for response variables to have different distributions, and each distribution has an appropriate link function to vary linearly with the predicted values.

Each comparison was made for two simulated groups from several sampling distributions with varying sample sizes. The comparisons regarded Type I error rates, power rates and estimates of the means. Overall, the *t*-test method with transformed data produced smaller Type I error rates and closer estimations. The GLM method, however, produced a higher power rate compared to *t*-test methods, though both reported acceptable power rates.

For gamma distribution, Type I error rates in the *t*-test case were very close to 0.05 (0.0497 to 0.0504), while the Type I error rates of the GLM method had a wider range (0.0490 to 0.0577). For most examples in the gamma-distributed data, the Type I error rates of the *t*-test method were smaller than the respective rates in the GLM method. Regarding power, the GLM rates were higher in about 85% of the settings than the ones using the *t*-test, with absolute values of differences, ranging from 0.000 to 0.363.

The back-transformed estimates of the mean differences in the *t*-test case were not significantly different from the estimates of the original data mean differences in the *t*-test method. The GLM estimates, in contrast, were significantly different from the estimates of the original data. So, if we are looking for lower Type I error and closer estimates, we can use the *t*-test method with transformed data. However, if we are looking for a method with higher power rates, we recommend choosing the GLM method.

In the exponentially distributed data, the GLM method has achieved a noticeably lower Type I error rate and higher power in most of the settings than the *t*-test method. Regarding the estimates, the *t*-test method gave closer estimates. Despite the closer estimates for the *t*-test method, our advice is to use the GLM method.

For beta distributed data, Type I error rates seem to favor the *t*-test method with transformed data. The power rates of the GLM method were higher than the power rates in the *t*-test method, with absolute values of differences ranging from 0 to 0.0884. Furthermore, by looking at Figure 4, we can see that the two methods have very close power rates. So, both methods seem to be good enough in this matter. Nevertheless, since the *t*-test method has lower Type I rates and closer estimates in the beta distributed data, we recommend it over GLM.

The missing rates for some of the parameters' combinations, especially in calculating power rates, are due to two reasons. First, in most cases, rates were not missing, but the counts for accepted simulated samples were less than 10,000. That caused the setting to be rejected. Particularly in the case of calculating power rates, the two groups are from the same distribution with different parameters, which made it harder to apply the two filters (both groups should not be normally distributed before the use of log transformation and normally distributed after the application of log transformation). Although being less than 10,000 caused the estimates to vary as a response to changing the random seed, it gave the same conclusion. For example, if the GLM had a higher power rate in one sitting of parameters, it kept having a higher power rate even if we changed the seed. Yet, we preferred not to include these settings because we needed the estimates to be reproducible.

Second, in rare cases, none of the samples' normality issues were resolved with log transformation, so we had zero accepted simulated samples. As a result, our comparison does not apply to that parameter combination. In conclusion, we did not consider missing rates as an issue since GLM had a higher power rate, as well as the *t*-test had closer mean difference estimates in all other accepted settings.

Our results were consistent across parameter settings and sample sizes ($N = 25, 50, 100$), so we expect that the difference in sample sizes will not affect the method choice no matter what the sample size effect is over the method performance itself.

After analyzing the data from our real-life examples, we recommend reporting the results from the *t*-test with log-transformed data for the lipid data example and catheters data example, since the best fit for both examples was a gamma distribution. Because the catheters data example had larger sample size ($n = 592$) than used in our simulations, we conducted additional simulations with sample size of 296 per group. Though not reported, these results concurred with our reported findings at lower sample sizes.

We followed the same steps for the third example (the pharmaceutical and computer data example), which had the exponential fit as the best fit. We conducted additional (though not reported) simulations with 16 subjects per group, and again observed results that agreed with our reported findings. Thus, our recommendation is to report the GLM method results.

Therefore, for any Bio-application research, studying the appropriate statistical distribution that fits the dependent variable can help us to determine if a parametric model can reasonably test the data after log transformation is used. Alternatively, it would probably be better to abandon the classic approach and switch to the GLM method.

Author Contributions: Conceptualization, H.M.H.; Investigation, H.M.H., R.T.S., R.A. and K.A.K.; Methodology, H.M.H.; Software, H.M.H. and R.A.; Writing—original draft, H.M.H., R.T.S., R.A. and K.A.K.; Writing—review and editing, H.M.H., R.T.S., R.A. and K.A.K. All authors have read and agreed to the published version of the manuscript.

Funding: This research received no external funding.

Conflicts of Interest: The authors declare no conflict of interest.

References

1. Al Garni, H.Z.; Awasthi, A. A Monte Carlo approach applied to sensitivity analysis of criteria impacts on solar PV site selection. In *Handbook of Probabilistic Models*, 1st ed.; Samui, P., Bui, D.T., Chakraborty, S., Deo, R.C., Eds.; Butterworth-Heinemann: Oxford, UK, 2020.
2. Martinez, W.L.; Martinez, A.R. *Computational Statistics Handbook with Matlab*, 2nd ed.; CRC Press: Boca Raton, FL, USA, 2007.
3. Morris, T.P.; White, I.R.; Crowther, M.J. Using simulation studies to evaluate statistical methods. *Stat Med.* **2019**, *38*, 2074–2102. [CrossRef] [PubMed]
4. Ghasemi, A.; Zahediasl, S. Normality tests for statistical analysis: A guide for non-statisticians. *Int. J. Endocrinol. Metabol.* **2012**, *10*, 486. [CrossRef] [PubMed]
5. Wang, C.C.; Lee, W.C. Evaluation of the normality assumption in meta-analyses. *Am. J. Epidemiol.* **2020**, *189*, 235–242. [CrossRef] [PubMed]
6. Feng, C.; Wang, H.; Lu, N.; Chen, T.; He, H.; Lu, Y. Log-transformation and its implications for data analysis. *Shanghai Arch. Psychiatry* **2014**, *26*, 105. [CrossRef] [PubMed]
7. Curran-Everett, D. Explorations in statistics: The log transformation. *Adv. Physiol. Educ.* **2018**, *42*, 343–347. [CrossRef] [PubMed]
8. Hassani, H.; Yeganegi, M.R.; Khan, A.; Silva, E.S. The effect of data transformation on singular spectrum analysis for forecasting. *Signals* **2020**, *1*, 2. [CrossRef]
9. Keene, O.N. The log transformation is special. *Stat. Med.* **1995**, *14*, 811–819. [CrossRef] [PubMed]
10. Nelder, J.A.; Wedderburn, R.W. Generalized linear models. *J. R. Stat. Soc. Ser. A* **1972**, *135*, 370–384. [CrossRef]
11. McCullagh, P.; Nelder, J.A. *Generalized Linear Models*; CRC Press: Boca Raton, FL, USA, 1989.
12. Song, L.; Langfelder, P.; Horvath, S. Random generalized linear model: A highly accurate and interpretable ensemble predictor. *BMC Bioinf.* **2013**, *14*, 5. [CrossRef]
13. Nelder, J.A.; Baker, R.J. *Generalized Linear Models*; Wiley Online Library: Hoboken, NJ, USA, 2006.
14. Dobson, A.J.; Barnett, A. *An Introduction to Generalized Linear Models*; CRC Press: Boca Raton, FL, USA, 2008.
15. Müller, M. Generalized linear models. In *Handbook of Computational Statistics*; Gentle, J., Härdle, W., Mori, Y., Eds.; Springer: Berlin, Germany, 2012; pp. 681–709.
16. Agresti, A. *Foundations of Linear and Generalized Linear Models*; John Wiley & Sons: Hoboken, NJ, USA, 2015.
17. Jørgensen, B. Generalized linear models. In *Encyclopedia of Environmetrics*, 2nd ed.; El-Shaarawi, A.H., Piegorsch, W.W., Eds.; Wiley: Hoboken, NJ, USA, 2013; Volume 3.
18. Fay, M.P.; Proschan, M.A. Wilcoxon-Mann-Whitney or *t*-test? On assumptions for hypothesis tests and multiple interpretations of decision rules. *Stat. Surv.* **2010**, *4*, 1. [CrossRef]
19. Claeskens, G.; Hjort, N.L. *Model Selection and Model Averaging*; Cambridge University Press: Cambridge, UK, 2008.
20. Lindsey, J.K.; Jones, B. Choosing among generalized linear models applied to medical data. *Stat. Med.* **1998**, *17*, 59–68. [CrossRef]
21. Mann, J.; Larsen, P.; Brinkley, J. Exploring the use of negative binomial regression modeling for pediatric peripheral intravenous catheterization. *J. Med. Stat. Inf.* **2014**, *2*, 6. [CrossRef]

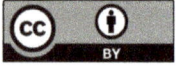

© 2020 by the authors. Licensee MDPI, Basel, Switzerland. This article is an open access article distributed under the terms and conditions of the Creative Commons Attribution (CC BY) license (http://creativecommons.org/licenses/by/4.0/).

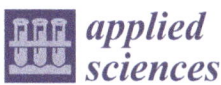

Commentary

Ten Points for High-Quality Statistical Reporting and Data Presentation

Pentti Nieminen

Medical Informatics and Data Analysis Research Group, University of Oulu, 90014 Oulu, Finland; pentti.nieminen@oulu.fi

Received: 5 May 2020; Accepted: 29 May 2020; Published: 3 June 2020

Featured Application: In this work, an applicable instrument is proposed to quickly evaluate the quality of the statistical reporting and data presentation in research papers.

Abstract: Background: Data analysis methods have become an essential part of empirical research papers, especially in health sciences and medical research. It has previously been reported that a noteworthy percentage of articles have flaws in their statistical reporting. Reporting problems have been a long-term issue, and despite continued efforts to improve the situation, improvements have been far from satisfactory. One explanation is an inadequate assessment of statistical reporting during peer review. This communication proposes a short instrument to assess the quality of data analysis reporting in manuscripts and published papers. Method: A checklist-type instrument was developed by selecting and refining items from previous reports about the quality of statistical reporting in medical journals and from published guidelines for reporting and data presentation. Items were pretested and modified during pilot studies. A total of 160 original medical research articles that were published in 4 journals were evaluated to test the instrument. Interrater and intrarater agreements were examined by comparing quality scores assigned to 40 articles published in a psychiatric journal. Results: The data analysis reporting test consists of nine questions that assess the quality of health research from a reader's perspective. The composed scale has a total score ranging from 0 to 10 and discriminated between journals and study designs. A high score suggested that an article had a good presentation of findings in tables and figures and that the description of analysis methods was helpful to readers. Interrater and intrarater agreements were high. Conclusion: An applicable checklist for quickly testing the statistical reporting quality of manuscripts and published research papers was developed. This instrument aims to improve the quality of empirical research in scientific fields where statistical methods play an important role.

Keywords: data analysis; statistics; reporting; data presentation; publications; medicine; health care

---

1. Introduction

Statistical reporting plays an important role in medical publications [1]. A high proportion of medical articles are essentially statistical in their presentation. For the reader, the main outward demonstration of a publication consists of statistical expressions that summarize the raw data used in the research. Regardless of the quality of the data and the variables chosen to express the results, the overt evidence of the research is produced as the lists of numbers, tables, plots, graphs, and other displays, i.e., the descriptive statistics. The communication of the descriptive statistics may also be combined with statistical inference procedures, such as test statistics and *p*-values [2].

The accurate communication of research results to the scientific community (i.e., other researchers) is essential providing reliable results [3,4]. Failure to report analysis methods or inadequate data presentation could lead to inaccurate inferences, even if the statistical analyses were performed correctly.

Several findings have demonstrated that a noteworthy percentage of articles, even those published in high-prestige journals, have flaws in their statistical reporting [3–8]. Methodological and reporting problems have been reported over several decades, and despite continued efforts to improve the situation [9], the improvements have been far from satisfactory. One explanation is the inadequate assessment of statistical reporting during peer review [8].

Author instructions and editorials alone have been insufficient to change the quality of statistical reporting. Numerous reporting guidelines offer tools or checklists to evaluate the reporting of health research [10]. The EQUATOR Network listed 424 such guidelines in March 2020 [11]. What is often problematic in these checklists is their extent. They try to evaluate all possible aspects of analysis from study design, settings, participants, description of measurements and variables, sample sizes, data analysis methods, specific methods, descriptive data, outcome data, and ancillary analysis. Often it is impossible to evaluate all these points. When reviewing and editing health care and medical papers, I have noticed that a few points will reveal the quality of reporting of data analysis. There is no need to read the whole manuscript and check all the statistical details to ensure that the manuscript contains all the information that readers need to assess the study's methodology and validity of its findings. Editorial processes of medical manuscripts often fail to identify obvious indicators of good and poor data presentation and reporting of results. Editors, reviewers and readers need new tools to quickly identify studies with inadequate descriptions of statistical methods and poor quality of data presentation.

I took on the challenge of compacting and refining the available quality criteria for statistical reporting and data presentation. I had three guiding starting points for assessing statistical reporting. The first key point was that if the data analysis methods are described with enough details, readers will be able to follow the flow of the analyses and to critically assess whether the data analyses provide reliable results. My second key point was the use of tables and figures in data presentation. Tables and figures are a fundamental means of scientific communications and they are included in most submitted and published medical and health care articles [12]. Most readers browse through tables and illustrations, but few read the whole article. Well-prepared tables and figures with proper titles, clear labeling, and optimally presented data will empower readers to scrutinize the data. I presume that the quality of tables and figures indicates the overall quality of data presentation. My third starting key point was that the new tool should be easy to use. I wanted to develop a short evaluation form with a low number of items.

In short, my objective was to develop a handy and reliable instrument to assess the quality of statistical reporting and data presentation that was applicable for a wide variety of medical and health care research forums, including both clinical and basic sciences. In this article, I define nine items for the proposed quality test. In addition, I report findings from an initial evaluation of its functionality and reliability.

2. Materials and Methods

2.1. Prework

My intention was to develop a test or checklist that would complement and not replicate other checklists. The construction of my quality evaluation tool began with a literature search. It included the following steps:

- Search for papers evaluating the use and misuse of statistics in medical articles.
- Search for papers evaluating statistical reporting and data presentation.
- Review medical statistics textbooks.
- Review statistical reporting guidelines, including journal guidelines for authors.
- Assess my experience as a handling editor and referee for medical and medicine-related journals.

After reading and reviewing the existing body of evidence, I discovered that including an assessment of statistical errors into a quality instrument would be very difficult. Several studies have reviewed medical papers and tried to find errors in the selection of statistical procedures [5,8,13]. Most of the statistical problems in medical journals reported in these reviews are related to elementary statistical techniques [14]. The errors in medical papers are probably more a matter of judgment. There is no general agreement on what constitutes a statistical error [6,15,16]. The recommended methods for a particular type of question may not be the only feasible methods, and may not be universally agreed upon as the best methods [17]. In addition, I decided to avoid any judgment of the content, such as the originality, ethics, or scientific relevance.

I found hundreds of journal guidelines for statistical reporting. I observed strong heterogeneity among the guidelines. Some journals have kept these guidelines to the minimum required for a decent manuscript presentation, whereas a large number of journals displayed too many instructions and journal-specific recommendations. Some recommendations regarding the test statistics (reporting of values, degrees of freedom and p-values) or the contents of tables were even contradictory (between journals). Most reporting guidelines said more about the presentation of methods than about the reporting of results. In addition, medical statistics textbooks did not cover the topic of statistical reporting.

By the end of the prework process, I had identified and formulated 20 items phrased as questions and grouped them into two domains (description of methods and data presentation). The draft questions were as follows:

Statistical analysis (or Data analysis) subsection in the Material and Methods section:

- Was Statistical analysis subsection included?
- Was there a sample size justification before the study?
- Did authors state how variables were described and summarized?
- Did authors state which methods were used to evaluate the statistical significances?
- Did authors identify the variables for each analysis and mentioned all the statistical methods used?
- Was extended description of some specific procedures provided?
- Did authors verify how data conformed to assumptions of the methods used?
- Was statistical software reported?
- Was missing data addressed?
- Were references to statistical literature provided?
- Was subject attrition or exclusion addressed?
- How any outlying data were treated in the analysis?

Data presentation:

- Was a table included where the basic characteristics of the study subjects were summarized with descriptive statistics?
- Were total and group sample sizes reported for each analysis in all tables and figures?
- Did all tables and figures have a clear and self-explanatory title?
- Were statistical abbreviations explained in all tables and figures?
- Were summary statistics, tests or methods identified and named in all tables and figures?
- Were p-values reported properly (e.g., no expressions like NS, $p < 0.05$, $p = 0.000$)
- Was the total number of reported p-values and confidence intervals in tables and figures less than 100?
- Were all tables and figures appropriate?

In line with my original key principles, the evaluation form should include two sections: (1) Material and Methods section and (2) tables and figures in Results section. In addition, the test form should be only one page long. I developed several pilot versions to structure the assessment of the quality of statistical reporting in an article or manuscript. Within these frames I reviewed the 20 draft questions for their importance and uniqueness with my health care students, who tested the instrument drafts during their studies. Further testing of the instrument, a review of the literature related to the topic and expert opinions from my colleagues resulted in the generation of 9 items pertaining to the description of statistical and data management procedures and the reporting of results in tables and figures. Following the pilot studies, several items were also reworded, rearranged, and consolidated in the test form for clarity. Because tables and figures should be self-explanatory, I decided to place the assessment of tables and figures at the beginning of the evaluation form. Thus, the assessment of the description of the statistical analysis in the Materials and methods section now follows the assessment of the tables and figures. The updated version of the instrument is included in as Table 1. In the evaluation form, questions 1–4 relate to basic guidelines for preparing effective tables and figures. Questions 5–9 evaluate the description of the data analysis methods.

Table 1. Statistical reporting and data presentation evaluation form.

TABLES AND FIGURES IN RESULTS SECTION:	No	Yes
1. Was a table included where the basic characteristics of the study participants were summarized with descriptive statistics?	0	1
2. Was the total number of participants provided in all tables and figures?	0	1
3. Were summary statistics, tests and methods identified and named in all tables and figures?	0	1
4. Were tables and figures well prepared?		
0 = more than 50% of the tables and figures had presentation issues		0
1 = 50% or fewer of the tables and figures had presentation issues		1
2 = no presentation issues in any of the tables and figures		2
MATERIALS AND METHODS SECTION:		
5. Was the statistical analysis (or data analysis) subsection provided in the Materials and Methods section?	0	1
6. Did authors identify the variables (and methods) for each analysis done in the study?	0	1
7. Was it verified that the data conformed to the assumptions and preconditions of the methods used to analyze them?	0	1
8. Were references to statistical literature provided?	0	1
9. Was the statistical software reported?	0	1
TOTAL SCORE:		

2.2. Ten Items to Assess the Quality of Statistical Reporting and Data Presentation

In the following chapter, I present the items as a sequence of 9 numbered questions and explain some of the reasoning behind the questions.

2.2.1. Item 1: Was a Table Included Where the Basic Characteristics of the Study Subjects Were Summarized with Descriptive Statistics?

Most papers reporting an analysis of health care and medical data will at some point use statistics to describe the sociodemographic characteristics, medical history and main outcome variables of the study participants. An important motive for doing this is to give the reader some idea of the extent to which study findings can be generalized to their own local situation [18]. The production of descriptive statistics is a straightforward matter, but often authors need to decide which statistics to present. The selected statistics should be included in a paper in a manner that is easy for readers to assimilate. When many patient characteristics are being described, the details of the statistics used and the number of participants contributing to analysis are best incorporated in tabular presentation [12,18,19].

I give one point if the main features of important characteristics of the participants were displayed in a table.

2.2.2. Item 2: Was the Total Number of Participants Provided in all Tables and Figures?

The medical literature shows a strong tendency to accentuate significance testing, specifically "statistically significant" outcomes. Most papers published in medical journals contain tables and figures reporting *p*-values [16,20,21]. Finding statistically significant or nonsignificant results depends on the sample size [22,23]. When evaluating the validity of the findings, the reader must know the number of study participants. Sample size is an important consideration for research. A larger sample size leads to a higher level of precision and thus a higher level of power for a given study to detect an effect of a given size. An excessively large number of study participants may lead to statistically significant results even when there is no clinical practicality; an inappropriately small number of study participants can fail to reveal important and clinically significant differences. The total number of participants or sample size of each group should be clearly reported.

I give one point if most of the tables and figures (at least 75%) have provided the total number of participants or number of participants in each subgroup.

2.2.3. Item 3: Were Summary Statistics, Tests, and Methods Identified and Named in all Tables and Figures?

Tables and figures should be able to stand alone [24]. That is, all information necessary for interpretation should be included within the table or figure, legend or footnotes [25]. This means that descriptive statistics, significance tests, and multivariable modeling methods used are named. Many readers will skim an article before reading it closely and identifying data analysis methods in the tables or figure will allow the readers to understand the procedures immediately. It is not necessary to define well known statistical abbreviations, such as SD, SE, OR, RR, HR, CI, r, R2, n, or NA, but the methods producing these statistics should be named.

I give one point if statistical summary statistics, tests, and methods in tables and figures were named.

2.2.4. Item 4: Were Tables and Figures Well Prepared?

High quality tables and figures increase the chance that readers can take advantage of an article's results. In effective scientific writing, it is essential to ensure that the tables and figures are flawless, informative, and attractive. Below is a list of a number of presentation issues that may prevent readers grasping the message quickly and will lower the overall quality of data presentation [12,24,26].

- Messy, inferior, or substandard overall technical presentation of data.

    - A table or a figure did not have a clear title.
    - The formatting of a table resembled a spreadsheet, and the lines of the same size between each row and each column did not help to clarify the different data presented in the table.
    - In a figure, data values were not clearly visible.
    - Data values were not defined.
    - Obvious errors in presented numbers or data elements.

- Tables or figures included unnecessary features:

    - In a figure, nondata elements (gridlines, shading, or three dimensional perspectives) competed with data elements and they did not serve a specific explanatory function in the graph.
    - A table or a figure was unnecessary because the data had too few values. Authors could have presented their results clearly in a sentence or two. For example, a sentence is preferred to a pie char.

- General guiding principles for reporting statistical results were not followed:

- *p*-Values were denoted with asterisks or with a system of letters in tables or figures, and actual *p*-values were not reported. Actual *p*-values should be reported, without false precision, whenever feasible. Providing the actual *p*-values prevents problems of interpretation related to *p*-values close to 0.05 [12,22]. Very small *p*-values do not need exact representation and $p < 0.001$ is usually sufficient.
- Numbers were not reported with an appropriate degree of precision in tables. In interpreting the findings, the reader cannot pay attention to the numbers presented with several decimals.
- The standard error of the mean (SE) was used to indicate the variability of a data set.
- Confidence intervals were not reported with the effect sizes (regression coefficients, ORs, HRs, or IRRs) in regression analyses or meta-analyses. The results of the primary comparisons should always be reported with confidence intervals [27].
- A table included only *p*-values. *p*-value cannot tell readers the strength or size of an effect, change, or relationship. In the end, patients and physicians want to know the magnitude of the benefit, change or association, not the statistical significance of individual studies [23,28].

I give zero points if more than 50% of the tables and figures included presentation issues.
I give one point if 50% or fewer of the tables and figures included presentation issues.
I give two points if all tables and figures were prepared efficiently and accurately, and the presentation issues mentioned above were avoided.

2.2.5. Item 5: Was a Statistical Analysis (or Data Analysis) Subsection Provided in the Methods Section?

Most general reporting guidelines and recommendations require that original research articles include a Methods section [10,24,29]. In these recommendations, it is stated that the Methods section should aim to be sufficiently detailed such that others with access to the data would be able to reproduce the results. This section should include at least the following subsections: Selection and description of participants, technical information about variables (primary and secondary outcomes, explanatory variables, other variables) and statistical methods. To many researchers, it seems quite obvious that a Statistical analysis (or Data analysis) subsection with a clear subheading should be provided in the Materials and Methods section when the manuscript contains some elements of statistical data analysis. However, in my experience, this is not obvious to all biomedical or health science researchers. I have reviewed several biomedical manuscripts for journals wherein the laboratory experiments were described in depth, but nothing was said about how the reported *p*-values were obtained. When statistical methods are described with enough detail in the Statistical analysis subsection, a knowledgeable reader can judge the appropriateness of the methods for the study and verify the reported methods.

I therefore give one point if the Methods section included a subsection headed with Statistical analysis (or Data analysis or Statistical methods).

2.2.6. Item 6: Did Authors Identify the Variables and Methods for Each Analysis?

Authors know their own work so well that some find it difficult to put themselves in the position of a reader encountering the study for the first time. As a reader, I often request more information about some aspect of the data analysis. Within the Statistical analysis section, authors need to explain which statistical methods or tests were used for each analysis, rather than just listing all the statistical methods used in one place [30]. In a well-written statistical analysis subsection, authors should also identify the variables used in each analysis. Readers should be informed which variables were analyzed with each method. Care must be taken to ensure that all methods are listed and that all tests listed are indeed applied in the study [31]. The statistical section should be consistent with the Results section.

I give one point if authors describe the goal (research question), the variables and the method used for each analysis done in the study.

2.2.7. Item 7: Was It Verified that the Data Conformed to the Assumptions and Preconditions of the Methods Used to Analyze Them?

All basic data analysis methods and multivariable techniques depend on assumptions about the characteristics of the data [32]. If an analysis is performed without satisfying the assumptions, incorrect conclusions may be made on the basis of erroneous results. For example, a widely applied analysis of variance depends at least on three assumptions [33]. In actual data analysis it is unlikely that all the assumptions for the analysis of variance will be satisfied. Some statistical assumptions are essential, while some assumptions are quite lenient. A normal distribution of main variables is a strong requirement in a number of statistical techniques and should be verified and reported. On the other hand, the use of a nonparametric significance test instead of a more powerful parametric test should be justified. If a brief justification is provided, readers may better understand why a specific data analysis method has been applied [14]. Regression modeling has several constraints or preconditions, such as linearity, independence between explanatory variables, and number of participants per variable. In an excellent description of multivariable methods, authors should describe possible limitations or preconditions.

I give one point if authors describe how the data satisfactorily fulfill the underlying assumptions and preconditions of the main analysis methods.

2.2.8. Item 8: Were References to Statistical Literature Provided?

The use of all the statistical methods in a study needs to be documented with a relevant description to help the readers to validate the findings described by the authors. References enable others to identify and trace the methods used in the data analyses. Common statistical methods can be described in brief, but some less common or obscure methods should be explained in detail. The International Committee of Medical Journal Editors (ICMJE) also instructs to give references to established methods [29]. Good scientific writing is includes references and brief descriptions for methods that have been published but are not well known or not commonly used, descriptions of new or substantially modified methods, reasons for using uncommon methods, and an evaluation of the method's limitations [34].

I give one point for providing statistical references.

2.2.9. Item 9: Was the Statistical Software Used in the Analysis Reported?

Identifying the statistical software package used in the data analysis is important because all statistical programs do not use the same algorithms or default options to compute the same statistics. As a result, the findings may vary from package to package or from algorithm to algorithm. In addition, privately developed algorithms may not be validated and updated [12].

I give one point for reporting statistical software if the name and version of the statistical program or package (name, version) is provided.

2.3. Total Score

Users of this tools can calculate a total score by summing all 9 items. The total score ranges from 0 to 10. I have assigned the following labels to the corresponding ranges of the total score:

9–10 Excellent
7–8 Good
5–6 Acceptable
3–4 Weak
0–2 Poor

Although this division is plain and unsophisticated, it does provide useful interpretation of the scores.

2.4. Set of Articles

I used original research articles published between 2017 and 2019 in 4 journals to test the instrument for published studies. I selected two highly visible medical journals (*Lancet* and *JAMA Psychiatry*), one dental journal (*Journal of Dentistry*) (*JD*), and one journal from environmental and public health subfields (*International Journal of Environmental Research and Public Health*) (*IJERPH*) for the evaluation. I chose these journals to cover the range of statistical reporting both in established journals, and in lower visibility journals. I analyzed 40 articles per journal. The starting articles for each journal were chosen randomly from the journal's chronological list of articles, with the only criteria being that there would be at least 39 eligible subsequent articles published that year in the journal in question. The following consecutive 39 articles were also included for the review. Editorials, letters, case reports and review articles were excluded from the evaluation.

2.5. Data Analysis

Cross-tabulation was used to report the differences in the study design and sample size of the evaluated articles by the publication journals. For the total score of statistical reporting and data presentation, the mean value with standard deviation and box plots were used to describe the distribution by study design, sample size, and journal. Analysis of variance (ANOVA) was applied to evaluate the statistical significance of possible differences in the mean values of the total score. The quality score was approximately normally distributed, and the normality assumption of the analysis of variance test was met by the data. The chi-squared test was applied to reveal the statistically significant differences in the distributions of the items of the statistical reporting and data presentation instrument across journals. All of the statistical analyses were executed using IBM SPSS Statistics (version 25) software.

When using quality evaluation forms, several methodological aspects can impact accuracy and reliability. For instance, to obtain an appropriate description of statistical methods, the basic statistical methods must be familiar. Additionally, the level of expertise reviewers have about scientific writing can affect their ability to accurately detect shortcomings in reporting. Therefore, it was important to determine the interrater and test-retest reliability of the proposed tool using raters with low (Rater 1) and moderate (Rater 2) medical statistics experience. I recruited a junior medical researcher to serve as an independent rater (Rater 1). I acted as Rater 2 myself. Rater 1 had minimal experience with medical data analysis but had been involved with medical writing for the previous 2 years. Rater 1 received training in the use of the assessment form, and general guidelines were given on the items of the instrument.

The reliability study started in parallel with a pilot study of the evaluation form. The reliability of the evaluation was checked by comparing Rater 1 ratings with the ratings of Rater 2. We independently read and evaluated 40 articles published in *JAMA Psychiatry*. These articles were selected from the previously described set of 160 articles.

First, agreement between the summary scores was assessed using an intraclass correlation coefficient ICC (with agreement definition, single measures, and mixed model) and Pearson correlation coefficient [35]. Generally, good agreement is defined as an ICC > 0.80. To evaluate the test-retest (or intrarater) performance, I read the 40 articles published in *JAMA Psychiatry* twice. The time interval between the scoring sessions was six months.

Second, the percentage agreement and Cohen's kappa coefficient were used to assess the degree of agreement for each item [35]. The simple percentage agreement is an adequate measure of agreement for many purposes, but it does not account for agreement arising from chance alone. Categorical agreement is often measured with the kappa coefficient, which attempts to account for the agreement that may arise from chance alone. A kappa score in the range of 0.81 to 1 was considered to represent high agreement.

3. Results

3.1. Characteristics of the Evaluated Articles

The articles in the validation sample came from a variety of specialties: general medicine, clinical topics, psychiatry, dentistry, environmental topics, public health, and dentistry. Table 2 shows the basic characteristics of the article set. Observational studies (cross-sectional surveys, longitudinal and case-control studies) were performed at a higher frequency in *JAMA Psychiatry* and *IJERPH*. The proportion of experimental studies (randomized clinical trials, non-randomized intervention studies) was highest in *Lancet* (67.5%). The test article set also included laboratory works that applied data analysis methods scantily and had low intensity of statistical methods. Sample sizes were larger in the more prominent journals.

Table 2. Distribution of study design and sample size of the evaluated articles by the publication journal.

	Lancet n (%)	*JAMA Psy* n (%)	*IJERPH* n (%)	*JD* n (%)	All n (%)
Study design					
Observational studies	11 (27.5)	27 (67.5)	27 (67.5)	13 (32.5)	78 (48.8)
Experimental studies	27 (67.5)	9 (22.5)	6 (15.0)	6 (15.0)	48 (30.0)
Reliability	1 (2.5)	0	2 (5.0)	2 (5.0)	5 (3.1)
Laboratory works	0	0	4 (10.0)	14 (35.0)	18 (11.3)
Meta-analysis	1 (2.5)	4 (10.0)	1 (2.5)	5 (12.5)	11 (6.9)
Sample size					
<99	0	3 (7.5)	14 (35.0)	20 (50.0)	37 (23.1)
100–499	5 (12.5)	12 (30.0)	12 (30.0)	8 (20.0)	37 (23.1)
500–2999	22 (55.0)	7 (17.5)	6 (15.0)	5 (12.5)	40 (25.0)
>3000	12 (30.0)	18 (45.0)	5 (12.5)	3 (7.5)	38 (23.8)
Missing	1 (2.5)	0	3 (7.5)	4 (10.0)	8 (5.0)
Total number of articles	40	40	40	40	160

JAMA Psy = JAMA Psychiatry, IJERPH = International Journal of Environmental Research and Public Health, and JD = Journal of Dentistry.

3.2. Distribution of the Total Quality Score

The total score assessing quality of statistical reporting ranges from 0 to 10. Figure 1 shows the distribution of the quality score among all 160 articles. A total of 14 (8.8%) articles were poor and 42 (26.3%) articles did not reach up to an acceptable level.

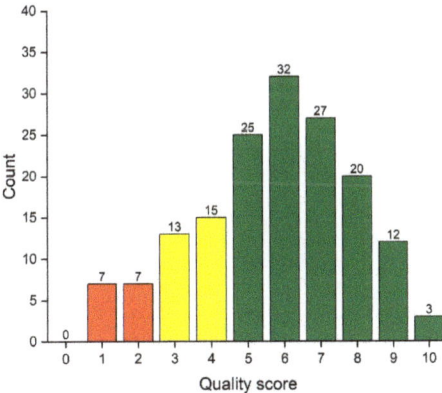

Figure 1. Column graph of the data analysis reporting quality score of 160 articles. Articles with poor quality (0–2) are denoted with red column color, those with weak quality (3–4) with yellow color and at least acceptable (5–10) articles with green color.

The distribution of the data analysis reporting score is summarized in Table 3 by article characteristics. The mean (SD) of quality score in all 160 evaluated reports was 5.7 (SD 2.2). The reporting quality was highest in the meta-analyses and lowest in laboratory works. The data analysis reporting quality was associated with the sample size of the evaluated study.

Table 3. Mean and standard deviation of the data analysis reporting score from 160 articles by study design and sample size.

	Number of Articles	Mean	Standard Deviation
Study design			
• Observational studies	78	5.5	2.2
• Experimental studies	48	6.5	1.8
• Reliability	5	5.4	2.6
• Laboratory works	18	3.9	1.9
• Meta-analysis	11	7.4	2.2
Sample size			
• <99	37	4.7	2.2
• 100–499	37	5.6	2.0
• 500–2999	40	7.2	1.5
• >3000	38	6.0	1.9
• Missing	8	2.9	1.0
All articles	160	5.7	2.2

p-Value of ANOVA < 0.001 for study design and sample size.

3.3. Quality of Statistical Reporting and Data Presentation by the Journal

Table 4 summarizes the distributions of the data analysis reporting test items in tables and figures by the journals. Neglecting to state the number of participants was the most common defect (65.6%). The quality of tables and figures was related to the journal; the failures to provide data and report findings was less common in the *Lancet*.

Table 4. The distributions of the data analysis reporting test items by the journals.

Item	Lancet n (%)	JAMA Psy n (%)	IJERPH n (%)	JD n (%)	All n (%)	p-Value of the Chi-Squared Test
Tables and figures in results section:						
Basic characteristics reported in a table	35 (87.5)	27 (77.5)	27 (67.5)	12 (30.0)	101 (63.1)	<0.001
Total number of participants provided	27 (67.5)	9 (22.5)	12 (30.0)	7 (17.5)	55 (34.4)	<0.001
Statistics, tests and methods identified	34 (85.0)	17 (42.5)	20 (50.0)	20 (50.0)	91 (56.9)	<0.001
Presentation issues: • several • 50% or less • no issues	2 (5.0) 16 (40.0) 22 (55.0)	6 (15.0) 14 (35.0) 20 (50.0)	10 (25.0) 18 (45.0) 12 (30.0)	10 (25.0) 20 (50.0) 10 (25.0)	28 (17.5) 68 (42.5) 64 (40.0)	0.029
Materials and methods section						
Statistical analysis subsection provided	37 (92.5)	37 (92.5)	30 (75.0)	28 (70.0)	132 (82.5)	0.011
Variables identified	23 (57.5)	35 (87.5)	22 (55.0)	22 (55.0)	102 (63.7)	0.005
Assumptions verified	14 (35.0)	14 (35.0)	11 (27.5)	15 (37.5)	54 (33.8)	0.858
Software reported	32 (80.0)	31 (77.5)	29 (72.5)	31 (77.5)	123 (76.9)	0.911
References to statistical literature	14 (35.0)	25 (62.5)	14 (35.0)	11 (27.5)	64 (40.0)	0.008
Software reported	32 (80.0)	31 (77.5)	29 (72.5)	31 (77.5)	123 (76.9)	0.911
Total number of articles	40	40	40	40	160	

JAMA Psy = JAMA Psychiatry, IJERPH = International Journal of Environmental Research and Public Health and JD = Journal of Dentistry.

Table 4 also compares the prevalence of adequate description of methods in the four journals. The failure to verify that the data conformed to the assumptions and preconditions of the methods used was very common (66.2%). A total of 28 articles (17.5%) did not provide a statistical analysis subsection; 60.0% (96 articles) did not provide references to statistical literature; and 23.1% (37 articles) did not report the statistical software.

Figure 2 shows how the quality score varies by journals. The high-impact general medical journal *Lancet* had mean score of 6.9 (SD 1.7) while the mean score in the leading psychiatric journal *JAMA Psy* was 6.1 (SD 1.4). The quality core also identified the journals (*IJERPH* and *JD*) that publish more laboratory studies with smaller sample sizes. Articles published in these journals had lower scores, with a mean score of 5.2 (SD 2.3) in *IJERPH* and a mean score of 5.0 (SD 2.3) in *JD*. The mean values were statistically significantly different (*p*-value of ANOVA < 0.001).

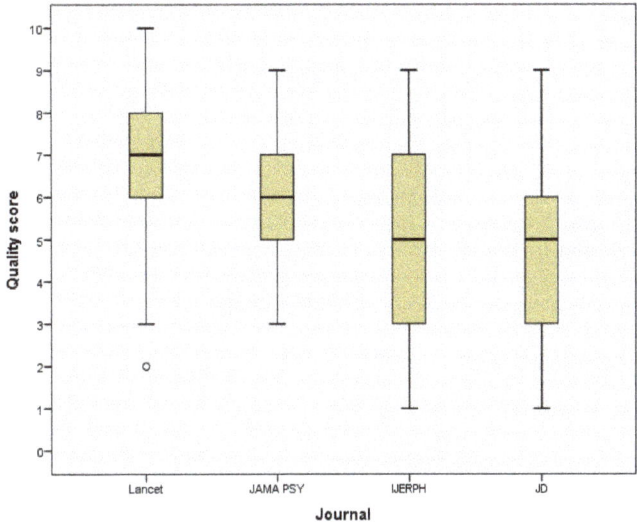

Figure 2. Box plot graph of the data analysis reporting quality score of 160 articles published in four journals. There were 40 articles from each journal. *JAMA Psy* = JAMA Psychiatry, *IJERPH* = International Journal of Environmental Research and Public Health, and *JD* = Journal of Dentistry.

3.4. Interrater and Test-Retest Reliability

The interobserver agreement measured by the ICC and Pearson correlation coefficient were 0.88 and 0.89, respectively. The test-retest reliability was excellent with identical mean scores for the first and second evaluations (Pearson's correlation coefficient was 0.95, and the intraclass correlation coefficient was 0.95).

The interrater reliability between Rater 1 and Rater 2 was also analyzed for each item. The overall percentage agreement ranged from 80% to 100% and kappa values ranged from 0.53 to 1. Individual item analyses showed very high agreement (100%) for items 5 (providing a statistical analysis subsection) and 9 (reporting software). The most common disagreement among Raters 1 and 2 was in the description of statistical methods. For Item 6 ("Did authors identify the variables with the methods for each analysis done in the study?"), the agreement was 92.5% and kappa was 0.53. For item 3 ("Were summary statistics, tests and methods identified and named in all tables and figures?") these values were 80% and 0.60, respectively.

The test-retest evaluation showed good agreement for each item: Agreement percentage ranged from 90% to 100% and the kappa coefficients ranged from 0.72 to 1. For items 1, 2, 5, 8, and 9, the reliability measures provided complete agreement. This preliminary intrarater validation analysis revealed that disagreement arose especially for item 6.

4. Discussion

My purpose was to help authors, editors, reviewers, and readers to evaluate the quality of statistical reporting and data presentation in research papers when data analysis procedures are invoked to clarify findings and to draw conclusions from raw data. I developed a test for quickly assessing the quality by selecting the checklist items from readers' and reviewers' perspectives. The composed scale from 0 to 10 assessed the selected reporting characteristics in the reviewed articles. A high value suggested that an article had a good presentation of findings in tables and figures and that the description of analysis methods was helpful to readers. This indicates an emphasis on analysis and reporting in the study and indicates that the methodological quality is high and understandable. The items included in the index also gave detailed information to reviewers and authors about the defects with respect to specific parts of the reporting of data analysis findings.

The problems in the reproducibility of biomedical research have received considerable attention in recent years [8,36–38]. One explanation is the poor presentation of statistical findings and inadequate reporting of data analysis techniques by authors. Low quality has been a long-term issue in medical research papers [4,8,36]. There seems to be a cultural component to these practices [39]. The reporting practices of senior scientists are transmitted to junior scientists. Authors will often copy inadequate reporting practices from previously published papers in their field and ignore the recommendations of current general guidelines. Another contributing factor is the disregard for medical biostatistics in biomedical and clinical education [36,40–43]. Many researchers clearly recognize the importance of data analysis concepts, but they continue to misunderstand elementary data analysis techniques and statistical concepts [44].

To clinicians and scientists, the literature is an important means for acquiring new information to guide health care research and clinical decision making. Poor reporting is unethical and may have serious consequences for clinical practice, future research, policy making, patient care, and ultimately for patients [10]. Securing the quality of the publications is an important activity of journals in their editorial policy. Journals need to be more proactive in providing information about the quality of what journals publish [10,45]. Journals should consider strategies and actions to verify that authors realize full responsibility for the statistical reporting quality of their manuscripts. Use of the short checklist proposed in this paper with reporting guidelines would be an important step towards quality-secured research.

Peer review provides the foundation for the scientific publishing system. During the editorial process peer reviewers are required to comment on whether the methods and findings are clearly reported [46]. This approach heavily relies on the statistical expertise of subject reviewers. In general, peer reviewers are competent in a specific range of statistical methods, but they may not necessarily be aware of more general statistical issues and best practices [16,36,47]. It has been claimed that due to the inadequate assessment of statistical reporting and data presentation during peer review and editorial processes, the quality of biomedical articles has not improved [8,36,47–49].

Medical journals often ask their subject reviewers if they are able to assess all statistical aspects of the manuscript themselves or whether they recommend an additional statistical review [47]. Leading medical journals, such as *Lancet*, *BMJ*, *Annals of Medicine* and *JAMA* have adopted statistical review. Despite demonstration of widespread statistical and data presentation errors in medical articles, increasing the use of statistical reviewers has been slow [50]. A recent survey found that only 23% of the top biomedical journals reported that they routinely employed statistical review for all original research articles [51]. Introduction of specialist statisticians to the peer review process has made peer review more specialized. In addition, statistical reviewing is time intensive, limited by both reviewer supply and expense.

In biomedical journals, there is no single model for statistical review in peer review strategies [51–53]. Some journals recruit statistical methodologists to the editorial board, some draw their statistical reviewers from an external pool. If all papers cannot be statistically reviewed, editors have to select which manuscripts should undergo statistical scrutiny. There are also models where subject reviewers are assisted to comment on the statistical aspects of a manuscript [47,48,54]. However, these checklists cover extensively all aspects of data analysis and are not straightforward for non-statistical reviewers to get an overall impression of the statistical quality. Some form of simplified checklist could be handy for editors and reviewers to spot the issues that might indicate more serious problems in the reporting of scientific articles. I hope that editors and reviewers could use the short quality test proposed in this paper for deciding when the presentation in a manuscript is clearly inadequate and they should recommend rejecting the manuscript. I agree with Kyrgidis and Triaridis [48] that if the reviewer cannot find the basic information and description related to the data analysis, the reviewer does not need to read the whole article. After checking tables and figures and reading through the statistical analysis subsection in the methods section, the reviewer can reject the manuscript on good grounds. When the proposed simple quality test shows that the statistical reporting and data presentation are appropriate, the whole article needs to be read and further reviewed.

In recent years, several journals have tried to improve peer review processes [55]. Their efforts have been focused on introducing openness and transparency to the models of peer review [56]. New strategies in peer review might help to address persistent statistical reporting and data presentation issues in the medical literature [55]. Software algorithms and scanners have been developed to assess internal consistency and validity of statistical tests in academic writing [57]. However, their use is still rare and limited to flag specific potential errors. The open peer review, where all peer reviews are made openly available brings into use new models where the quality of a paper may be assessed by the whole scientific community. The pre- and post-publication peer review models include commenting systems for the readership. Readers could use tools, such as proposed in this paper, to give feedback to authors. Subsequently, authors prepare a second version of the manuscript reflecting the comments and suggestions proposed by the scientific community.

My validation set of articles included four journals with different levels of prestige and visibility. The reporting of data analysis information was more detailed and useful for the reader in the more visible journals (*Lancet* and *JAMA Psychiatry*). This is in line with previous studies [5,6]. High-impact journals have more rigorous review process, including extensive statistical reviews. Several researchers in scientific communication have recommended sending out all manuscripts with numerical data for statistical review [8,58,59]. In addition, the strict monitoring of revisions made in manuscripts is important.

The proposed quality test is short. It includes only nine items. These items measure the data presentation quality and the description of data analysis methods. It does not include items about study design, justification of sample size, potential sources of bias, common statistical methodological issues, or interpretation of results. Several reporting guidelines and checklists are available to ensure that authors have paid attention to these other aspects [10,11]. However, these checklists have had little impact on the quality of statistical reporting, and they have not been sufficient for ensuring that issues related to poor statistical reporting and inadequate data presentation are eliminated from manuscripts [3,8,60]. In addition, the general checklists do not include detailed recommendations for reporting how statistical analyses were performed and how to present data.

The article set for pilot testing the proposed instrument included only published studies. Editors and reviewers can use the proposed tool to judge whether manuscripts should be accepted for publication. Educators can utilize it when educating researchers about how to improve statistical reporting and data presentation. A future study is required to apply the instrument at the initial submission of manuscripts to scientific journals and to test how applicable it is in the peer review process. In addition, content and construct validity properties [61] need to be evaluated in future studies.

It should be noted that the instrument was specifically developed for health care, biomedical and clinical studies, and limitations may arise if it is used in nonmedical fields that apply statistical methods.

5. Conclusions

In summary, I have developed an applicable checklist for quickly testing the statistical reporting quality of manuscripts and published research papers. One aim of this work was to help authors prepare manuscripts. Good research deserves to be presented well, and good presentation is as much a part of the research as the collection and analysis of the data. With this instrument authors could test the effectiveness of their presentations (tables and figures) for their readers. In addition, they could check that they have not described statistical methods too briefly or superficially.

Competent editors and scientific reviewers should be able to identify errors in basic statistical analysis and reporting. However, there is accumulative evidence that inadequate reporting of basic statistics is a persistent and ubiquitous problem in published medical studies. Editors and reviewers can improve the quality of reporting by identifying submitted manuscripts with poor-quality statistical reporting and data presentation. I hope that the editors and reviewers of scientific journals will incorporate the proposed test instrument in their editorial process. For a manuscript to be considered for full review, its statistical presentation has to be good enough for readers, subject reviewers, and statistical reviewers to understand what statistical methods have been applied and what data are presented in tables and figures. Manuscripts with poor-quality statistical reporting (total score ranges from 0 to 2) should be rejected. Giving detailed comments in review reports to improve the reporting may not be straightforward in those cases.

Readers can use the proposed data analysis reporting test as an initial indicator of research quality. They can easily check whether, based on numerical data analyses, a published research article is readable, understandable and accessible to healthcare professionals who might wish to use similar techniques in their future work or to those who are not experts in a particular subfield. A high score indicates that the authors have focused on reporting and readers should be able to express an opinion about the results after reading the main text.

Further refinement of the data analysis reporting instrument will continue, and I invite feedback.

Author Contributions: P.N. has undertaken all the works of this paper.

Funding: This research received no external funding.

Acknowledgments: I am grateful to Jasleen Kaur who provided useful comments on the draft of the instrument items. I wish to thank all health since students at the University of Oulu who participated in the piloting of the instrument.

Conflicts of Interest: The authors declare no conflict of interest.

References

1. Sato, Y.; Gosho, M.; Nagashima, K.; Takahashi, S.; Ware, J.H.; Laird, N.M. Statistical Methods in the Journal—An Update. *N. Engl. J. Med.* **2017**, *376*, 1086–1087. [CrossRef] [PubMed]
2. Nieminen, P.; Miettunen, J.; Koponen, H.; Isohanni, M. Statistical methodologies in psychopharmacology: A review. *Hum. Psychopharmacol. Clin. Exp.* **2006**, *21*, 195–203. [CrossRef] [PubMed]
3. Norström, F. Poor quality in the reporting and use of statistical methods in public health—The case of unemployment and health. *Arch. Public Health* **2015**, *73*, 56. [CrossRef] [PubMed]
4. Diong, J.; Butler, A.A.; Gandevia, S.C.; Héroux, M.E. Poor statistical reporting, inadequate data presentation and spin persist despite editorial advice. *PLoS ONE* **2018**, *13*, e202121. [CrossRef] [PubMed]
5. Altman, D.G. Poor-quality medical research: What can journals do? *JAMA* **2002**, *287*, 2765–2767. [CrossRef]
6. Nieminen, P.; Carpenter, J.; Rucker, G.; Schumacher, M. The relationship between quality of research and citation frequency. *BMC Med. Res. Methodol.* **2006**, *6*, 42. [CrossRef]
7. McClean, M.; Silverberg, J. Statistical reporting in randomized controlled trials from the dermatology literature: A review of 44 dermatology journals. *Br. J. Dermatol.* **2015**, *173*, 172–183. [CrossRef]

8. Dexter, F.; Shafer, S.L. Narrative Review of Statistical Reporting Checklists, Mandatory Statistical Editing, and Rectifying Common Problems in the Reporting of Scientific Articles. *Anesth. Analg.* **2017**, *124*, 943–947. [CrossRef]
9. Vandenbroucke, J.P.; Von Elm, E.; Altman, D.G.; Gøtzsche, P.C.; Mulrow, C.D.; Pocock, S.J.; Poole, C.; Schlesselman, J.J.; Egger, M. Strengthening the Reporting of Observational Studies in Epidemiology (STROBE): Explanation and elaboration. *PLoS Med.* **2007**, *4*, 1628–1654. [CrossRef]
10. Moher, D.; Altman, D.G.; Schultz, K.F.; Simera, I.; Wager, E. *Guidelines for Reporting Health Research. User's Manual*; John Wiley & Sons, Ltd.: Chichester, UK, 2014.
11. EQUATOR Network. Available online: https://www.equator-network.org/ (accessed on 30 March 2020).
12. Lang, T.A.; Michelle, S. *How to Report Statistics in Medicine: Annotated Guidelines for Authors, Editors and Reviewers*, 2nd ed.; American College of Physicians: Philadelphia, PA, USA, 2006.
13. Strasak, A.M.; Zaman, Q.; Pfeiffer, K.P.; Gobel, G.; Ulmer, H. Statistical errors in medical research—A review of common pitfalls. *Swiss Med. Wkly.* **2007**, *137*, 44–49.
14. Lee, S. Avoiding negative reviewer comments: Common statistical errors in anesthesia journals. *Korean J. Anesthesiol.* **2016**, *69*, 219–226. [CrossRef] [PubMed]
15. Altman, D.G. Statistical reviewing for medical journals. *Stat. Med.* **1998**, *17*, 2661–2674. [CrossRef]
16. Nieminen, P.; Virtanen, J.I.; Vähänikkilä, H. An instrument to assess the statistical intensity of medical research papers. *PLoS ONE* **2017**, *12*. [CrossRef] [PubMed]
17. Bland, M. *An Introduction to Medical Statistics*; Oxford University Press: Oxford, UK, 2015; ISBN 0199589925.
18. Pickering, R.M. Describing the participants in a study. *Age Ageing* **2017**, *46*, 576–581. [CrossRef] [PubMed]
19. Lang, T.A.; Altman, D.G. Basic statistical reporting for articles published in Biomedical Journals: "The Statistical analyses and methods in the published literature" or the SAMPL guidelines. *Int. J. Nurs. Stud.* **2015**, *52*, 5–9. [CrossRef]
20. Nieminen, P.; Kaur, J. Reporting of data analysis methods in psychiatric journals: Trends from 1996 to 2018. *Int. J. Methods Psychiatr. Res.* **2019**, *28*. [CrossRef]
21. Nieminen, P.; Vähänikkilä, H. Use of data analysis methods in dental publications: Is there evidence of a methodological change? *Publications* **2020**, *8*, 9. [CrossRef]
22. Thiese, M.S.; Ronna, B.; Ott, U. P value interpretations and considerations. *J. Thorac. Dis.* **2016**, *8*, E928–E931. [CrossRef]
23. Motulsky, H. *Intuitive Biostatistics*, 3rd ed.; Oxford University Press: New York, NY, USA, 2014; ISBN 9780199946648.
24. American Medical Association. *AMA Manual of Style: A Guide for Authors and Editors*, 11th ed.; Oxford University Press: New York, NY, USA, 2020; ISBN 978-0190246556.
25. Oberg, A.L.; Poland, G.A. The process of continuous journal improvement: New author guidelines for statistical and analytical reporting in VACCINE. *Vaccine* **2012**, *30*, 2915–2917. [CrossRef]
26. American Psychological Assiciation. *Publication Manual of the American Psychological Assiciation*, 6th ed.; American Psychological Assiciation: Washington, DC, USA, 2017; ISBN 978-1-4338-0561-5.
27. Gardner, M.J.; Altman, D.G. Confidence intervals rather than P values: Estimation rather than hypothesis testing. *Br. Med. J. (Clin. Res. Ed.)* **1986**, *292*, 746–750. [CrossRef]
28. Spector, R.; Vesell, E.S. Pharmacology and statistics: Recommendations to strengthen a productive partnership. *Pharmacology* **2006**, *78*, 113–122. [CrossRef] [PubMed]
29. ECMJE Recommendations for He Conduct, Reporting, Editing, and Publication of Scolarly Work in Medical Journals. Available online: http://www.icmje.org/recommendations/ (accessed on 25 May 2020).
30. Lang, T.A.; Altman, D.G. Statistical Analyses and Methods in the Published Literature: The SAMPL Guidelines. In *Guidelines for Reporting Health Research: A User's Manual*; John Wiley & Sons, Ltd.: Oxford, UK, 2014; pp. 264–274. ISBN 9780470670446.
31. Simundic, A.-M. Practical recommendations for statistical analysis and data presentation in Biochemia Medica journal. *Biochem. Med.* **2012**, *22*, 15–23. [CrossRef] [PubMed]
32. Mayo, D. *Statistical Inference as Severe Testing. How to Get beyond the Statistical Wars*; Cambridge University Press: Cambridge, UK, 2018; ISBN 978-1-107-66464-7.
33. Indrayan, A.; Malhotra, R.K. *Medical Biostatistics*, 4th ed.; CRC Press: Cambridge, UK, 2018; ISBN 1498799531.
34. Indrayan, A. Reporting of Basic Statistical Methods in Biomedical Journals: Improved SAMPL Guidelines. *Indian Pediatr.* **2020**, *57*, 43–48. [CrossRef] [PubMed]

35. Gwet, K.L. *Handbook of Inter-Rater Reliability*, 4th ed.; Advances Analytics, LLS: Gaithersburg, MD, USA, 2014; ISBN 9780970806284.
36. Glasziou, P.; Altman, D.G.; Bossuyt, P.; Boutron, I.; Clarke, M.; Julious, S.; Michie, S.; Moher, D.; Wager, E. Reducing waste from incomplete or unusable reports of biomedical research. *Lancet* **2014**, *383*, 267–276. [CrossRef]
37. *The Academy of Medical Sciences Reproducibility and Reliability of Biomedical Research: Improving Research Practice*; The Academy of Medical Sciences: London, UK, 2015.
38. Vetter, T.R.; McGwin, G.; Pittet, J.F. Replicability, Reproducibility, and Fragility of Research Findings-Ultimately, Caveat Emptor. *Anesth. Analg.* **2016**, *123*, 244–248. [CrossRef]
39. Smaldino, P.E.; McElreath, R. The natural selection of bad science. *R. Soc. Open Sci.* **2016**, *3*, 9. [CrossRef]
40. Shetty, A.C.; Al Rasheed, N.M.; Albwardi, S.A. Dental professionals' attitude towards biostatistics. *J. Dent. Oral Hyg.* **2015**, *7*, 113–118.
41. Hannigan, A.; Hegarty, A.C.; McGrath, D. Attitudes towards statistics of graduate entry medical students: The role of prior learning experiences. *BMC Med. Educ.* **2014**, *14*, 70. [CrossRef]
42. Batra, M.; Gupta, M.; Dany, S.S.; Rajput, P. Perception of Dental Professionals towards Biostatistics. *Int. Sch. Res. Not.* **2014**, *2014*, 1–6. [CrossRef]
43. Altman, D.G.; Goodman, S.N.; Schroter, S. How statistical expertise is used in medical research. *JAMA* **2002**, *287*, 2817–2820. [CrossRef]
44. Belia, S.; Fidler, F.; Williams, J.; Cumming, G. Researchers misunderstand confidence intervals and standard error bars. *Psychol. Methods* **2005**, *10*, 389–396. [CrossRef]
45. Moher, D. Reporting guidelines: Doing better for readers. *BMC Med.* **2018**, *16*, 18–20. [CrossRef]
46. Glonti, K.; Cauchi, D.; Cobo, E.; Boutron, I.; Moher, D.; Hren, D. A scoping review on the roles and tasks of peer reviewers in the manuscript review process in biomedical journals. *BMC Med.* **2019**, *17*, 1–14. [CrossRef] [PubMed]
47. Greenwood, D.C.; Freeman, J.V. How to spot a statistical problem: Advice for a non-statistical reviewer. *BMC Med.* **2015**, *13*, 1–3. [CrossRef] [PubMed]
48. Kyrgidis, A.; Triaridis, S. Methods and Biostatistics: A concise guide for peer reviewers. *Hippokratia* **2010**, *14*, 13–22. [PubMed]
49. Patel, J. Why training and specialization is needed for peer review: A case study of peer review for randomized controlled trials. *BMC Med.* **2014**, *12*, 1–7. [CrossRef] [PubMed]
50. Horbach, S.P.J.M.; Halffman, W. The changing forms and expectations of peer review. *Res. Integr. Peer Rev.* **2018**, *3*, 1–15. [CrossRef]
51. Hardwicke, T.E.; Goodman, S.N. How often do leading biomedical journals use statistical experts to evaluate statistical methods? The results of a survey. *MetArXiv Prepr.* **2020**, 1–29.
52. Hardwicke, T.E.; Frank, M.C.; Vazire, S.; Goodman, S.N. Should Psychology Journals Adopt Specialized Statistical Review? *Adv. Methods Pract. Psychol. Sci.* **2019**, *2*, 240–249. [CrossRef]
53. Overgaard, K.; Roberts, J.; Schaeffer, M.B.; Pessin, R. the Trenches. *Sci. Ed.* **2015**, *38*, 2015.
54. Curtis, M.J.; Alexander, S.; Cirino, G.; Docherty, J.R.; George, C.H.; Giembycz, M.A.; Hoyer, D.; Insel, P.A.; Izzo, A.A.; Ji, Y.; et al. Experimental design and analysis and their reporting II: Updated and simplified guidance for authors and peer reviewers. *Br. J. Pharmacol.* **2018**, *175*, 987–993. [CrossRef]
55. Fresco-Santalla, A.N.A.; Hernández-Pérez, T. Current and evolving models of peer-review. *Ser. Libr.* **2014**, *67*, 373–398. [CrossRef]
56. Vercellini, P.; Buggio, L.; Vigano, P.; Somigliana, E. Peer review in medical journals: Beyond quality of reports towards transparency and public scrutiny of the process. *Eur. J. Intern. Med.* **2016**, *31*, 15–19. [CrossRef]
57. Nuijten, M.B.; Hartgerink, C.H.J.; van Assen, M.A.L.M.; Epskamp, S.; Wicherts, J.M. The prevalence of statistical reporting errors in psychology (1985–2013). *Behav. Res. Methods* **2016**, *48*, 1205–1226. [CrossRef] [PubMed]
58. Vahanıkkıla, H.; Tjaderhane, L.; Nieminen, P. The statistical reporting quality of articles published in 2010 in five dental journals. *Acta Odontol. Scand.* **2015**, *73*, 76–80. [CrossRef] [PubMed]
59. Lukic, I.; Marusic, M. Appointment of statistical editor and quality of statistics in a small medical journal. *Croat. Med. J.* **2001**, *42*, 500–503. [PubMed]

60. Pouwels, K.B.; Widyakusuma, N.N.; Groenwold, R.H.H.; Hak, E. Quality of reporting of confounding remained suboptimal after the STROBE guideline. *J. Clin. Epidemiol.* **2016**, *69*, 217–224. [CrossRef]
61. Mokkink, L.B.; Terwee, C.B.; Patrick, D.L.; Alonso, J.; Stratford, P.W.; Knol, D.L.; Bouter, L.M.; de Vet, H.C.W. The COSMIN study reached international consensus on taxonomy, terminology, and definitions of measurement properties for health-related patient-reported outcomes. *J. Clin. Epidemiol.* **2010**, *63*, 737–745. [CrossRef]

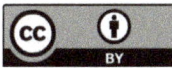

© 2020 by the author. Licensee MDPI, Basel, Switzerland. This article is an open access article distributed under the terms and conditions of the Creative Commons Attribution (CC BY) license (http://creativecommons.org/licenses/by/4.0/).

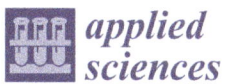

Article
Stretched Exponential Survival Analysis for South Korean Females

Byung Mook Weon [1,2,3]

1. Soft Matter Physics Laboratory, School of Advanced Materials Science and Engineering, SKKU Advanced Institute of Nanotechnology (SAINT), Sungkyunkwan University, Suwon 16419, Korea; bmweon@skku.edu
2. Research Center for Advanced Materials Technology, Sungkyunkwan University, Suwon 16419, Korea
3. Department of Biomedical Engineering, Johns Hopkins University, Baltimore, MD 21218, USA

Received: 7 September 2019; Accepted: 30 September 2019; Published: 10 October 2019

Featured Application: The stretched exponential survival analysis enables quantitative and comparative study of female lifespan between South Korea and other countries, particularly quantifying the survival rate, the characteristic life, and the maximum lifespan.

Abstract: South Korea has recently exhibited a remarkable rapid increase in female lifespan. Here, a mathematical analysis is suggested for a clear interpretation of current trends in female lifespan in South Korea. To mathematically analyze life tables, a modified stretched exponential function is employed and demonstrated to estimate current trends of female lifespan in South Korea based on reliable life tables from 1987 to 2016 taken from the Korean Statistical Information Service. This methodology enables us to perform quantitative and comparative analyses of female lifespan in South Korea with representative industrialized countries such as Japan, France, Australia, Switzerland, UK, Sweden, and USA. This analysis provides quantitative and comparative evidence that South Korea has the highest increase rate of female lifespan over the past three decades. Further application would be feasible for a better estimation of human aging statistics.

Keywords: modified stretched exponential function; age-dependent stretched exponent; characteristic life; maximum lifespan; South Korean female

---

1. Introduction

Statistical analysis of human lifespan is a central topic in demography and gerontology. Life expectancy of humans has risen steadily and rapidly over the past 150 years in most countries and keeps increasing in the 21st century [1–3]. A recent study of 35 industrialized countries shows an interesting projection: there is more than 50% probability that by 2030, female life expectancy is likely to break the 90-year barrier [4]. Interestingly, South Korea is predicted to have the highest female life expectancy at birth by 2030 [4]. This prediction is achieved by applying a mathematical ensemble of 21 forecasting models to reliable statistics data about life tables for humans [4]. South Korean females are an important model to understand current trends in human lifespan and a better survival analysis is required for a better understanding of human lifespan.

To achieve a more reliable prediction, a mathematical model of human survival curves is helpful in quantifying current trends in human lifespan for human aging and demography research [5–8]. In fact, many mathematical models for survival curves have been proposed, including the Gompertz, Weibull, Heligman-Pollard, Kannisto, quadratic, and logistic models [5]. In a recent work, a mathematical model has been suggested owing to a usefulness to describe survival curves with complexity in shape by adopting a modified function from the stretched exponential (Weibull or Kohlrausch–Williams–Watts) function [9–14]. Flexibility of a modified stretched exponential function, originating from an age-dependent stretched exponent, enables us to mathematically describe plasticity and rectangularity of survival curves [5,13]. In this work, by incorporating this mathematical model to the reliable life table datasets taken from the Korean Statistical Information Service (KOSIS, http://kosis.kr/eng), a practical application is demonstrated to quantify current trends in female lifespan for South Korea over three recent decades, from 1987 to 2016. This analysis for South Korea is compared with that for Japan, France, Australia, Switzerland, UK, Sweden, and USA, which are the representative leading countries in longevity [4].

In this study, a mathematical analysis with a modified stretched exponential model is demonstrated to interpret the recent survival curves for South Korean female, taken from the Korean Statistical Information Service. The current trends for 1987–2016 are estimated from the female survival curves in South Korea based on the estimates of the characteristic life and the maximum lifespan.

2. Methods

The stretched exponential survival analysis is summarized as follows. The methodology is based on the modified stretched exponential function to describe the human survival curves, which has been developed for the past decade [5,12–14]. This section briefly introduces into the mathematical approach. The survival rate, $s(x)$, is a function of age, x. Mathematically the mortality rate (equivalently the hazard function or the force of mortality), $\mu(x) = -d\ln(s(x))/dx$, is the derivative of the survival rate with respect to age. As a mathematical constraint, $s(x)$ is a monotonic decrease function with age, starting from 1 and ending to 0. To mathematically describe the survival curves, a modified stretched exponential function is quite flexible by applying a form of $s(x) = \exp(-(x/\alpha)^{\beta(x)})$ where the stretched exponent, $\beta(x)$, is an age-dependent term as $\beta(x) = \ln[-\ln(s(x))]/\ln(x/\alpha)$ and the characteristic life, α, is a reference age, determined at $s(\alpha) = \exp(-1)$ that equals to the interception point between $s(x)$ and $s(\alpha) = \exp(-1)$ [5,12–14]. The characteristic life is an alternative to the life expectancy at birth, ε [14,15]. The age dependence of the stretched exponent is the critical feature of the modified stretched exponential function, which is fundamentally different from the classical stretched exponential function [5,12–14]. The characteristic life and the stretched exponent are useful to respectively describe the scale effect (associated with *living longer*, characterized by α) and the shape effect (associated with *growing older*, characterized by $\beta(x)$) of the individual survival curve [14]. For old-age patterns, the quadratic formula of $\beta(x) = \beta_0 + \beta_1 x + \beta_2 x^2$ is applicable [5,12], which leads to the occurrence of the (mathematical) maximum lifespan, ω, which is obtained at the age for $\beta(x) = -x\ln(x/\alpha)\frac{d\beta(x)}{dx}$ by the mathematical constraint of $\frac{ds(x)}{dx} \to 0$ [12]. This methodology is beneficial in modeling the human mortality curves in very old age [5].

3. Results and Discussion

3.1. Survival Analysis

The survival curves for women were obtained at the complete life tables taken from the Korean Statistical Information Service (http://kosis.kr/eng). Figure 1 shows how we evaluate the survival curves for Korean female in the most recent decades, 1987–2016. The summarized survival curves in Figure 1a show the historic trends in the survival rates for Korean female over three recent decades. The survival curves for Korean female show that $s(x)$ gradually decreases with age and historically shifts rightwards and towards a rectangular shape over three recent decades, as consistent with Swedish female [5,14].

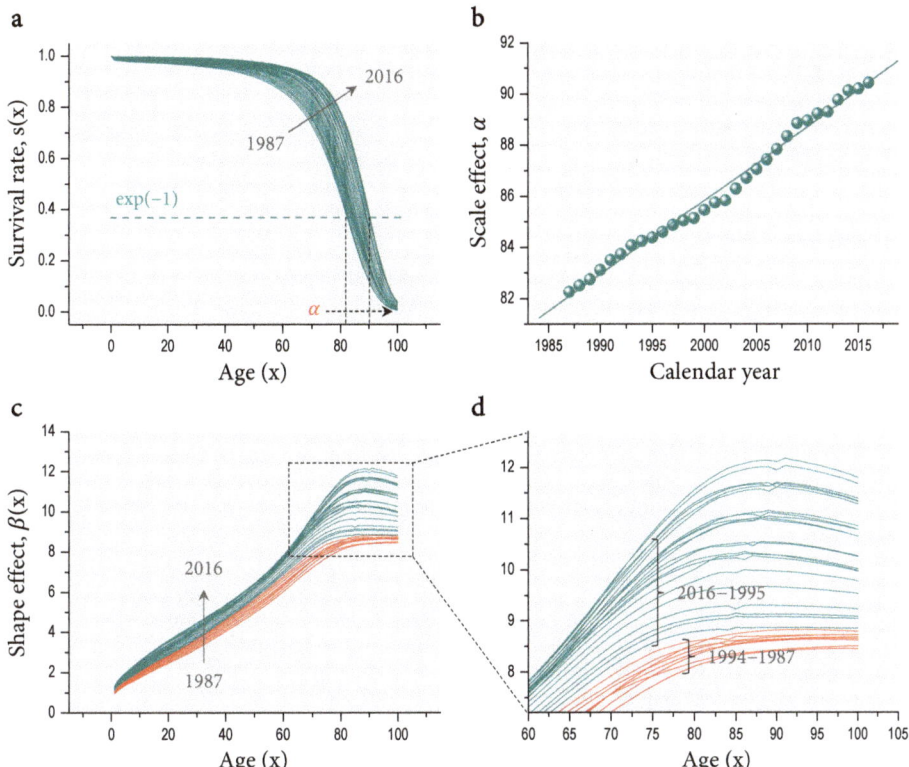

Figure 1. Survival analysis. (**a**) The survival curves for Korean female in recent decades, 1987–2016, were obtained at the complete life tables taken from the Korean Statistical Information Service (http://kosis.kr/eng). (**b**) The characteristic life of the given survival curve. (**c**) The age-dependent stretched exponent. (**d**) The old-age patterns of the stretched exponent at ages over 60 years could be fitted with the quadratic formula of age. The phase transition in the stretched exponent with age appears for 1995–2016 but not for 1987–1994.

The characteristic life, α, indicating the scale effect of the individual survival curve, was measured for each survival curve through the graphical analysis at $s(\alpha) = \exp(-1) \approx 0.367879$. The recent historic trends in the α values were summarized in Figure 1b. The characteristic life for Korean female was depicted as a function of the calendar year (1987–2016) in Figure 1b. This result shows that the α value linearly increases at a constant rate of ~2.88 years per decade (as marked by the solid line in Figure 1b). This steady increase rate for South Korean female is much higher than the rate of ~1.20 years per decade for Swedish female in the previous analyses (data from the Human Mortality Database, http://www.mortality.org) [5,14]. The historic trends in the characteristic life clearly demonstrate that South Korean women have lived longer in the past three decades.

The $\beta(x)$ value, indicating the shape effect of the individual survival curve, was obtained from $\beta(x) = -x \ln(x/\alpha) \frac{d\beta(x)}{dx}$ as shown in Figure 1c. Particularly as demonstrated in Figure 1d, old-age patterns of $\beta(x)$ at ages over 60 years could be empirically fitted with the quadratic formula as $\beta(x) = \beta_0 + \beta_1 x + \beta_2 x^2$ as suggested previously [5,12,13]. The modified stretched exponential function is successfully applicable to the survival curves and to the age-dependent stretched exponents for all ages (Figure 1c) and for old ages over 60 years (Figure 1d). Most remarkably, the $\beta(x)$ curve smoothly varies with age at old ages over 60 years and old-age $\beta(x)$ patterns over 90 years can be depicted with the quadratic function of age. As found previously, the $\beta(x)$ patterns for old-age populations undergo the phase transition with age: $\beta(x)$ increases with age at $x < \alpha$ and decreases with age at $x > \alpha$ [12]. The phase transition appears in South Korean female datasets after the calendar year of 1995: there are phase transitions for 1995–2016 and no transitions for 1987–1994, as separately marked in Figure 1d. Considering old-age $\beta(x)$ patterns, the female lifespan of South Korea would experience the critical phase change through the calendar year of 1995. The historic trends in age dependence in $\beta(x)$ clearly show how the female lifespan in South Korea has been growing older during 1987–2016.

3.2. Characteristic Life Analysis

The comparison in the increase rate of α for South Korea with that for major industrialized countries is shown in Figure 2. The increase rate in α was obtained from Figure 1b for South Korea, 1987–2016 (data from the Korean Statistical Information Service, http://kosis.kr/eng), and from literature [14] for other countries, 1980–2010 (data from the Human Mortality Database, http://www.mortality.org). The error bars were taken from the standard errors by linear fits. The increase rate in α per decade was evaluated as ~2.88 years for South Korea, ~2.71 years for Japan, ~1.96 years for France, ~1.85 years for Australia, ~1.61 years for Switzerland, ~1.49 years for UK, ~1.24 years for Sweden, and ~0.76 years for USA. This analysis result confirms the highest increase rate of the characteristic life for women in South Korea among the representative high-income countries including Japan, France, Australia, Switzerland, UK, Sweden, and USA.

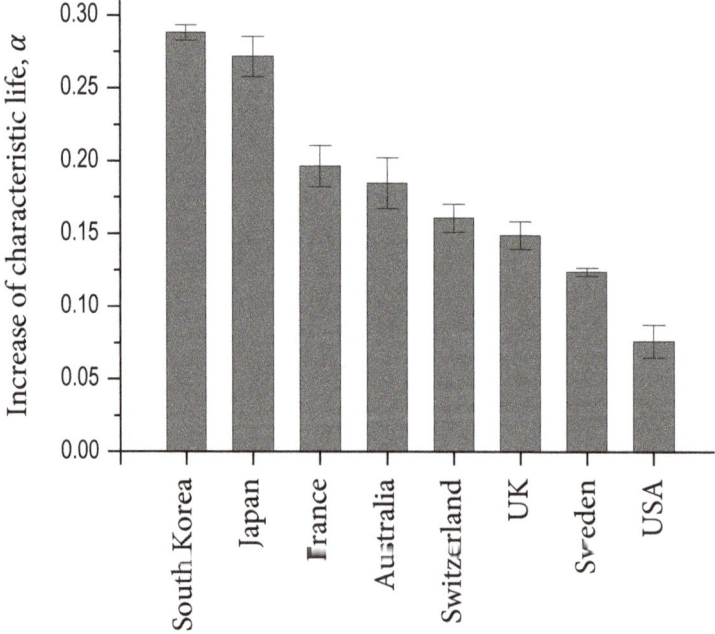

Figure 2. Comparison in the increase rate of the characteristic life per decade among representative industrialized countries. The data were taken for South Korea (1987–2016) from the Korean Statistical Information Service (http://kosis.kr/eng) and for other countries (1980–2010) from the Human Mortality Database (http://www.mortality.org).

To demonstrate the association of the characteristic life (α), taken from Figure 2, with the life expectancy at birth (ε), the annual increase rates of α and ε are compared in Figure 3. The ε values for 1980–2015 were taken from the Organization for Economic Cooperation and Development [16] and the increase rates of the ε values were achieved by linear fits (the error bars taken from the standard errors: some of the error bars are smaller than the symbol sizes). The increase rates of the ε values per decade were evaluated as ~4.15 years for South Korea, ~2.33 years for Japan, ~2.15 years for France, ~1.96 years for Australia, ~1.78 years for Switzerland, ~1.93 years for UK, ~1.43 years for Sweden, and ~1.06 years for USA. The annual increase rate of the ε values (marked by m) is proportionally correlated with the annual increase rate of the α values (marked by n) as $n \approx 1.173\,m - 0.046$ (adj. $R^2 \sim 0.85243$) except for South Korea. This analysis result suggests that the annual increase rate of the ε values for South Korea looks an extraordinary case among the representative high-income countries.

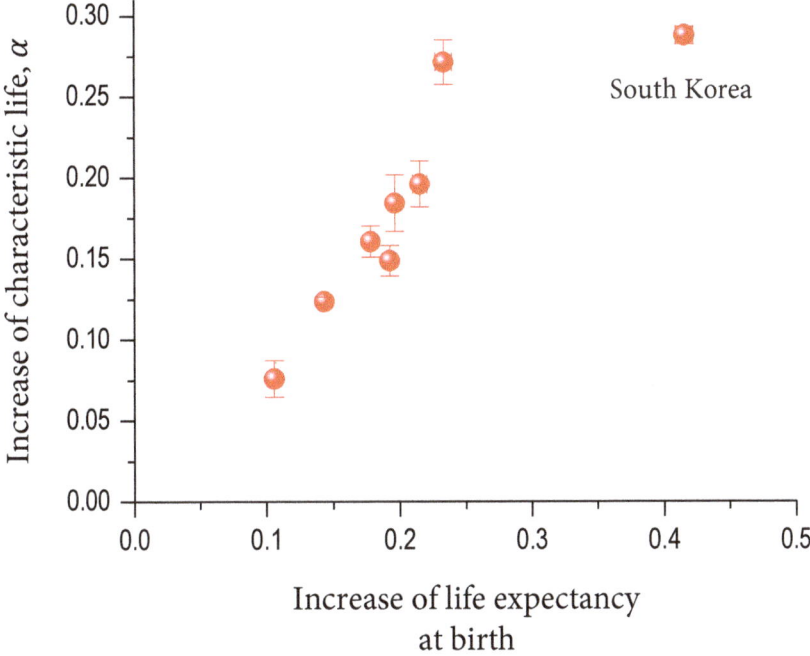

Figure 3. Association of the characteristic life, taken from Figure 2, with the life expectancy at birth per decade in representative industrialized countries, taken from the Organization for Economic Cooperation and Development [16].

The highest increase rate in the female lifespan (in both α and ε) for South Korea in Figure 3 is consistent with that the female life expectancy at birth in South Korea is the sixth ranked in 2010 and expected to be the first ranked in 2030 among the 35 industrialized countries [4]. So far, little attention has been given to South Korea in research on human health and longevity except for a few reports [4]. This analysis supports that South Korea has the highest increase rate in the female lifespan in the world in the past three decades.

3.3. Maximum Lifespan Analysis

The term *lifespan* describes how long an individual can live and the (observed) maximum lifespan is the age reached by the longest-lived member of a species, while the life expectancy is a population-based estimate of expected duration of life for individuals at any age, based on a statistical life table [3]. Our methodology enables us to estimate the characteristic life (α) and the (mathematical) maximum lifespan (ω) as good measures of the human lifespan. The estimates of α and ω for Korean female (data from the Korean Statistical Information Service, http://kosis.kr/eng) are summarized in Figure 4. The estimates of ω are obtained by the mathematical constraint of $\frac{ds(x)}{dx} \to 0$ [5,14]. The fitting of $\beta(x)$ with the quadratic formula enables us to determine the estimates of ω at the specific age of $\gamma(x) = -x \ln(x/\alpha) \frac{d\beta(x)}{dx}$ which corresponds to the intercept point $\beta(x) = \gamma(x)$ [5]. This estimation is practically available if and only if the phase transition exists in old-age $\beta(x)$ curves. Indeed, the estimates of ω are significant over the calendar year of 2002, as shown in Figure 4.

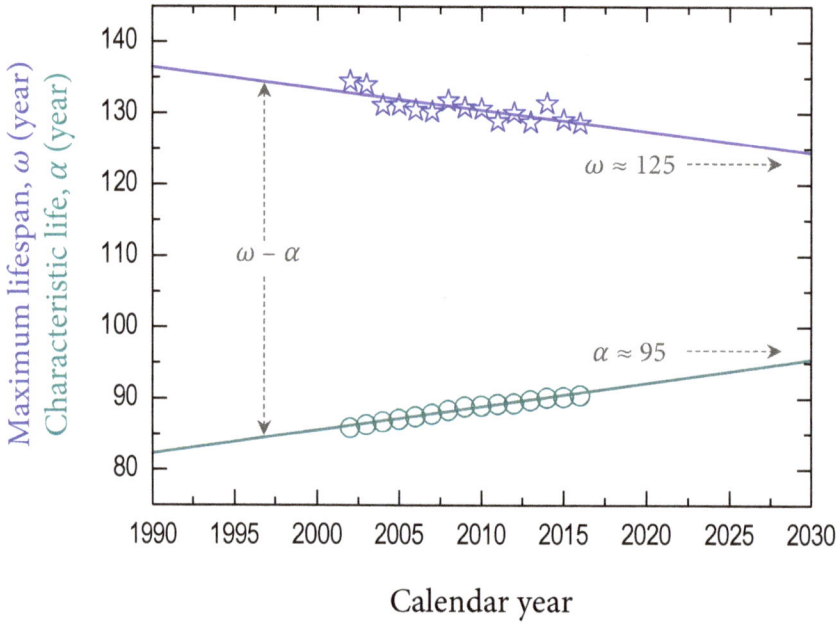

Figure 4. Estimation of the maximum lifespan and the characteristic life for Korean female (data from the Korean Statistical Information Service, http://kosis.kr/eng). The maximum lifespan gradually decreases at a constant rate of ~2.99 years per decade and the characteristic life gradually increases at a constant rate of ~3.30 years per decade.

Looking at the recent trends in ω and α for the South Korean female in Figure 4, the estimates of ω gradually decrease at a constant rate of ~2.99 years per decade and the estimates of α gradually increase at a constant rate of ~3.30 years per decade. Assuming continuity in the increments, the estimates of ω and α are predicted to reach ~125 years and ~95 years respectively around 2030. The change rates for South Korean female are much higher than those of ~1.6 years per decade in the ω values and ~1.2 years per decade in the α values for Swedish female [5]. The estimates of ω and α eventually become closer together over time; this tendency for South Korean female is consistent with Swedish female [5]. This result indicates that the survival curves have been increasingly concentrated at old ages, demonstrating the population aging [17,18]. As α becomes closer to ω (Figure 4), the survival curves tend to become strongly concentrated at very old ages, corresponding to the retangularization of survival curves [13,19]. This result would be relevant to the compression of morbidity, which is responsible for the accumulation of the very old populations in the population configuration [5].

3.4. Discussion

Now, it is noteworthy that the stretched exponential survival analysis enables the quantitative and comparative study of female lifespan between South Korea and other countries, particularly quantifying the survival rate, the characteristic life, and the maximum lifespan. All evidence suggests that South Korea has a remarkable rapid increase in female lifespan during the three recent decades (from 1987 to 2016), as demonstrated from the characteristic life analysis in Figures 2 and 3. An interesting question is why South Korea exhibits the highest increase rate in female lifespan. Economic development in South Korea is supposed to be beneficial to health care improvement, presumably provoking many potential social or cultural changes that are favorable for healthy daily habits and welfare. Obviously, health is the result of a combination of individual, social, and environmental factors [20]. In general, the recent increase in the numbers of older people in developed countries is a consequence of advances in hygiene and biomedicine as well as an artefact of human civilization [21]. In particular, South Korea has experienced rapid economic development and a substantial increase in life expectancy in an extremely short period, between 1970 and 2010, mainly due to the rapid processes of industrialization and urbanization [22,23].

Specifically, South Korea is expected to become the first country where the life expectancy at birth will exceed 90 years for women [24]. The recent industrialization and the subsequent improvements in living standards, nutrition, and health care have often been cited as major contributions to the remarkable improvements in health for South Korea [25]. The rapid increases in life expectancy in South Korea could be mostly achieved by reductions in infant mortality and in decreases related to infections and blood pressure [25]. More recent gains in South Korea have been largely due to postponement of death from chronic diseases [25]. These gains were mainly due to broad-based inclusive improvements in economic status and social capital (including education), which improved childhood and adolescent nutrition [26], expanded access to primary and secondary health care, and facilitated rapid scale-up of new medical technologies [25]. South Korea has also maintained lower body-mass index and blood pressure than other industrialized countries [27,28], and lower smoking in women. Additionally, South Korea might have lower health inequalities (for cancer and cardiovascular disease mortality, and for self-reported health status) than some of their western counterparts, especially for women [24,29,30]. The death rates from all causes in South Korea decreased significantly in both genders in the last three decades except for a period following the economic crisis in the late 1990s [31]. Looking at the trends in infectious disease mortality for South Korea, 1983−2015, infant mortality caused by infectious diseases has substantially decreased, while death rates from infectious disease for elderly populations with lower education levels and subgroups susceptible to respiratory infections and sepsis has not decreased overall [32]. The potential reasons for South Korea may be plausible but not for other countries.

Finally, the lifespan trends for Korean female may give a clue for the question regarding if there is a biological or social limit to human lifespan [3,33–36]. The heterogeneity in population and the dynamics of heterogeneous populations would become important in interpreting human lifespan [37,38]. The question about whether the upper limit to the maximum lifespan is fixed or flexible has been topics of continuous debate [34,39–45]. The decrease of the ω estimate in Figure 4 means that more people can reach the biological lifespan limit as expected to be 125 years [12]. The mathematical evaluation for female survival curves would be useful in achieving reliability and reproducibility in aging research [6–8] as well as in demonstrating the effectiveness of anti-aging therapies to slow the aging process [46]. Finding the appropriate mathematical model is quite important to accurately evaluate the human survival curves that exhibit a variety of heterogeneity and complexity. The practical implication of this study is that the potential reasons of South Korea may be useful to improve human lifespan, suggesting a further application of the stretched exponential survival analysis to identify personal, social, and environmental factors on human lifespan.

4. Conclusions

A steady increase in female lifespan is obvious in recent decades for most industrialized countries. This study shows the quantitative and comparative evidence for a remarkable rapid increase of female lifespan in South Korea during three recent decades, from 1987 to 2016, by applying the stretched exponential survival analysis. Based on the estimation of the increase rate of female lifespan for South

Korea, the comparative analysis with Japan, France, Australia, Switzerland, UK, Sweden, and USA implies that South Korea would have the highest increase rate of female lifespan during recent three decades. This result suggests that Korean female datasets would be a representative population dataset for further study on what contributions would be essential to human longevity. Further application would be feasible for a better estimation of human aging statistics, which will be useful for future population prediction and policy making.

Funding: This research was supported by Basic Science Research Program through the National Research Foundation of Korea (NRF) funded by the Ministry of Education (Grant No. NRF-2016R1D1A1B01007133 and Grant No. 2019R1A6A1A03033215).

Conflicts of Interest: The author declares no conflict of interest. The funders had no role in the design of the study; in the collection, analyses, or interpretation of data; in the writing of the manuscript, or in the decision to publish the results.

References

1. Wilmoth, J.R.; Deegan, L.J.; Lundström, H.; Horiuchi, S. Increase of maximum life-span in Sweden, 1861–1999. *Science* **2000**, *289*, 2366–2368. [CrossRef] [PubMed]
2. Oeppen, J.; Vaupel, J.W. Broken limits to life expectancy. *Science* **2006**, *296*, 1029–1031. [CrossRef] [PubMed]
3. Olshansky, S.J. Ageing: Measuring our narrow strip of life. *Nature* **2016**, *538*, 175–176. [CrossRef] [PubMed]
4. Kontis, V.; Bennett, J.E.; Mathers, C.D.; Li, G.; Foreman, K.; Ezzati, M. Future life expectancy in 35 industrialised countries: Projections with a Bayesian model ensemble. *Lancet* **2017**, *389*, 1323–1335. [CrossRef]
5. Weon, B.M. A solution to debates over the behavior of mortality at old ages. *Biogerontology* **2015**, *16*, 375–381. [CrossRef] [PubMed]
6. Petrascheck, M.; Miller, D.L. Computational analysis of lifespan experiment reproducibility. *Front. Genet.* **2017**, *8*, 92. [CrossRef] [PubMed]
7. Ruby, J.G.; Smith, M.; Buffenstein, R. Naked mole rat mortality rates defy Gompertzian laws by not increasing with age. *eLife* **2018**, *7*, e31157. [CrossRef] [PubMed]
8. Beltrán-Sánchez, H.; Finch, C. Life expectancy: Age is just a number. *eLife* **2018**, *7*, e34427. [CrossRef] [PubMed]
9. Weibull, W.A. A statistical distribution function of wide applicability. *J. Appl. Mech.* **1951**, *18*, 293–297.
10. Kohlrausch, R. Theorie des elektrischen rückstandes in der leidener flasche. *Pogg. Ann. Phys. Chem.* **1854**, *91*, 179–214. [CrossRef]
11. Williams, G.; Watts, D.C. Non-symmetrical dielectric relaxation behavior arising from a simple empirical decay function. *Trans. Faraday Soc.* **1970**, *66*, 80–85. [CrossRef]
12. Weon, B.M.; Je, J.H. Theoretical estimation of maximum human lifespan. *Biogerontology* **2009**, *10*, 65–71. [CrossRef] [PubMed]
13. Weon, B.M.; Je, J.H. Plasticity and rectangularity in survival curves. *Sci. Rep.* **2011**, *1*, 104. [CrossRef] [PubMed]
14. Weon, B.M.; Je, J.H. Trends in scale and shape of survival curves. *Sci. Rep.* **2012**, *2*, 504. [CrossRef] [PubMed]
15. Wrycza, T.; Baudisch, A. The pace of aging: Intrinsic time scales in demography. *Demogr. Res.* **2014**, *30*, 1571–1590. [CrossRef]
16. OECD. *Health at a Glance 2017: OECD Indicators*; OECD Publishing: Paris, France, 2017. [CrossRef]
17. Anderson, G.F.; Hussey, P.S. Population aging: A comparison among industrialized countries. *Health Aff.* **2000**, *19*, 191–203. [CrossRef] [PubMed]
18. Robine, J.M.; Michel, J.P. Looking forward to a general theory on population aging. *J. Gerontol. A Biol. Sci. Med. Sci.* **2004**, *59*, 590–597. [CrossRef]
19. Fries, J.F. Aging, natural death, and the compression of morbidity. *N. Engl. J. Med.* **1980**, *303*, 130–135. [CrossRef]
20. Shkrabtak, N.; Frolova, N.; Kiseleva, T.; Sergeeva, I.; Pomozova, V. Impact of environmental conditions on the health of the Far Eastern region population. *Appl. Sci.* **2019**, *9*, 1354. [CrossRef]

21. Hayflick, L. The future of ageing. *Nature* **2000**, *408*, 267–269. [CrossRef]
22. Kim, I.K.; Liang, J.; Rhee, K.O.; Kim, C.S. Population aging in Korea: Changes since the 1960s. *J. Cross Cult. Gerontol.* **1996**, *11*, 369–388. [CrossRef] [PubMed]
23. Bahk, J.; Lynch, J.W.; Khang, Y.H. Forty years of economic growth and plummeting mortality: The mortality experience of the poorly educated in South Korea. *J. Epidemiol. Community Health* **2017**, *71*, 282–288. [CrossRef] [PubMed]
24. Khang, Y.H.; Bahk, J.; Yi, N.; Yun, S.C. Age- and cause-specific contributions to income difference in life expectancy at birth: Findings from nationally representative data on one million South Koreans. *Eur. J. Public Health* **2016**, *26*, 242–248. [CrossRef] [PubMed]
25. Yang, S.; Khang, Y.H.; Harper, S.; Davey Smith, G.; Leon, D.A.; Lynch, J. Understanding the rapid increase in life expectancy in South Korea. *Am. J. Public Health* **2010**, *100*, 896–903. [CrossRef] [PubMed]
26. NCD-RisC. A century of trends in adult human height. *eLife* **2016**, *5*, e13410. [CrossRef] [PubMed]
27. NCD-RisC. Trends in adult body-mass index in 200 countries from 1975 to 2014: A pooled analysis of 1698 population-based measurement studies with 19.2 million participants. *Lancet* **2016**, *387*, 1377–1396. [CrossRef]
28. NCD-RisC. Worldwide trends in blood pressure from 1975 to 2015: A pooled analysis of 1479 population-based measurement studies with 19.1 million participants. *Lancet* **2017**, *389*, 37–55. [CrossRef]
29. Di Cesare, M.; Khang, Y.H.; Asaria, P.; Blakely, T.; Cowan, M.J.; Farzadfar, F.; Guerrero, R.; Ikeda, N.; Kyobutungi, C.; Msyamboza, K.P.; et al. Inequalities in non-communicable diseases and effective responses. *Lancet* **2013**, *381*, 585–597. [CrossRef]
30. OECD. *Health at a Glance 2015: OECD Indicators*; OECD Publishing: Paris, France, 2015. [CrossRef]
31. Lim, D.; Ha, M.; Song, I. Trends in the leading causes of death in Korea, 1983–2012. *J. Korean Med. Sci.* **2014**, *29*, 1597–1603. [CrossRef]
32. Choe, Y.J.; Choe, S.A.; Cho, S.I. Trends in infectious disease mortality, South Korea, 1983–2015. *Emerg. Infect. Dis.* **2018**, *24*, 320–327. [CrossRef]
33. Carnes, B.A.; Witten, T.M. How long must humans live? *J. Gerontol. A Biol. Sci. Med. Sci.* **2014**, *69*, 965–970. [CrossRef]
34. Dong, X.; Milholland, B.; Vijg, J. Evidence for a limit to human lifespan. *Nature* **2016**, *538*, 257–259. [CrossRef] [PubMed]
35. Newman, S.; Easteal, S. The dynamic upper limit of human lifespan [version 1; referees: 1 approved, 1 approved with reservations]. *F1000Research* **2017**, *6*, 569. [CrossRef] [PubMed]
36. Marck, A.; Antero, J.; Berthelot, G.; Saulière, G.; Jancovici, J.M.; Masson-Delmotte, V.; Boeuf, G.; Spedding, M.; Le Bourg, E.; Toussaint, J.F. Are we reaching the limits of homo sapiens? *Front. Physiol.* **2017**, *8*, 812. [CrossRef] [PubMed]
37. Carnes, B.A.; Olshansky, S.J. Heterogeneity and its biodemographic implications for longevity and mortality. *Exp. Gerontol.* **2001**, *36*, 419–430. [CrossRef]
38. Vaupel, J.W. Biodemography of human ageing. *Nature* **2010**, *464*, 536–542. [CrossRef]
39. Ben-Haim, M.S.; Kanfi, Y.; Mitchel, S.J.; Maoz, N.; Vaughan, K.; Amariglio, N.; Lerrer, B.; de Cabo, R.; Rechavi, G.; Cohen, H.Y. Breaking the ceiling of human maximal lifespan. *J. Gerontol. A Biol. Sci. Med. Sci.* **2018**, *73*, 1465–1471. [CrossRef]
40. Brown, N.J.L.; Albers, C.J.; Ritchie, S.J. Contesting the evidence for limited human lifespan. *Nature* **2017**, *546*, E6–E7. [CrossRef]
41. De Beer, J.; Bardoutsos, A.; Janssen, F. Maximum human lifespan may increase to 125 years. *Nature* **2017**, *546*, E16–E17. [CrossRef]
42. Hughes, B.G.; Hekimi, S. Many possible maximum lifespan trajectories. *Nature* **2017**, *546*, E8–E9. [CrossRef]
43. Lenart, A.; Vaupel, J.W. Questionable evidence for a limit to human lifespan. *Nature* **2017**, *546*, E13–E14. [CrossRef] [PubMed]
44. Rozing, M.P.; Kirkwood, T.B.L.; Westendorp, R.G.J. Is there evidence for a limit to human lifespan? *Nature* **2017**, *546*, E11–E12. [CrossRef] [PubMed]

45. Rootzen, H.; Zholud, D. Human life is unlimited–but short. *Extremes* **2017**, *20*, 713–728. [CrossRef]
46. De Magalhães, J.P.; Stevens, M.; Thornton, D. The business of anti-aging science. *Trends Biotechnol.* **2017**, *35*, 1062–1073. [CrossRef] [PubMed]

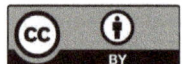 © 2019 by the authors. Licensee MDPI, Basel, Switzerland. This article is an open access article distributed under the terms and conditions of the Creative Commons Attribution (CC BY) license (http://creativecommons.org/licenses/by/4.0/).

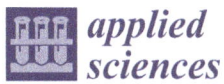

Article

Using the Importance–Satisfaction Model and Service Quality Performance Matrix to Improve Long-Term Care Service Quality in Taiwan

Shun-Hsing Chen [1], Fan-Yun Pai [2,*] and Tsu-Ming Yeh [3,*]

[1] Department of Marketing and Distribution Management, Oriental Institute of Technology, New Taipei City 220, Taiwan; chen88@mail.oit.edu.tw
[2] Department of Business Administration, National Changhua University of Education, Changhua 500, Taiwan
[3] Department of Industrial Engineering and Management, National Quemoy University, Kinmen 892, Taiwan
* Correspondence: fypai@cc.ncue.edu.tw (F.-Y.P.); tmyeh@nqu.edu.tw (T.-M.Y.);
  Tel.: +886-47-232105 (ext. 7415) (F.-Y.P.); +886-82-313585 (T.-M.Y.)

Received: 11 October 2019; Accepted: 19 December 2019; Published: 20 December 2019

Abstract: The present study integrates the importance–satisfaction (I-S) model and service quality performance matrix (SQPM) to examine long-term care (LTC) service demands and satisfaction improvement. Many scholars have used a single model to explore project improvement. Each model has advantages, but we think they are too subjective and suggest that it is best to integrate models to determine what should be improved. We established quality attributes of service demands based on more than two sessions of discussions and expert consultations with LTC service users (older adults). The final questionnaire was divided into three parts: a demand survey, satisfaction survey, and demographics survey, and 292 valid questionnaires were collected. The questionnaire items were summarized with means and standard deviations. In this study, if only the I-S model was used to examine LTC in Taiwan, then seven service elements of the system would need to be improved. However, if only the SQPM method was used, then 16 service elements would need to be improved. Only seven service elements were identified by both methods. When time and resources are limited, it is not feasible to take comprehensiveness into account. When many projects must be improved and it is impossible to implement them at the same time, improvement priorities need to be developed. Taiwan lacks sufficient LTC resources, so it is impossible to provide enough resources for all those who need care. To use resources efficiently, the I-S model and SQPM were integrated in this study to identify areas for improvement.

Keywords: Long-term care (LTC); importance-satisfaction (I-S) model; performance evaluation matrix (PEM); service quality performance matrix (SQPM); voice of customer (VOC)

1. Introduction

An aging population and changes in population structure directly impact social systems, such as the labor market, retirement planning, and the medical care system, and can lead to an economic crisis, such as a recession or government bankruptcy [1]. Therefore, population factors have become closely watched important issues in developed countries [2]. Taiwan's population of older adults exceeded 7% in 1993, making it an aging society [3], exceeded 14% in 2018, categorizing it as an aged society [4], and will exceed 20% in 2025, making Taiwan a super-aged society [5].

Long-term care (LTC) involves a variety of services designed to meet people's health or personal care needs during a short or long period of time. These services help people live as independently and safely as possible when they can no longer perform everyday activities on their own [6]. LTC is a very important issue for everyone in an aging society [5]. With the advancement of technology and medical treatments, the global average age has been extended to 75 years [7]. Taiwan is no exception. The continuous extension of life has resulted in changes in population structures [8]. The aging phenomenon is a problem that developed countries must face, along with related problems regarding the care of older adults [9]. In recent years, late marriage, bachelorism, and infertility have continued to intensify. Coupled with extended average life expectancy, low fertility, and population aging, they have also become concerning and unavoidable issues [10].

The implementation of LTC policies is based on the manager perspective rather than the user or customer point of view. In other words, LTC implementation ignores the voice of the customer (VOC). In the present study, the user point of view was used to explore service demands in LTC in Taiwan. Those who require LTC were divided into two groups: healthy older people, who are only interested in living happily, and older people with disabilities or dementia, who require medical interventions [11]. As the demands of these two groups are different, a service demand design would be ineffective, and could even affect national life, if it was viewed from an official perspective. Furthermore, the Taiwanese government has limited resources, and the needed resources would not necessarily be utilized at the same time. To address these issues and prioritize the efficient use of LTC resources, the importance-satisfaction (I-S) model and the revised performance evaluation matrix (PEM) can be used. Such a practice could fulfill LTC service demands by building a complete set of service design measurement methods.

Yang [12] developed the I-S model with reference to the importance performance analysis (IPA) method. The I-S model is the best tool for quality improvement [12,13]. Lambert and Sharma [14] proposed the performance evaluation matrix (PEM) to determine the importance of logistical service quality factors and the performance of companies based on these factors. PEM-related applications have been used in the machinery industry and in education; few applications have been used in long-term care. The PEM can help industries find service items that need improvement. The present study found no analyses on combining the I-S model and the PEM method for LTC service demands in the relevant literature. Due to insufficient studies and that the fact that currently LTC service demand policies are considered to be very important and urgent, the I-S model and PEM are introduced in the present study. It is hoped that this will provide more accurate quality service design and improve the essentials of LTC services to better meet the needs and expectations of the older adult population in Taiwan.

We conducted in-depth interviews in more than two sessions of discussions with experts and scholars through a focused discussion method to understand the LTC demands of the public and further confirm the service demands of caregivers, and we distributed 350 questionnaires. We also used the I-S model and the revised PEM method to find LTC users of corresponding management strategies to serve as a transmission basis for decision makers to adjust their services. This was to ensure that user service demands could be fully satisfied. In general, the purposes of this study can be summarized as follows:

1. To perform in-depth interviews with experts and scholars in focused discussions to confirm user service demands and service resources
2. To use the I-S model and the revised PEM method to confirm the importance and priority levels of various service demands in order to serve as a basis for decision makers to adjust LTC service quality design and improve care for older adults.

The rest of this study is organized as follows: Section 2 reviews the literature related to long-term care in Taiwan, long-term care service demands of older adults, the service quality evaluation model, the I-S model, the service quality evaluation model, and related research methods. Section 3 presents the research process, methodology, questionnaire design, data collection method, and statistical analysis methods. The results of the analysis and discussion are given in Section 4. Finally, the conclusions of this study and suggestions are presented in Section 5.

2. Literature Review

2.1. Long-Term Care Act 2.0 of Taiwan

The advent of an aging society has brought about new challenges [11]. In the past, people around the world looked upon older adults as vulnerable and in need of care [8]. Through solutions provided by social welfare programs, we have gradually changed the traditional image that older adults are dependent towards a more positive image [15]. In addition to providing social benefits, such as nursing and medical care, we assist older adults in matters of self-reliance and self-esteem. Therefore, older adults do not become a social burden but instead can share their wisdom and contribute to national competitiveness [16].

Taiwan's LTC industry has taken a significant step forward due to assistance from the government. We must take further preventative measures to cope with the expected rise in the number of older people in Taiwan in the next 10 years. To ease the burden on young people, the Long-Term Care Act 2.0 (LTCA 2.0) is imperative [17]. The overall goal of LTCA 2.0 is to establish a high-quality, affordable, and universal LTC service system that has a community-based spirit, provides disabled people with basic care services, helps older adults to enjoy old age comfortably in familiar environments, and eases the burden of family care [18]. Therefore, a budget of NT$20.079 billion (0.11% of gross domestic product (GDP)) is expected to be allocated to LTCA 2.0, which is over four times the size of the NT$5.126 billion budget in 2016. The LTC Management Center has indicated that the linking of social resources such as medical treatment, LTC, and life support can be carried out through an overall community care model by connecting various service systems to provide needed care, while also saving LTC resources [19]. According to the long-term care policy blueprint proposed by Taiwan's Ministry of Health and Welfare [20], older adults who live at home and get sick and need to see a doctor can go through the medical system, older adults who are healthy and able to live on their own can go through the life support system, and older adults who are unhealthy or even disabled can go through the long-term system. The medical/long-term/life support care model can be seen in Figure 1.

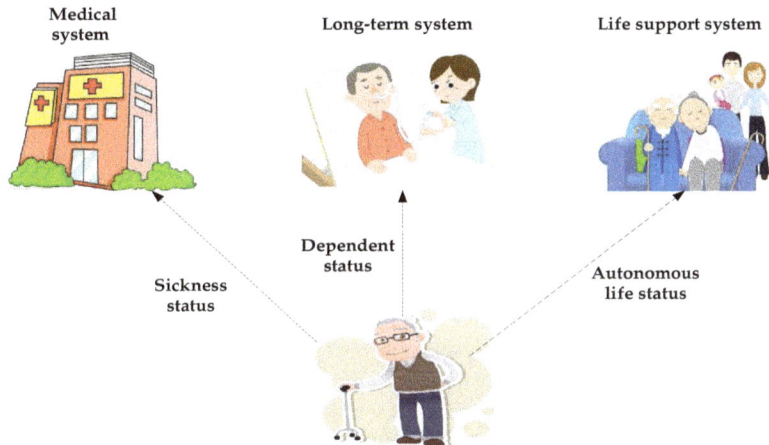

Figure 1. Medical/long-term/life support care model. Source: Ministry of Health and Welfare, Taiwan [20].

LTCA 2.0 is an extension of Taiwan's LTC political views. To address Taiwan's increasingly aging society, LTCA 2.0 proposes improving the strategies of three projects [20].

2.1.1. Widen Service Targets

Besides widening the care level of existing service targets, LTCA 2.0 also covers the following targets: (1) older people over 50 years old with dementia and disabled lowland aboriginals over 55 years old, and (2) disabled people younger than 49 years old and frail older people over 65 years old.

2.1.2. Provide Easily Accessible Service Units for the Public

For older people who could not find ways to get help in the past, the government introduced an innovative system by proposing an "ABC" long-term community-based care model (see Figure 2). It is described as follows: Tier A is referred to as the LTC flagship store, tier B as the LTC specialty store, and tier C as the LTC corner store. These "stores" are located within small communities, local neighborhoods, counties, and townships, and the different levels provide different services. For example, if you want to chat with someone, you should go to a tier C LTC corner store. If you want to receive day care, you should go to a tier B LTC specialty store. Finally, if you want to receive complete services, you should go to a tier A LTC flagship store.

2.1.3. Relax Subsidy Approval Regulations

In the past, the LTC Center paid subsidies in advance before asking for payment. This practice often affected service quality due to long processing times. However, under LTCA 2.0, the subsidy approval regulations have been relaxed to allow more institutions to invest in LTC services.

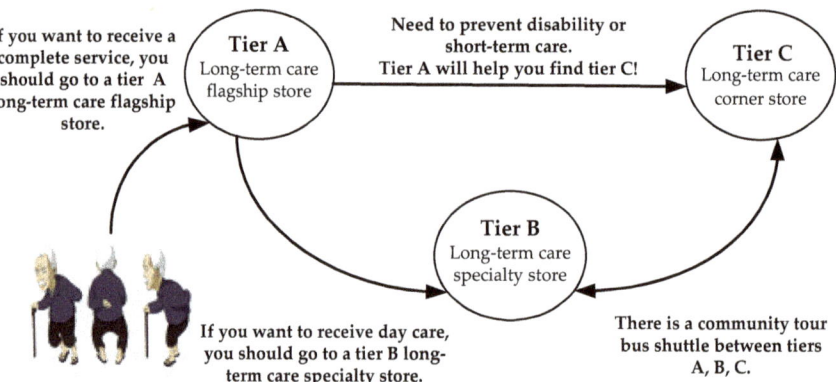

Figure 2. ABC long-term community-based care model. Source: Ministry of Health and Welfare, Taiwan [20].

2.2. Long-Term Care Service Demands of Older Adults

Older people who need care are divided into three categories: retired, demented, and disabled [8]. The physical and mental conditions of older adults in these categories are inherently different, and their demands for services are also different [11]. Since the older adult population continues to grow, along with reduced family capabilities to provide assistance, the demand for care services continues to rise [21]. Furthermore, although physiological differences between older adults are predictable, their mental, psychological, and behavioral conditions are not. The basic demands of older adults include economic, living, safety, health, leisure, and other types of support [22]. Lin and Chen [23] pointed out that the service demands of older adults include medical treatment, economic support, retirement, and reemployment, social participation, family care, interpersonal relationships, psychological adjustment, LTC, housing arrangements, annuity insurance, transportation, education and learning, leisure and entertainment, and other types of support. Shih et al. [24] divided older adult care services into home-based, community-based, and institution-style. The first two are for older adults living in communities. Home-based services include the following 10 services: health care, rehabilitation, physical care, housework, care visits, telephone-based care, catering, emergency rescue, home environment improvement, and other. Community-based services include the following 15 services: health care, medical care, rehabilitation, psychological counseling, day care, catering, family care, education, legal, transportation, retirement preparation, leisure, provision of information, referrals, and other.

2.3. Service Quality Evaluation Model

2.3.1. Importance Performance Analysis

Martilla and James [25] proposed importance performance analysis (IPA) (see Figure 3). IPA is a technique that prioritizes the relevant attributes of a particular service product by measuring its importance and degree of performance [26]. The IPA framework was first put forward in an attribution study on the motorcycle industry by plotting the average scores of importance and degree of performance in a 2D matrix and proposing different manufacturing/service strategies, depending on the position of each element, to resolve the production process faced by the enterprise [27].

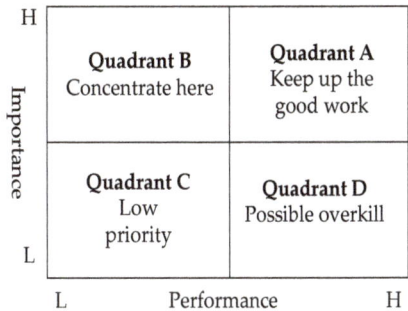

Figure 3. Importance performance analysis. Source: Martilla and James [25].

2.3.2. Importance-Satisfaction Model

Businesses generally determine enhancement priorities based on attributes with low satisfaction rather than considering actual customer requirements [28,29]. Although this approach has removed some unsatisfactory quality attributes, these attributes are not the main areas that customers focus on [30]. Yang [12] considered that low-quality attributes should not be the only consideration when designing an improvement plan. In accordance with this rationale, Yang [12] developed the importance–satisfaction (I-S) model, with reference to the IPA method. This model is illustrated in Figure 4. The quadrants are designated as excellent (high importance, high satisfaction), to be improved (high importance, low satisfaction), surplus (low importance, high satisfaction), and unimportant (low importance, low satisfaction). Improvement strategies are based on the area in which each quality attribute is placed.

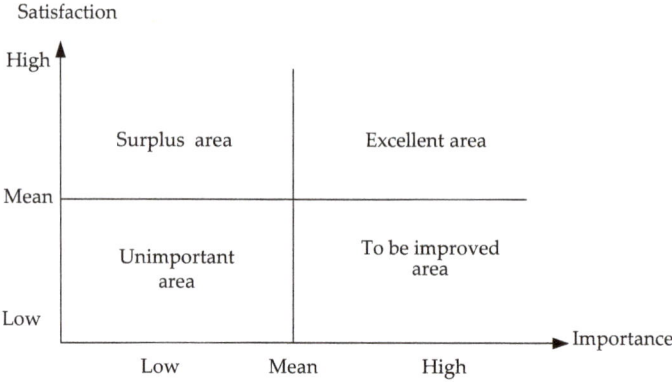

Figure 4. Importance–satisfaction model. Source: Yang [31].

2.3.3. Performance Evaluation Matrix

Lambert and Sharma [14] proposed the performance evaluation matrix (PEM) to determine the importance of logistical service quality factors and the performance of companies based on these factors. Performance variables are placed on the horizontal axis, and importance variables on the vertical axis [31]. Improvement strategies are then suggested based on evaluating these two factors in response to different positions (see Figure 5).

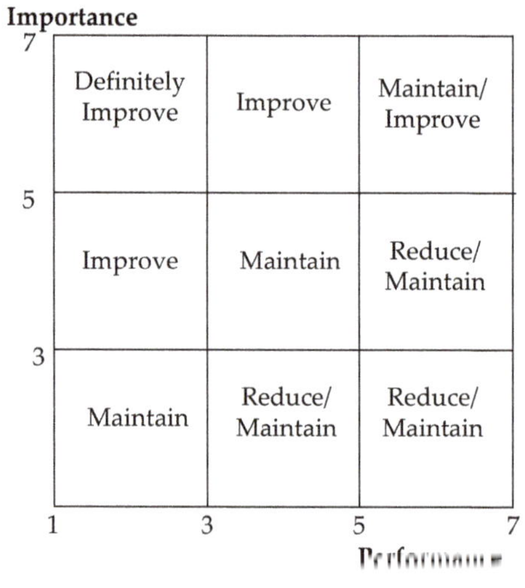

Figure 5. Performance evaluation matrix. Source: Lambert and Sharma [32].

From this matrix analysis, the current performance and competition status of the examined organizations can serve as directions for future development. PEM provides a reference for whether or not business owners should adjust their performance and response strategies [32]. Due to different perspectives explored by scholars, the viewpoints vary. Chen and Yeh [13] proposed amending the variables by placing importance variables on the horizontal axis and satisfaction variables on the vertical axis. The revised PEM was developed from these changes (see Figure 6).

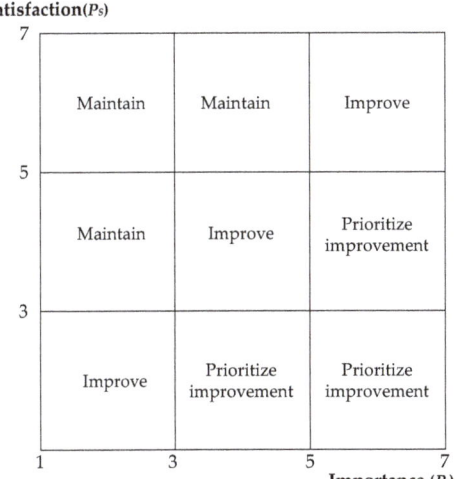

Figure 6. Revised performance evaluation matrix. Sources: Chen and Yeh [13].

2.3.4. Establishment of Service Quality Performance Matrix

Lambert and Sharma [14] proposed the PEM as a reference for quality improvement, but this matrix lacks generalization and standardization and is limited to a 7-point Likert scale [33]. Many subsequent scholars, such as Lin et al. [34] and Chen [28], proposed a revised PEM and applied it to the management method of quality improvement in enterprises. Scholars have not implemented this model as a basis for quality improvement in the LTC industry. In light of the views of previous scholars, this study applied a revised PEM to the quality management strategy of the LTC industry (see Figure 7). To generalize and standardize this model, a 5-point Likert scale, which is considered to be the most reliable scaling tool in the literature and widely used by scholars, was adopted in this study [35].

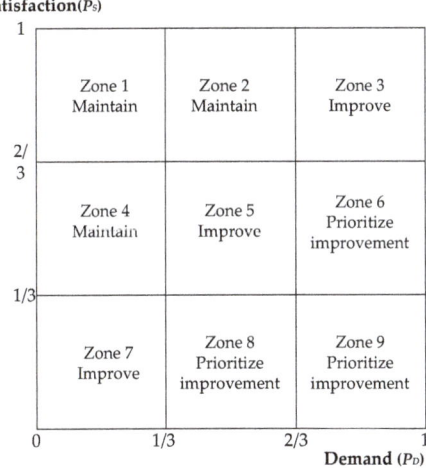

Figure 7. The service quality performance matrix.

Below, according to the theory of Hung et al. [33], the random variable D denotes demand, and S denotes satisfaction. A 5-point scale was adopted to evaluate the demand and satisfaction of each item. The indices of demand and satisfaction are defined as follows:

$$P_D = \frac{\mu_D - min}{R} \qquad (1)$$

$$P_S = \frac{\mu_S - min}{R} \qquad (2)$$

where P_D is the index of demand, P_S is index of satisfaction, min is the minimum value of scale k, and R is the full range of scale k. Furthermore, μ_D and μ_S are the means of demand (D) and satisfaction (S), respectively, min = 1 represents the minimum of scale k, and $R = k - 1$ is the full range of scale k.

Based on the literature review, we know that PEM has been used extensively in recent years and can be applied to decision-making practices [32]. This method is mostly used in logistics and in the semiconductor, financial, and service industries, and its application in relevant studies of LTC is still rare. Hence, we chose PEM as one of the research methods. In this study, the resource allocation for the LTC concept was used as the basis to explore service satisfaction levels for older people who require care. The corresponding strategies of maintenance, improvement, and priority improvement of the revised PEM put forward by Chen and Yeh [13] were re-proposed. This matrix is called the service quality performance matrix (SQPM). Zones 1, 2, and 4 are areas where older adults' cognitive satisfaction exceeds demand. Therefore, service resources should be maintained at their current status, and the strategy is to maintain service quality. Zones 3, 5, and 7 are areas where satisfaction is equal to demand, indicating that the service does not exceed user expectations; therefore, organizations must improve their existing service quality by investing in more resources, and the proposed strategy is to improve. Zones 6, 8, and 9 are areas where demand exceeds satisfaction, indicating that older adults are well aware of service projects, but they are not satisfied with the services provided. As a result, governments and organizations must actively make improvements to correct these issues, and the response strategy is to prioritize improvement. All factors that prioritize improvement are the response strategies that this study puts forward and are regarded as factors that should be prioritized.

In the relevant literature, most PEM-related applications were in the machinery industry [34] and education [36], and few were applied in the service industry, and PEM was not formally applied to LTC service demand and resource allocation at all. In this study, the literature and relevant practical experience were used to identify the elements of LTC service demands, and the SQPM method was used to determine the priority of these demands to optimize resource allocation and implement care for older adults' retirement.

3. Research Methods

3.1. Research Process

This study aimed to explore issues related to aging and long-term care services in Taiwan. First, the relevant literature was analyzed and sorted to serve as a conceptual framework for the construction of LTC service demands. Second, relevant impacts of LTC on national development, politics, culture, and the quality of the population were explored to confirm the status of and problems faced by LTC. According to the long-term care policy blueprint proposed by Taiwan's Ministry of Health and Welfare and more than two sessions of discussions and expert consultations with LTC users (older adults) to ensure the service elements of LTCA 2.0, the 20 quality attributes of service demands were established as follows. We used these 20 quality attributes for demand and satisfaction surveys.

1. Retirement pension or living allowance subsidies
2. Health-promoting physical fitness activities
3. Visits or telephone care services by social welfare agencies
4. Catering delivery services

5. Emergency medical care and rescue services
6. Transportation services
7. Older people eating meals together
8. Retirement planning
9. Employment services
10. Day care center services
11. Family companionship
12. Financial planning
13. Hospice care
14. Prices charged (older people eating meals together or class fees)
15. Service staff attitudes
16. Institutional accessibility
17. Community/residential institution environmental cleanliness
18. Community/institution activity planning
19. Community/institution dining comfort
20. Community/institution emergency response.

3.2. Design and Size of the Questionnaire

The questionnaire was based on: (i) a review of the literature [22,23,37] and (ii) discussions with experts (including LTC consultants and scholars) and older adults. The final questionnaire included 40 items (20 quality attributes for demand and satisfaction surveys) and was divided into three parts:

1. Demand survey: included 20 quality attributes, responses requested on a 5-point Likert-type scale, with 1 representing extremely low demand and 5 representing extremely high demand; we used a mean value of these items.
2. Satisfaction survey: included 20 quality attributes, responses requested on a 5-point Likert-type scale, with 1 representing extremely dissatisfied and 5 representing extremely satisfied; we also used a mean value of these items.
3. Demographics survey: gender, marital status, age, living status, education degree, and occupation prior to retirement.

The samples for this research were people older than 55 years (service targets of LTC) who lived in a long-term institution or attended a senior citizens' learning camp. Taiwanese older people residing in Taipei and New Taipei were the participants in this study. In addition, in the process of questionnaire distribution, some older people were found to be much older or illiterate. In these cases, the questionnaire was administered verbally to make the questions more comprehensive.

3.3. Data Analysis

In this study, we first reported the frequency and percentage distributions of the participants' basic characteristics (such as gender, marital status, age, living status, education and occupation before retirement). Descriptive statistics were used to summarize the respondents' profiles and then the mean and standard deviation of service demand and satisfaction. Cronbach's alpha was calculated for the sums of demand items and satisfaction items surveys as an estimate of the reliability of a psychometric test. Finally, we put all 20 service elements into the Importance–satisfaction (I-S) model and Service Quality Performance Matrix to determine the items that need to improve. Improvement strategies are then suggested based on evaluating these two factors in response to different positions. We used SPSS version 18 (SPSS, Chicago, IL, USA) to execute all analyses.

4. Research Results

4.1. Sample Narrative Statistical Analysis

The samples of this research were people older than 55 years (service targets of LTC) who lived in a long-term institution or attended a senior citizens' learning camp. Out of the 350 questionnaires distributed from January to May 2018, 315 were collected, for a recovery rate of 90.0%. A total of 23 questionnaires were found to be invalid, making the total valid responses 292. The results of the questionnaire indicated that 267 respondents were married (91.44%); 189 were female (64.73%); 115 lived in residential institutions (39.38%); 84 had a university education background (28.77%); 87 were in the military, government employees, or teachers before retirement (29.79%); and 87 were in the age range 65–70 years old (29.79%), as shown in Table 1.

Table 1. Descriptive statistics of the sample population.

Category	Items	No.	%	Category	Items	No.	%
Gender	Male	103	35.27%	Education degree	Illiterate	17	5.82%
	Female	189	64.73%		Elementary school	60	20.55%
Marital status	Unmarried (divorced)	25	8.56%		Junior high school	51	17.47%
	Married	267	91.44%		High school	78	26.71%
Age	55–64	52	17.81%		College/university	84	28.77%
	65–70	87	29.79%		Above master	2	0.68%
	71–75	51	17.47%	Occupation before retirement	Office holder	87	29.79%
	76–80	80	27.40%		Service industry	61	20.89%
	Above 80	22	7.53%		Industry	49	16.78%
Living status	Living with children/couples	106	36.30%		High-tech industry	12	4.11%
	Living with relatives	51	17.47%		Agriculture industry	7	2.40%
	Living in a residential institution	115	39.38%		Household	61	20.89%
	Living alone	20	6.85%		Self-employed	15	5.14%

A service needs survey was conducted to examine the demand level of older adults for essential elements. The higher the demand level, the more important these elements are to older adults; therefore, the government should pay attention to them in its administrative measures. The results are shown in Table 2. The average value of the demand survey was found to be 4.16, with a standard deviation of 0.99, showing that older adults have a very high awareness of all the elements, and each element is vital to them. The three items with the highest demand were retirement pension or living allowance subsidies, emergency medical care and rescue services, and retirement planning.

The survey was meant to understand the service demands of older adults and confirm whether their demands were satisfied. The lower the satisfaction level, the higher the dissatisfaction with services provided by the government and service providers, indicating that these items should be improved. The average value of the satisfaction survey was found to be 2.93, with a standard deviation of 0.78, indicating that older adults are less satisfied with all elements. The three items with the lowest satisfaction levels were retirement pension or living allowance subsidies, emergency medical care and rescue services, and family companionship. These elements must be listed in the improvement priorities.

Table 2. The mean and standard deviation of service demand and the satisfaction survey (N = 292).

	Item	Demand		Satisfaction	
		ME	S.D.	ME	S.D.
1.	Retirement pension or living allowance subsidies	4.89	0.95	2.19	0.49
2.	Health-promoting physical fitness activities	4.67	0.81	2.67	0.65
3.	Visits or telephone care services by social welfare agencies	4.01	1.01	2.70	0.68
4.	Catering delivery services	4.10	1.11	2.68	1.12
5.	Emergency medical care and rescue services	4.79	0.91	2.48	0.54
6.	Transportation services	4.33	1.05	2.61	0.91
7.	Older people eating meals together	4.61	0.99	2.72	0.56
8.	Retirement planning	4.72	1.08	2.97	0.54
9.	Employment services	4.06	1.11	2.66	0.83
10.	Day care center services	3.91	1.18	2.64	1.13
11.	Family companionship	4.24	0.91	2.56	0.75
12.	Financial planning	3.99	1.04	2.65	0.82
13.	Hospice care	4.34	1.10	2.64	1.03
14.	Prices charged (older people eating meals together or class fees)	4.69	1.02	3.05	1.07
15.	Service staff attitudes	3.51	0.98	3.92	0.71
16.	Institutional accessibility	4.18	0.87	3.46	0.93
17.	Community/residential institution environmental cleanliness	3.58	0.75	3.37	0.87
18.	Community/institution activity planning	3.32	0.91	3.86	0.77
19.	Community/institution dining comfort	3.28	0.85	3.40	0.69
20.	Community/institution emergency response	4.01	1.07	3.32	0.59
	Total of all 20 items	4.16	0.99	2.93	0.78

Note: ME = mean; S.D. = standard deviation.

4.2. Reliability Analysis

A reliability test is used to measure whether a tool is consistent and reliable, and Cronbach's alpha is generally used as a benchmark to measure the reliability of a questionnaire. If Cronbach's alpha is greater than 0.7, it has high reliability, while if it falls between 0.35 and 0.7, the reliability is barely acceptable [38,39]. In this study, Cronbach's alpha for service demand was 0.82, and for satisfaction was 0.89. As the overall reliability value of 0.91 is greater than 0.7, it shows high reliability and indicates that the scale has good consistency and reliability.

4.3. Importance-Satisfaction Model Results

When all the service elements were placed in the I-S model, as shown in Figure 8, those in the excellent area were items 8, 14, and 16. Service demand and service satisfaction are above the average, which indicates that customers need these services, and older adults feel satisfied about services provided by the government or service providers. This also shows that the resources can be used effectively.

The service elements in the to be improved area were items 1, 2, 5, 6, 7, 11, and 13, indicating that service demand is above the average, and satisfaction is below the average. This indicates that customers highly need these services, but they are not offered by service providers or have not been provided at a level found to be satisfactory by older adults. Given the low level of satisfaction, it is recommended that service providers should improve these services first.

The service elements in the surplus area were items 15, 17, 18, 19, and 20, indicating that service demand is below the average, and customers are not concerned with these services. Service satisfaction is higher than the average, indicating that resources are being misplaced or wasted. Therefore, surplus resources should be reallocated to service items with high demand and low satisfaction.

The service elements in the unimportant area were items 3, 4, 9, 10, and 12, indicating that service demand and satisfaction are lower than the average. Customers do not value these services but accept the performance of service providers. Therefore, as long as these elements are provided appropriately, it is not necessary to enhance the service quality. In fact, increasing resources in this area could be considered a waste.

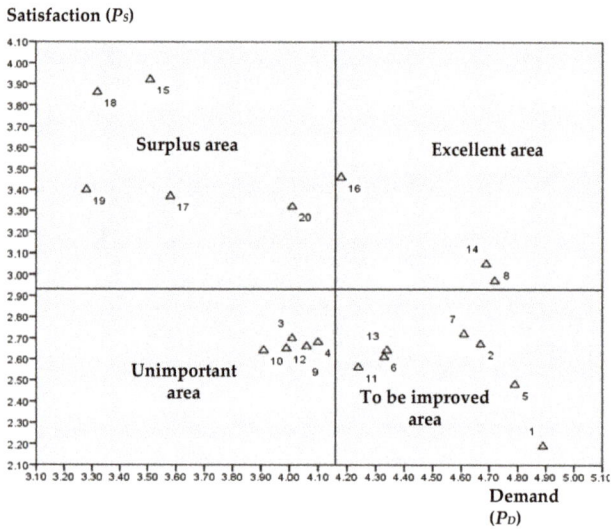

Figure 8. Importance–satisfaction (I-S) model results.

4.4. Service Quality Performance Matrix Results

The average value and index of each question were calculated through Formulas (1) and (2), as shown in Table 3, and the relevant values were introduced into the SQPM, as shown in Figure 9. The service elements in the priority improvement area were items 1–16 and 20, indicating that the demand for these services exceeds satisfaction, and older adults are unsatisfied with them. Therefore, they need to be improved. The service elements in the improvement area were items 17 and 19, indicating that the demand for these services is equal to the satisfaction, and they are accepted by older adults. Therefore, service providers can list surplus resources as secondary improvement items. The service elements in the maintenance area were items 15 and 18, indicating that satisfaction for those services is higher than the demand, and older adults are happy about them and highly satisfied. Therefore, service providers can maintain the current service quality.

Table 3. Relative values for I-S model and service quality performance matrix (SQPM).

No.	μ_D	μ_P	P_D	P_P	I-S Model	SQPM
1	4.89	2.19	0.97	0.30	To be improved	Prioritize improvement
2	4.67	2.67	0.92	0.42	To be improved	Prioritize improvement
3	4.01	2.70	0.75	0.43	Unimportant	Prioritize improvement
4	4.10	2.68	0.78	0.42	Unimportant	Prioritize improvement
5	4.79	2.48	0.95	0.37	To be improved	Prioritize improvement
6	4.33	2.61	0.83	0.40	To be improved	Prioritize improvement
7	4.61	2.72	0.90	0.43	To be improved	Prioritize improvement
8	4.72	2.97	0.93	0.49	Excellent	Prioritize improvement
9	4.06	2.66	0.77	0.42	Unimportant	Prioritize improvement
10	3.91	2.64	0.73	0.41	Unimportant	Prioritize improvement
11	4.24	2.56	0.81	0.39	To be improved	Prioritize improvement
12	3.99	2.65	0.75	0.41	Unimportant	Prioritize improvement
13	4.34	2.64	0.84	0.41	To be improved	Prioritize improvement
14	4.69	3.05	0.92	0.51	Excellent	Prioritize improvement
15	3.51	3.92	0.63	0.73	Surplus	Maintain
16	4.18	3.46	0.80	0.61	Excellent	Prioritize improvement
17	3.58	3.37	0.65	0.59	Surplus	Improve
18	3.32	3.86	0.58	0.71	Surplus	Maintain
19	3.28	3.40	0.57	0.60	Surplus	Improve
20	4.01	3.32	0.75	0.58	Surplus	Prioritize improvement

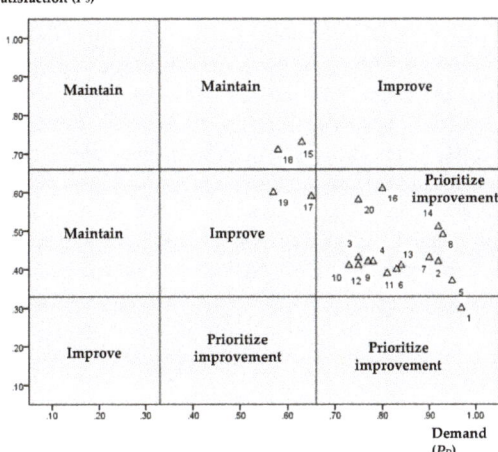

Figure 9. SQPM results.

4.5. Discussion

Many scholars have used a single model or tool, such as IPA, the I-S model, or the PEM, to explore projects that organizations need to improve. Each model has its advantages, but we think they are too subjective. Instead, it is best to use several models to repeatedly determine the areas that need to be improved before proposing an improvement strategy. The present study integrates the importance-satisfaction (I-S) model and service quality performance matrix (SQPM) to examine long-term care (LTC) service demands and satisfaction improvement.

Japan's LTC system was established in 2000 to support older people with LTC demands and alleviate the burden of caregiving on family members [40]. People choosing to use LTC services, including in-home, facility, and community services, reduce their financial expenses and improve their quality of care [41]. Taiwan established LTCA 1.0 in 1998, and amended it to develop LTCA 2.0 in 2018. The implementation schedule in Taiwan was earlier than in Japan, but its effectiveness has not been high. Therefore, the Taiwanese government and service providers must actively emphasize implementing the LTC system and making improvements regarding older adults' demands.

Generally speaking, when time and resources are limited, it is not feasible to take comprehensiveness into account. When many projects must be improved and it is impossible to implement them at the same time, improvement priorities are developed [42]. In this study, if only the I-S model was used to examine LTC in Taiwan, then seven elements of the system would need to be improved: items 1, 2, 5, 6, 7, 11, and 13. However, if only SQPM were used, 16 elements would need to be improved: items 1–16 and 20. In other words, the outcomes are different when using different models.

As mentioned earlier, Taiwan lacks sufficient LTC resources, so it is impossible to provide enough resources for all those who need care. To use resources efficiently, the I-S model and SQPM were integrated in this study to identify areas for improvement, and items 1, 2, 5, 6, 7, 11, and 13 were identified by both methods.

From the empirical analysis, it was found that the average demand score is approximately 4 and the average satisfaction score is approximately 3, showing that older adults have a very high demand level, but their tendency for satisfaction is low. Regarding improvements, it was found that older adults are most dissatisfied with pensions and living allowances. Therefore, the results of this study are consistent with the viewpoints of other scholars [22,43]. After all, adequate pensions or government subsidies would allow older adult retirees without income and/or in poor health to feel more assured.

Taiwan's declining birthrate and aging population have become more severe. In 2018, more than 14% of the populations were older adults, making the nation an aged society. This has forced some people to rely on foreign workers to help provide care, companionship, and other support for older adults. However, the improper foreign labor management system and language barriers have caused frequent incidents of abuse of older adults by foreign workers. Therefore, four service elements (items 5, 6, 11, and 13) related to these issues were generated due to older adults' helplessness and loneliness. In addition to satisfaction about materials and money, spiritual sustenance and care for older adults are equally crucial.

Items that need improvement, except for pensions and living allowances, cannot be improved due to financial difficulties, but for emergency medical care and rescue services and transportation services, it is recommended that government agencies and hospitals provide transportation resources for the elderly. For travel to emergency medical care, private sector operators should be encouraged to invest in transport services for the elderly and provide appropriate subsidies to enhance emergency medical services.

The results also shows that most of the older people lived in residential institutions were male, their education level were mainly university, their economic status were better, and their work were mainly in the military, government employees, or teachers before retirement. In a Chinese society, many older people were unwilling to live in residential institutions. In addition to considering financial planning factors, they were also afraid of giving others a feeling that they have been abandoned by their children. Therefore, the proportions of living with their families were also high. The interview found that the older people living families alone have poor financial support, their need government subsidies, and transportation services. The older people lived in residential institutions have a stable pension or their children provide financial assistance therefore, the needs were family companionship and health-promoting physical fitness activities.

Finally, this study attempts to analyze the differences from the sample background information, such as gender, age, education, occupation, living status, marital status, etc., to compare the differences in the needs of different people for LTC. After analysis of I-S model and SQPM, the research results show that there is no significant difference between different background samples and the overall sample. It is speculated that the reason for this might be that the samples for this research were Taiwanese older people residing in Taipei and New Taipei who lived in a long-term institution or attended a senior citizens' learning camp. And Taipei and New Taipei City are the two largest Taiwanese Cities, the population is evenly distributed, and older adults' views are also converging, which were also likely to be factors in the results.

5. Conclusions and Suggestions

5.1. Conclusions

The advancement of medical science and technology has extended the average life expectancy and brought about changes in social structure and values and, together with the declining birthrate, has accelerated the advent of aged societies. To cope with the current global aging population, LTC for older adults is an essential goal of government administrations. To meet older people's needs, it is unwise to construct aid devices or service needs from a managerial perspective instead of listening to them and customizing relevant services based on a user perspective. It is also important to encourage healthy older people to continue being active, such as by performing volunteer work, participating in community services, and acting as guides, to enrich their retirement lives and simultaneously increase their contribution to society. Older adults who are in poor health, suffering from illnesses such as dementia, or facing disabilities can be provided with medical care to reduce their pains, ensuring that all older people receive proper care. The government is responsible for appropriately allocating the necessary resources.

During the implementation process, the I-S model and SQPM were mainly used to evaluate resource allocation, followed by a secondary consideration of service quality improvement. Seven services were found to be in urgent need of improvement by this study after integrating the I-S model and SQPM. This research results can serve as a basis for quality improvement for the Taiwanese government and service providers investing in resources. If government resources are limited and cannot be allocated simultaneously, it is suggested to prioritize the improvement projects in order.

5.2. Suggestions and Research Limitations

Rapid population aging has made the burden of caring for older adults relatively heavy. Following an extension of the average life expectancy of older adults, their demand for care services has also intensified. Advances in medical technology have led to the control of many diseases, but such advances still cannot fully restore the original state of health, and many older people suffer from physical and mental disabilities. With the continuous growth of the older adult population and the decline of family function, the demand for care services continues to rise, along with the need to rely on foreign workers to handle these jobs. Therefore, it is imperative to strengthen professional training for foreign workers.

There are significant differences in physical and mental health among older people who need care, and the nonuniformity of care resources has created a high variance in care needs. Therefore, healthy older people who could move freely in the community or institutions were chosen as the objects of this study, and those with physical and mental disabilities were excluded. Based on the empirical research, the study proposes the following suggestions:

1. Although the government has established the ABC LTC model, the new system has not properly implemented departmental linkages and integrated resources. Therefore, it is recommended that the government, nongovernment organizations, and social welfare groups coordinate and integrate their communications as soon as possible.

2. From the outside, the LTC industry has the impression of being low-paid, humble work focused on helping older adults with their toileting routines. As a result, young people are not very interested in entering this field. As an alternative, it is suggested to hire foreign workers for this kind of work. It is also the government's responsibility to urgently encourage young people to join and manage this industry, making it into a respectful and dignified profession.

The samples for this research were Taiwanese older people residing in Taipei and New Taipei who lived in a long-term institution or attended a senior citizens' learning camp. The follow-up researchers can expand the sample size to compare the LTC needs. They may find significant differences between different background samples.

Author Contributions: S.-H.C. and T.-M.Y. developed the idea, motivation, and question of the paper and contributed to the discussion. F.-Y.P. outlined and revised the manuscript and made substantial contributions to the design of this study. All authors have read and agreed to the published version of the manuscript.

Funding: The Article Processing Charge was funded by the Ministry of Science and Technology of Taiwan under grant number MOST 108-2221-E-507-004-MY3.

Acknowledgments: The authors would like to express their sincere gratitude to the editor and the anonymous reviewers for their insightful and constructive comments.

Conflicts of Interest: The authors declare no conflict of interest.

References

1. Lin, C.S.; Jeng, M.Y.; Yeh, T.M. The elderly perceived meanings and values of virtual reality leisure activities: A means-end chain approach. *Int. J. Environ. Res. Public Health* **2018**, *15*, 663. [CrossRef] [PubMed]
2. Wang, Z.H.; Yang, Z.H.; Dong, T. A review of wearable technologies for elderly care that can accurately track indoor position.recognize physical activities and monitor vital signs in real time. *Sensors* **2017**, *17*, 341. [CrossRef] [PubMed]
3. Jeng, M.Y.; Pai, F.Y.; Yeh, T.M. The virtual reality leisure activities experience on elderly people. *Appl. Res. Qual. Life* **2017**, *12*, 49–65. [CrossRef]
4. Lin, T.C. Discussion on the Health Promotion Management and the Demand of Life Support in Senior Citizen: A Case study with Taiwan. *CSR Summit Entrep. Cross Strait Coop.* **2019**, *4*, 36–52.
5. Lee, I.; Chiou, C.J.; Su, H.S. Comparison of Caring Status and Needs between Elderly and Non-Elderly Family Caregivers. *J. Long-term Care* **2017**, *21*, 149–164.
6. Lehnert, T.; Heuchert, M.; Hussain, K.; König, H. Stated preferences for long-term care: A literature review. *Ageing Soc.* **2019**, *39*, 1873–1913. [CrossRef]
7. Huang, F.S. The Rise, Trends and Recent Developments of Elder Education in Taiwan. *J. Adult Lifelong Educ.* **2012**, *43*, 2–14.
8. Lin, Y.Y. Strategies of enhancing capacity of long-term care policy by government: A case study of taichung city government. *J. Long-Term Care* **2017**, *21*, 19–25.
9. Kim, J.; Han, W. Improving Service Quality in Long-term Care Hospitals: National Evaluation on Long-term Care Hospitals and Employees Perception of Quality Dimensions. *Osong Public Health Res. Perspect.* **2012**, *3*, 94–99. [CrossRef]
10. Chen, S.H. Determining the service demands of an aging population by integrating QFD and FMEA method. *Qual. Quant.* **2016**, *50*, 283–298. [CrossRef]
11. Chen, S.F.; Teng, S.W. The Development of the Long-Term Care Service System in Taiwan. *J. Nurs.* **2010**, *57*, 5–10.
12. Yang, C.C. Improvement actions based on the customers' satisfaction survey. *Total Qual. Manag. Bus. Excell.* **2003**, *14*, 919–930. [CrossRef]
13. Chen, S.H.; Yeh, T.M. Integration PEM and AHP methods to determine service quality improvement strategy for the medical industry. *Appl. Math. Inf. Sci.* **2015**, *9*, 3073–3082.
14. Lambert, D.M.; Sharma, A. A customer based competitive analysis for logistics decisions. *Int. J. Phys. Distrib. Logist. Manag.* **1990**, *20*, 17–24. [CrossRef]
15. Shieh, M.D.; Hsiao, H.C.; Lin, Y.H.; Lin, J.Y. A study of the elderly people's perception of wearable device forms. *J. Interdiscip. Math.* **2017**, *20*, 789–804. [CrossRef]
16. Helbostad, J.L.; Vereijken, B.; Becker, C.; Todd, C.; Taraldsen, K.; Pijnappels, M.; Aminian, K.; Mellone, S. Mobile health applications to promote active and healthy ageing. *Sensors* **2017**, *17*, 622. [CrossRef]
17. Huang, Y.C.; Chang, T.Y. A Study of Long-term Care Policy 2.0 Edition: An Example for Pingtung County. *J. Manag. Syst.* **2019**, *26*, 241–269.
18. Chung, C.C. Reflect on for long-term care 2.0 from the view point of quality of medical life. *Qual. Mag.* **2017**, *53*, 5–11.

19. Lee, M.C.; Kuo, T.C.; Ueng, W.N. Perspectives on Long-Term Care in Taiwan-Integration of Health Care and Welfare services. *HOSPITAL* **2019**, *52*, 1–5.
20. Ministry of Health and Welfare. *Long Term Care Plan for Ten Years 2.0 Report*; Ministry of Health and Welfare: Taiwan, China.
21. Sun, W.J.; Chu, D.C.; Huang, S.J. Medical Home Care and National Long-Term Care Integration. *J. Med.* **2018**, *22*, 278–282.
22. Liu, Y.H. Older clinical psychology lecture (1). *Consult. Couns.* **2010**, *289*, 56–60.
23. Lin, Y.G.; Chen, P.W. The application of community consultation model in the service of the elderly. *Couns. Q.* **2009**, *45*, 49–60.
24. Shih, Y.; Lo, H.T.; Chen, C.Y. Study on Quality of Services and Satisfaction for Elderly Day Care Centers: A Case Study of a Hospital in Southern Taiwan. *J. Gerontechnol. Serv. Manag.* **2018**, *6*, 121–136.
25. Martilla, J.A.; James, J.C. Importance-Performance Analysis. *J. Mark.* **1997**, *41*, 77–79. [CrossRef]
26. Sampson, S.E.; Showalter, M.J. The performance-importance response function: Observations and implications. *Serv. Ind. J.* **1999**, *19*, 1–25. [CrossRef]
27. Guo, D.S.; Su, S.C. An IPA Analysis of Customer Value. *Manag. Sci. Res.* **2016**, *10*, 83–96.
28. Chen, S.H. A performance matrix for strategies to improve satisfaction among faculty members in higher education. *Qual. Quant.* **2011**, *45*, 75–89. [CrossRef]
29. Cheng, C.C.; Tsai, M.C.; Lin, S.P. Developing strategies for improving the service quality of casual-dining restaurants: New insights from integrating IPGA and QFD analysis. *Total Qual. Manag. Bus. Excell.* **2015**, *26*, 415–429. [CrossRef]
30. Wong, K.; Tunku, U.; Rahman, A. Constructing a survey questionnaire to collect data on service quality of business academics. *Eur. J. Soc. Sci.* **2012**, *29*, 209–221.
31. Yeh, T.M.; Lai, H.P. Evaluating the effectiveness of implementing quality management practices in the medical industry. *J. Nutr. Health Aging* **2015**, *19*, 102–112. [CrossRef]
32. Chen, S.H.; Liu, A.C.; Chen, F.Y. Using the PEM method to determine service quality improvement strategies of medical industry. *Int. J. Manag. Stud. Res.* **2014**, *2*, 41–46.
33. Hung, Y.H.; Huang, M.L.; Chen, K.S. Service quality evaluation by service quality performance matrix. *Total Qual. Manag. Bus. Excell.* **2003**, *14*, 79–89. [CrossRef]
34. Lin, W.T.; Chen, S.C.; Chen, K.S. Evaluation of performance in introducing CE marking on the European market to the machinery industry in Taiwan. *Int. J. Qual. Reliab. Manag.* **2005**, *22*, 503–517. [CrossRef]
35. Wu, M.L. *Paper Writing and Quantitative Research*; Wu-Nan Publishing Company: Taipei, Taiwan, 2018.
36. YuCMChang, H.T.; Chen, K.S. Developing a performance evaluation matrix to enhance the learner satisfaction of an e-learning system. *Total Qual. Manag. Bus. Excell.* **2018**, *29*, 727–745.
37. Kim, S.H.; Kim, D.H.; Kim, W.S. Long-Term Care Needs of the Elderly in Korea and Elderly Long-Term Care Insurance. *Soc. Work Public Health* **2010**, *25*, 176–184. [CrossRef] [PubMed]
38. Nunnally, J.C. *Psychometric Theory*; McGraw-Hill: New York, NY, USA, 1987.
39. Cuieford, J.P. *Fundamental Statistics in Psychology and Education*, 4th ed.; McGraw Hill: New York, NY, USA, 1965.
40. Iwagami, M.; Tamiya, N. The Long-Term Care Insurance System in Japan: Past, Present 2019, and Future. *JMA J.* **1965**, *2*, 67–69.
41. Araia, A.; Ozakib, T.; Katsumatac, Y. Behavioral and psychological symptoms of dementia in older residents in long term care facilities in Japan: A cross-sectional study. *Aging Ment. Health* **2017**, *21*, 1099–1105. [CrossRef]
42. Chen, S.H.; Yang, C.C.; Shiau, J.Y.; Wang, H.H. The development of an employee satisfaction model for higher education. *TQM Mag.* **2006**, *18*, 484–500. [CrossRef]
43. Liao, W.C.; Chiu, L.A.; Yueh, H.P. A study of rural elderly's health information needs and seeking behavior. *J. Libr. Inf. Stud.* **2012**, *10*, 155–204.

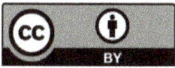 © 2019 by the authors. Licensee MDPI, Basel, Switzerland. This article is an open access article distributed under the terms and conditions of the Creative Commons Attribution (CC BY) license (http://creativecommons.org/licenses/by/4.0/).

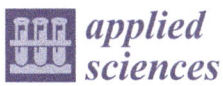

Article

Investigation of Vocal Fatigue Using a Dose-Based Vocal Loading Task

Zhengdong Lei [1], Laura Fasanella [1], Lisa Martignetti [2] and Nicole Yee-Key Li-Jessen [2] and Luc Mongeau [1,*,†]

1 Department of Mechanical Engineering, McGill University, Montreal, QC H3A 0C3, Canada; zhengdong.lei@mail.mcgill.ca (Z.L.); laura.fasanella@mail.mcgill.ca (L.F.)
2 School of Communication Sciences and Disorders, McGill University, Montreal, QC H3A 1G1, Canada; lisa.martignetti@mail.mcgill.ca (L.M.); nicole.li@mcgill.ca (N.Y.-K.L.-J.)
* Correspondence: luc.mongeau@mcgill.ca
† Current address: 845 Sherbrooke Street West, Montreal, QC H3A 0G4, Canada.

Received: 7 January 2020; Accepted: 6 February 2020; Published: 10 February 2020

Abstract: Vocal loading tasks are often used to investigate the relationship between voice use and vocal fatigue in laboratory settings. The present study investigated the concept of a novel quantitative dose-based vocal loading task for vocal fatigue evaluation. Ten female subjects participated in the study. Voice use was monitored and quantified using an online vocal distance dose calculator during six consecutive 30-min long sessions. Voice quality was evaluated subjectively using the CAPE-V and SAVRa before, between, and after each vocal loading task session. Fatigue-indicative symptoms, such as cough, swallowing, and voice clearance, were recorded. Statistical analysis of the results showed that the overall severity, the roughness, and the strain ratings obtained from CAPE-V obeyed similar trends as the three ratings from the SAVRa. These metrics increased over the first two thirds of the sessions to reach a maximum, and then decreased slightly near the session end. Quantitative metrics obtained from surface neck accelerometer signals were found to obey similar trends. The results consistently showed that an initial adjustment of voice quality was followed by vocal saturation, supporting the effectiveness of the proposed loading task.

Keywords: vocal fatigue; vocal distance dose; neck surface accelerometer

1. Introduction

Vocal fatigue may be diagnosed through a series of voice symptoms, which include, for example, hoarse and breathy vocal qualities, pitch breaks, reduced pitch and loudness ranges, throat discomfort, and unsteady voice [1]. Vocal fatigue may be experienced by any individuals during their life time, but it is more frequently encountered by professional voice users in occupational settings. Vocal fatigue increases vocal effort and decreases speaking stamina. Ultimately, vocal fatigue can lead to voice disorders, such as vocal hyperfunction or vocal nodules. Vocal fatigue is difficult to define because many factors, such as self-reported feelings, doctor-rated symptoms, and instrumental measures, could be criteria for its determination. For example, a self-reported feeling of vocal fatigue might be due to psychological stress, thereby not causing much detectable change in physiological measures [2]. Standards for assessing vocal fatigue are therefore difficult to establish. Nevertheless, most current research adopted the definition of vocal fatigue as a sense of increased vocal effort [3].

Considerable progress has been made in the evaluation of voice quality. Perceptual, acoustic, and aerodynamic measurements, along with self-administered tests, have been used to characterize changes in voice quality and performance in laboratory settings [4,5]. The most commonly used method of voice quality evaluation in clinics is auditory perception, which relies on listeners' personal experience and expertise. Commonly used subjective evaluation tools included the GRBAS (Grade,

Roughness, Breathiness, Asthenia and Strain) proposed by the Japan Society of Logopedics and Phoniatrics, the CAPE-V (Consensus Auditory-Perceptual Evaluation of Voice) proposed by the American Speech-Language and Hearing Association, and the SAVRa (Self-Administered Voice Rating) proposed by the National Center for Voice and Speech in the United States. These tools require specific vocal stimuli. For example, the CAPE-V requires the completion of three defined phonation tasks assessed through perceptual rating. This therefore limits the applicability of these tools in situations where the vocal stimuli are varied or unspecified. Many studies have investigated uncertainties in subjective judgment methodologies for voice quality evaluation. Kreiman and Gerratt investigated the source of listener disagreement in voice quality assessment using unidimensional rating scales, and found that no single metric from natural voice recordings allowed the evaluation of voice quality [6]. Kreiman also found that individual standards of voice quality, scale resolution, and voice attribute magnitude also significantly influenced intra-rater agreement [7]. Objective metrics obtained using various acoustic instruments have been investigated, and attempts have been made to correlate these with perceptual voice quality assessments [8–12].

A plethora of temporal, spectral, and cepstral metrics have been proposed to evaluate voice quality [13,14]. Commonly used features or vocal metrics include fundamental frequency ($f0$), loudness, jitter, shimmer, vocal formants, harmonic-to-noise ratio (HNR), spectral tilt (H1-H2, harmonic richness factor), maximum flow declination rate (MFDR), duty ratio, cepstral peak prominence (CPP), Mel-frequency cepstral coefficients (MFCCs), power spectrum ratio, and others [15–19]. Self-reported feelings of decreased vocal functionality have been used as a criterion for vocal fatigue in many previous studies [1,4,20–22]. Standard self-administered questionnaires, such as the SAVRa and the Vocal Fatigue Index (VFI), have been used to identify individuals with vocal fatigue, and to characterize their symptoms [23–25]. Hunter and Titze used the SAVRa to quantify vocal fatigue recovery based on 86 participants' tracking reports. The results showed a self-reported 50% recovery within 4–6 h, and 90% recovery within 12–18 h [24]. Halpern et al. used one of the three dimensions in SAVRa, i.e., the inability to produce soft voice (IPSV), to track vocal changes in school teachers. The SAVRa scores were then compared with two clinicians' ratings of the participants' $f0$, and loudness [26]. The overall correlation between self-ratings and clinician ratings was not significant. The average absolute difference score was 1.7. This showed that the clinicians and the teachers had different rating standards.

Prolonged or inappropriate voice use is commonly regarded as one of the causes of vocal fatigue. Vocal loading tasks (VLTs) are often used to investigate the relationship between voice use and vocal fatigue in laboratory settings [1]. Previous VLT studies have typically instructed participants to complete standardized reading tasks of prescribed durations at specific loudness levels [1,4,24]. Perceptual, acoustic, and aerodynamic measurements have been used to evaluate changes in voice quality and performance before and after VLTs [4]. Unfortunately, the findings from these studies were often reported as inconsistent. Comparisons across different studies have been at times contradictory. This may have been caused by multiple factors: (1) the prescribed VLT might not have induced a detectable level of vocal fatigue across individuals, (2) the amount of vocal loading across participants may not have been consistent due to the lack of a universal method to quantify vocal loading, and (3) there may have been variability in experimental settings. A more robust vocal loading protocol for VLT is therefore needed to improve consistency, and to allow comparisons across different studies.

Amongst methods of quantifying voice use for vocal fatigue assessment, the vocal distance dose, D_d, first proposed by Titze et al., was adopted in the present study [27]. The vocal distance dose attempts to approximately quantify the distance traveled by vocal folds during vocal oscillation [27,28]. It is usually calculated in terms of the fundamental frequency, the sound pressure level, the voicing duration, and the vocal duty ratio. Whether D_d correspondes to the true cumulative vocal fold displacement has not yet been verified. But, as a four-parameter estimates, vocal distance dose is more comprehensive than other metrics that are based on one single parameter. Svec et al. described the procedures to calculate the distance dose using synchronized microphone and EGG data [29]. The EGG signal was used to locate the peak position for each vocal cycle in the time domain. The microphone signal was used to quantify loudness. Carroll et al. used cumulative vocal dose data correlations with subjective measurements in vocal fatigue experiments. An abrupt increase in vocal loading was closely related to a harsher subjective self-reported rating [30]. Echternach et al. found that a 10-min intensive VLT with a >80 dB loudness level was comparable to a 45-min teaching task in terms of vocal dose [31]. Remacle et al. showed that kindergarden teachers had significantly greater distance doses than elementary school teachers based on an investigation of 12 kindertarten and 20 elementary school female teachers [5]. Bottalico and Astolfi calculated the vocal distance dose and the sound pressure level (SPL) for school teachers during their daily teaching assignments. They found that female teachers had on average a higher (>3.4 dB) loudness level than male teachers, but vocal distance doses did not differ very much between female and males teachers [32]. Morrow and Connor used an ambulatory phonation monitor to record and calculate the SPL and the distance dose for elementary music teachers with and without voice amplification [33]. The results showed that voice amplification significantly decreased the average SPL and the distance dose. These studies used the vocal distance dose as a quantitative measure of voice use in the VLTs or routine phonation tasks. Despite progress, no definitive correlations have been yet made between subjective assessments and objective measures in vocal fatigue studies. The distance dose prospectively offers a quantitative metric for vocal loading. Such framework is essential for cross-participants or cross-sessions comparisons to be meaningful and reasonable.

In the present study, a uniquely designed VLT was investigated. Ten human subjects were recruited and participated in the study. The vocal distance dose was used to quantify the participants' vocal loading online during the experiment. Subjective and objective measures were used to assess participants' voice qualities. A cross-session comparison was made to investigate the relationship between total distance dose and voice quality.

2. Research Hypothesis and Objective

We hypothesized that vocal fatigue during dose-based VLT varies with the vocal distance dose, D_d. The objective of this study was to investigate possible correlations between auditory-perceptual ratings, self-reported ratings, and acoustic measures during a dose-monitored VLT.

3. Participant Recruitment

The human research ethics protocol (A09-M46-11A) was approved by the Institutional Review Board at McGill University. No occupational voice users such as singers, teachers, and voice actors were recruited, because previous studies showed that their voice had greater endurance for vocal loadings than normal voice users [1,34]. The purpose of the study was not communicated to the participants before the experiment was concluded. The participants were only informed that they had to perform reading sessions. This was to help reduce the participants' biases towards the SAVRa ratings. For example, if the participants were aware that the study was measuring vocal fatigue, they would expect their voice quality to degrade throughout the sessions. This may increase the risk of biased ratings through the introduction of a psychological variable into the cross-session analysis of the participants' voice quality.

Participants were recruited in Montreal, Canada. The inclusion criteria were that the participants should be female, native English speakers with no history of voice disorders. Sex and gender differences in voice performance were found to be significant by Hunter et al. [35,36]. The present study only used female participants to exclude sex as a variable in the pilot study. Male participants will be used in future experiments. The participants' demographic information is shown in Table 1. The experiments were conducted in a sound-proof voice recording studio located in the Centre for Interdisciplinary Research in Music Media and Technology (CIRMMT). All experiments took place in the morning, around 9:00 a.m. The participants were instructed not to use their voice often over a period of 8 h before the experiments. The participants were required to withdraw from the study if they were found to have a voice problem, such as cough and cold, in the early morning. During the experiment, participants who reported any severe physical discomforts, such as unceasing cough and voice loss, were asked to withdraw from the recording session.

Table 1. Personal information about the participants.

ID	Age	Occupation
1	32	SLP
2	22	psychology student
3	38	psychology student
4	25	engineering student
5	23	SLP student
6	22	nutrition student
7	24	SLP student
8	26	engineering student
9	31	arts student
10	26	psychology student

4. Experimental Protocol Design and Data Acquisition

4.1. Vocal Loading Protocol

The VLT protocol is illustrated in Figure 1. Before the formal recording, the participants were required to attend a preparation session, during which they learned how to use a voice biofeedback monitor for the experiment. The VLT was structured as a series of six successive sessions ($S_i (i = 1, 2, .., 6)$). The participants were asked to read loudly the novel "Harry Potter and the Sorcerer's Stone" [37]. For each session, the participants were required to reach a D_d of 500 m within 25 min. After this reading task, the participants were required to finish a voice quality evaluation test with in 5 min. In preliminary study, a D_d of 500 m in 25 min was found to be intensive enough to induce vocal fatigue on participants, as self-reported. All the participants' voice was fully recovered after one day. This indicated that the selected D_d level did not induce any long-term vocal damage to the participants. The preliminary study also showed that the distance dose was sensitive to $f0$, loudness and phonatory style. A reading task using a habitual $f0$ and SPL yielded a distance dose of approximately 5 m per 20 s. But a note sung with similar $f0$ and SPL yielded a distance dose over 20 m per 20 s. Therefore, singing was prohibited in this experiment. The participants were asked to use a daily speech communication style.

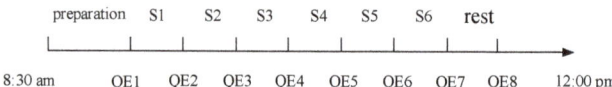

Figure 1. Measurement protocol of the vocal loading task in the vocal fatigue study. $QE_i (i = 1, 2, .., 8)$: Quality Evaluation; $S_i (i = 1, 2, .., 6)$ represents each vocal loading task session.

4.2. Voice Biofeedback Monitoring

The participants were seated in front of a microphone, and wore a neck surface accelerometer (NSA) mounted using adhesive (*Tensive*) [38]. The NSA recorded the neck surface vibration and streamed it on a hard disk [39–41]. During recording, the participants were asked to remain stationary, with the microphone at a distance of 50 cm from their mouth. The VLT sessions were monitored using a short-time (20 s long) distance dose calculator and a accumulative distance dose calculator in *LabView* (2018, NI, TX, US). A screenshot of the tool is shown in Figure 2. When the cumulative distance dose reached 500 m, the circular progress LED indicator turned from green to red, indicating the completion of one VLT session. The square-shaped LED indicator turned from green to red if the participant's previous 20 s distance dose did not reach a threshold value of 11 m. The threshold value was adjusted by trial-and-error to be high enough to induce vocal fatigue while ensuring that all participants could complete the VLT sessions. The participants were asked to keep an eye on the two indicators during the VLT sessions, so that they could adjust their vocal effort online, in real time. The virtual vocal distance dose monitoring tool prompted participants to read intensively throughout the VLT sessions. The 20 s distance dose calculation algorithm is illustrated in Figure 3. The total distance dose was calculated as the sum of all previous 20 s distance doses. The recording devices were a condenser acoustic microphone (Type 4178, Brüel & Kjær, Denmark) and the NSA. The microphone sensitivity was verified using a calibrated precision sound pressure level meter (Type 2250-L, Brüel & Kjær, Denmark).

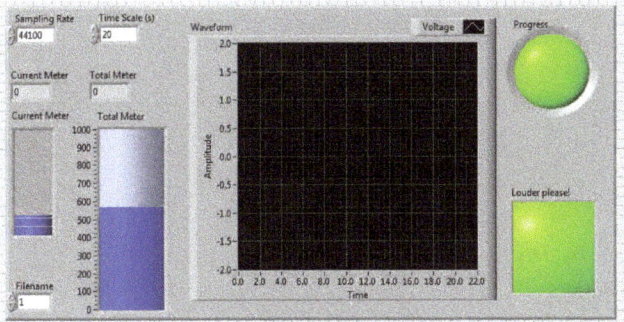

Figure 2. Virtual vocal distance dose monitor.

1: segment the entire recording into uniform-length (100 ms) frames;
2: remove unvoiced utterances from each frame using a zero-cross-rate based vocal activity detection method;
3: locate the position (x_i, y_i) of the vocal cycle peak for each frame, $i = [1, 2, ..., n]$ where n is the number of cycles for each frame;
4: calculate the SPL (dB ref. 20μ Pa) for each peak value using the formula: SPL $= 1.108 \times 20 \times \log10(|y_i|) + 89.25$;
5: calculate $f0$ in Hz using $44100/(x_{i+1} - x_i)$;
6: calculate the phonation threshold pressure in kPa using $P_{th} = 0.14 + 0.06(f0/f_{0N})^2$, where f_{0N} was 190 Hz for females [48];
7: calculate the lung pressure in kPa using $P_L = P_{th} + 10^{(SPL-78.5)/27.3}$ [40];
8: calculate the amplitude of vocal fold vibration in m using $A_i = 0.05 \times 0.01 \times [(P_L - P_{th})/P_{th}]^{1/2}$ [33];
9: calculate the distance dose in m for each frame using $D_d = \sum_{i=1}^{n-1} 4A_i$ [35].

Figure 3. Procedure for the 20 s distance dose calculation.

4.3. Subjective and Objective Measures of Vocal Fatigue

Three subjective methods of voice quality assessment were used in the experiment. They were the fatigue-indicative symptom documentation, the CAPE-V rating, and the SAVRa. Fatigue-indicative symptoms, such as cough, swallowing, and voice break, were recorded manually. Before, between, and after each VLT session, the participants performed a voice quality evaluation (QE) task, rated using the CAPE-V rating [42] and the SAVRa rating [23]. The CAPE-V ratings included six dimensions: overall severity, roughness, breathiness, strain, pitch, and loudness. The SAVRa ratings included three dimensions: speaking effort level (EFFT), laryngeal discomfort level (DISC), and inability to produce soft voice (IPSV). The QE took less than 5 min to complete. After completion, the participants remained silent until the start of the next session. A fixed volume (100 mL) of water was given to the participants immediately before each QE. No drinking was allowed during the VLT sessions. After the experiment, the microphone recordings of the CAPE-V task were sent to four certified speech language pathologists (SLPs) for auditory-perceptual rating. The four SLPs had more than 3 years of experience on voice research and clinical diagnosis, and they used the CAPE-V on voice patients and experimental participants quite often during the past three years. Three of them were voice doctors in the McGill University Health Centre, and the other one was a voice research associate in

McGill University. The CAPE-V recordings were blindly rated by the SLPs. There were eight audio recordings for each participant. The order of within-participant files was randomized to reduce the SLPs' rating bias. The audio files were rated participant by participant, so that the SLPs could identify the participant-specific baseline of voice quality for each rating task.

Voice features, such as $f0$, SPL, duty ratio, CPP, spectral tilt, HRF, jitter, and shimmer extracted from the recorded NSA and microphone signals, were labeled with the corresponding session numbers. These voice features were compared across sessions to track the variations between the participants' voice qualities. These vocal metrics were also compared with the CAPE-V and SAVRa ratings.

4.4. Data Analysis

The mean values and standard deviations of the normalized SAVRa and the original CAPE-V rating scores were calculated. The SAVRa scores were first normalized for each participant, and then the normalized scores were clustered for statistical analysis. The scores in the SAVRa and CAPE-V ratings are inversely related to the voice quality, i.e., a higher score implies lower voice quality and vice-versa. This rule applies to all dimension ratings of the SAVRa and CAPE-V. For correlation analysis, all voice quality data were assumed to obey a Gaussian distribution. A rigorous validation of this assumption would require a larger data set, which was beyond the scope of the present study. A Pearson correlation analysis was done between each pairs of dimensions of the SAVRa rating scores and the CAPE-V rating scores.

Fifteen acoustic features were calculated from the microphone and the NSA data using Matlab (2018a). The symbols and a description of the features are shown in Table 2. Features commonly used in previous vocal fatigue studies were selected. The original microphone and NSA signals were segmented into uniform frames of duration 100 ms (20–40 vocal cycles). Frames that were too short (20–30 ms) were insufficient for extracting effective jitter and shimmer, and frames that were too long (>500 ms) could not satisfactorily resolve $f0$ variations. The unvoiced frames were detected and removed using the zero-cross rate method [43].

Table 2. List of features extracted from the microphone and NSA signals.

Symbols	Explanation	Source
$f0$	fundamental frequency	microphone
SPL	sound pressure level	microphone
duty ratio	voicing percentage in recording time	microphone
CPP_MIC	cepstral peak prominence	microphone
jitter_MIC	pitch perturbation	microphone
shimmer_MIC	loudness perturbation	microphone
CPP_NSA	cepstral peak prominence	NSA
jitter_NSA	pitch perturbation	NSA
shimmer_NSA	loudness perturbation	NSA
TILT_MIC	spectral tilt	microphone
HRF_MIC	harmonic richness factor	microphone
H1H2_MIC	different between H1 and H2 magnitudes	microphone
TILT_NSA	spectral tilt	NSA
HRF_NSA	harmonic richness factor	NSA
H1H2_NSA	different between H1 and H2 magnitudes	NSA

The procedure of multivariate analysis in the present study was that a trend was searched in SAVRa scores at first to build a baseline of identifying vocal fatigue. A similar trend in the CAPE-V scores was then searched to verify the consistency between self-administered and SLP-rated methods. Finally, this trend was searched in the fifteen acoustic features to demonstrate some specific features have the potential of indicating vocal fatigue.

5. Data Analysis Results and Discussions

5.1. SAVRa and CAPE-V Rating Results

The mean values and standard deviations of the normalized SAVRa and the original CAPE-V rating scores are shown in Figures 4 and 5, respectively. The Pearson correlation coefficients for SAVRa rating results (mean values) were 0.957 (EFFT vs. DISC), 0.834 (EFFT vs. IPSV), and 0.852 (DISC vs. IPSV), respectively. The average variation trajectories of these three dimensions are well correlated with each other. The EFFT and the DISC scores increased rapidly from QE1 to QE2, as shown in Figure 4. The IPSV score increased mildly at the beginning of the VLT sessions, which indicated that the soft phonation quality decreased slightly for S1. The average score increased for the EFFT, DISC, and IPSV from QE1 to QE2 were 0.52, 0.38, and 0.07, respectively. The effect of rest on self-reported voice quality ratings was notable for all dimensions. The mean and the standard deviation values of the three dimensions of the SAVRa ratings are shown in Table 3. The EFFT, the DISC, and the IPSV decreased by 50.0%, 59.3%, and 50.9%, respectively, from QE7 to QE8. In general, the high score ratings for all three dimensions occurred late in the sessions. The maximum (0.88) EFFT scores occurred at QE6, the maximum (0.88) DISC scores occurred at QE7, and the maximum (0.82) IPSV scores occurred at QE5. This indicated a cumulative effect, i.e., vocal fatigue increased over time during VLT sessions. In general, all three dimensions of the SAVRa ratings followed a similar trend across sessions.

Table 3. SAVRa mean and deviation values in terms of VLT session. The display format was $x(y)$, where x was the mean and y was the standard deviation. QE_i (i = 1...8): quality evaluation. EFFT: speaking effort level. DISC: laryngeal discomfort level. IPSV: inability to produce soft voice.

	EFFT	DISC	IPSV
QE1	0.08 (0.25)	0.02 (0.07)	0.23 (0.39)
QE2	0.61 (0.38)	0.40 (0.27)	0.30 (0.28)
QE3	0.54 (0.20)	0.52 (0.27)	0.46 (0.28)
QE4	0.66 (0.27)	0.48 (0.22)	0.71 (0.31)
QE5	0.80 (0.14)	0.76 (0.13)	0.82 (0.19)
QE6	0.88 (0.25)	0.83 (0.14)	0.67 (0.30)
QE7	0.84 (0.26)	0.88 (0.26)	0.72 (0.36)
QE8	0.42 (0.38)	0.36 (0.32)	0.35 (0.45)

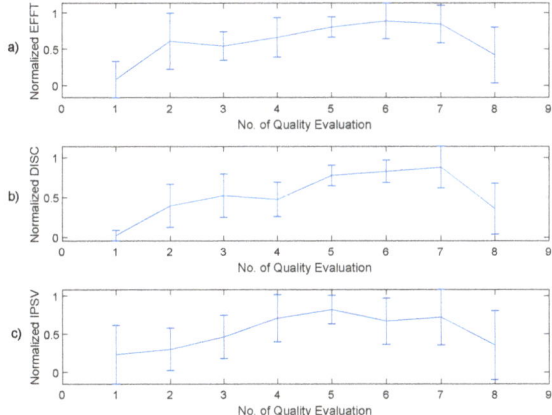

Figure 4. Cross-session variations mean and standard deviation values of SAVRa ratings for all participants (n = 10). (**a**) speaking effort level (EFFT); (**b**) laryngeal discomfort level (DISC); (**c**) inability to produce soft voice (IPSV).

The Pearson correlation coefficients between the overall severity trace and other dimensions in the CAPE-V ratings are shown in Table 4. This indicated that the overall severity, roughness, and strain variations were well correlated. The mean values of the overall severity, the roughness, and the strain scores followed a trend similar to that of the SAVRa results, as shown in Figure 5. They increased rapidly after S1 (QE1–QE3), remained constant for several sessions, and decreased over the remainder of the session. This trend was generally consistent with those of all three dimensions in SAVRa ratings, which showed a vocal 'transition' or 'adjustment' period in the first session and a vocal 'recovery' period during the final session. The maximum values of these three dimensions, shown in Figure 5, occurred at QE6. The mean and deviation values of the three dimensions of the SAVRa ratings are shown in Table 5. Other dimensions in the CAPE-V ratings followed different trends. The standard deviations of the CAPEV ratings across SLPs were larger than those of SAVRa ratings.

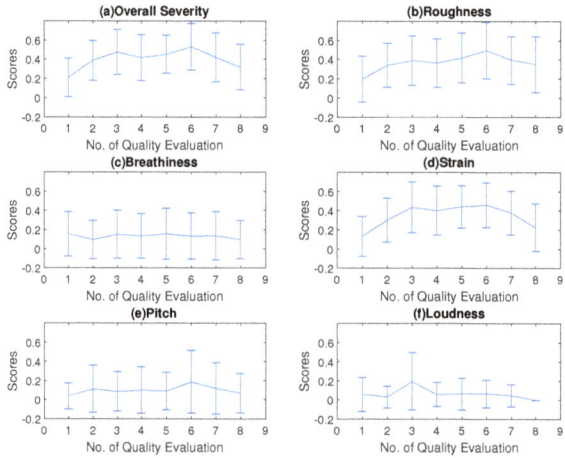

Figure 5. Cross-session variations mean and standard deviation values of CAPE-V ratings for all participants (n = 10).

Table 4. Pearson correlation coefficients between the overall severity and other dimensions.

With Overall Severity	r	p
Roughness	0.948	0.00
Breathiness	0.103	0.81
Strain	0.969	0.00
Pitch	0.810	0.01
Loudness	0.402	0.32

Table 5. CAPEV mean and deviation values in terms of VLT session. The display format was $x(y)$, where x was the mean and y was the standard deviation. OS: overall severity, RG: Roughness, BT: Breathiness, ST: Strain, PT: Pitch, LD: Loudness.

	OS	RG	BT	ST	PT	LD
QE1	0.22 (0.20)	0.20 (0.24)	0.16 (0.23)	0.14 (0.21)	0.04 (0.14)	0.06 (0.18)
QE2	0.39 (0.21)	0.34 (0.23)	0.10 (0.20)	0.31 (0.23)	0.12 (0.25)	0.03 (0.12)
QE3	0.48 (0.23)	0.39 (0.26)	0.15 (0.25)	0.44 (0.27)	0.09 (0.21)	0.20 (0.30)
QE4	0.42 (0.24)	0.37 (0.25)	0.14 (0.23)	0.41 (0.25)	0.11 (0.24)	0.06 (0.13)
QE5	0.46 (0.20)	0.42 (0.26)	0.16 (0.27)	0.44 (0.22)	0.10 (0.20)	0.07 (0.17)
QE6	0.53 (0.24)	0.50 (0.29)	0.14 (0.24)	0.46 (0.23)	0.19 (0.33)	0.07 (0.15)

5.2. Vocal Fatigue Symptoms Recordings

The participants' vocal fatigue-indicative symptoms during the six VLT session are shown in Figure 6. The cross-participant discrepancy in the vocal symptoms is notable. For example, participant No. 4 was found to display much more (+47) symptoms than participant No. 8. One cough by participant No. 5 occurred for 4 VLT sessions, but no cough was observed for participants No. 3, No. 7, and No. 8 during any VLT sessions. The mean counts of vocal fatigue symptom appearances for all participants are shown in Figure 6. The average counts of swallowing increased by a factor of 1.8 from S1 to S2, then decreased to a relatively stable level (4–4.5 times). This trend is consistent with that of the overall severity, the roughness, and the strain in the CAPE-V ratings, and the EFFT in the SAVRa ratings. This finding validated the previous study results, which showed that re-hydration could relieve vocal fatigue, and allow voice to be sustained over longer time periods [44,45]. No similar trends were observed for any other symptoms, nor any dimensions in the CAPE-V and the SAVRa.

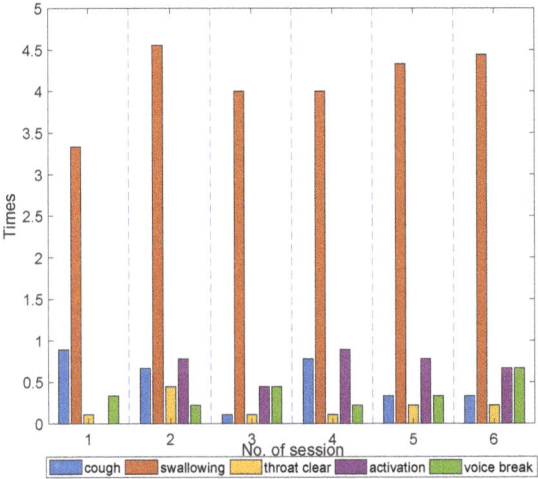

Figure 6. Mean counts of vocal fatigue symptom appearances for all participants during the VLTs in terms of session. The vertical blue dash lines separate different VLT sessions.

5.3. Acoustic Feature Analysis

The cross-session variations of the mean and confidence level (95%) of the features for all participants are shown in Figure 7. The NSA data of participant No.1 was unavailable due to sensor failure. The $f0$, SPL, and duty ratio in Figure 7 follow a similar trend. They increase rapidly at the beginning, reach a certain saturation level over the remaining sessions. $f0$, SPL, and duty ratio indicated a vocal adjustment over session S1. The mean value variations of these three features from S1 to S2 were at least 100% larger than those of any other following VLT session. The $f0$ had the minimal mean value variation (<2 Hz) in the last three sessions. The SPL mean value decreased by 2 dB after S4 and increased by 1 dB after S5. The duty ratio mean value increased by 2% from one plateau (S2–S4) to another (S5–S6). The trends in $f0$, SPL and duty ratio were largely consistent with the trends in CAPE-V and SAVRa ratings.

A considerable decrease in CPP was found to be related to the presence of dysphonia by Heman-Ackah [16]. The CPP_MIC in Figure 7 showed a slight increase (0.15 dB) from S1 to S2, and a decrease (0.3 dB) from S3 to S4. The fluctuation of the CPP_MIC from S1 to S6 was less than 2%, which means that the variation of CPP_MIC was not significant. The CPP_NSA showed a sharp increase (2 dB) in the late session after sustaining a relatively low level for the first three sessions. The jitter_MIC increased rapidly from S1 to S4 by 10% but decreased by 5% afterwards, which was not well correlated with the subjective rating results for the VLT sessions. The jitter_NSA showed a trend similar to jitter_MIC, but with a larger decrease after S3. The mean values of the shimmer_MIC and shimmer_NSA were well correlated ($r = 0.91, p = 0.987$). Their progressions were similar to that of the $f0$. This indicates that the loudness perturbation increased rapidly in the early sessions, and saturated at a high level over the last sessions.

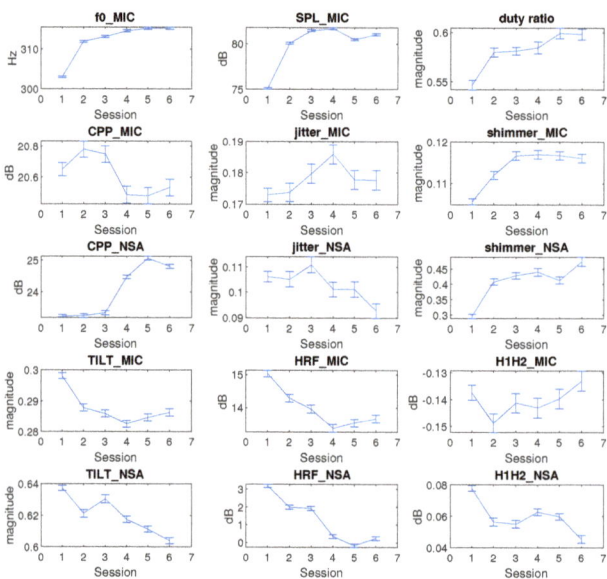

Figure 7. Cross-session variations of means and confidential levels in terms of feature for all participants.

A decrease in spectral tilt slope was found to correlate with stressed phonation by Sluijter and Heuven [46]. A decrease in spectral tilt slope indicates that higher frequencies are increased more than lower frequencies. In Figure 7, the TILT_MIC slopes and the TILT_NSA slopes decreased from S1 to S6 in general. Thus, the high frequencies of both the microphone and NSA spectra increased throughout VLT sessions. Childers and Lee found that vocal fry had a higher HRF value than modal and breathy voice [47]. The HRF_MIC and the HRF_NSA obeyed similar trends than TILT_MIC and TILT_NSA. The HRF_MIC was well correlated ($r = 0.94, p = 0.98$) with HRF_NSA. These two features showed identical trends. The HRF mean values decreased from S1 and converged to S6. The H1H2_NSA decreased by 50% from S1 to S6, and remained constant from S2 to S5. A comprehensive analysis of the Pearson correlation between each pair of features is shown in Table 6. There are two groups of well correlated (>90%) features. The first group includes $f0$, SPL_MIC, duty ratio, shimmer_MIC, and shimmer_NSA. The first group shows a rapid increase in early session followed by saturation. The second group includes TILT_MIC, TILT_NSA, HRF_MIC, and HRF_NSA and shows a general decrease from S1 to S6.

Table 6. Pearson correlation coefficients for each pair of features. The fi (i = 1,..., 15) represents f_0, SPL, duty ratio, CPP_MIC, jitter_MIC, shimmer_MIC, CPP_NSA, jitter_NSA, shimmer_NSA, TILT_MIC, HRF_MIC, H1H2_MIC, TILT_NSA, HR_NSA, and H1H2_NSA, respectively.

	f1	f2	f3	f4	f5	f6	f7	f8	f9	f10	f11	f12	f13	f14	f15
f1	1	*	*	*	*	*	*	*	*	*	*	*	*	*	*
f2	0.95	1	*	*	*	*	*	*	*	*	*	*	*	*	*
f3	0.97	0.86	1	*	*	*	*	*	*	*	*	*	*	*	*
f4	−0.39	−0.20	−0.45	1	*	*	*	*	*	*	*	*	*	*	*
f5	0.61	0.69	0.44	−0.51	1	*	*	*	*	*	*	*	*	*	*
f6	0.96	0.96	0.90	−0.40	0.74	1	*	*	*	*	*	*	*	*	*
f7	0.68	0.46	0.76	−0.91	0.46	0.63	1	*	*	*	*	*	*	*	*
f8	−0.44	−0.24	−0.56	0.70	−0.15	−0.30	−0.78	1	*	*	*	*	*	*	*
f9	0.95	0.94	0.90	−0.28	0.59	0.91	0.57	−0.51	1	*	*	*	*	*	*
f10	−0.96	−0.97	−0.87	0.37	−0.75	−0.96	−0.59	0.29	−0.89	1	*	*	*	*	*
f11	−0.95	−0.89	−0.89	0.62	−0.79	−0.95	−0.79	0.49	−0.87	0.95	1	*	*	*	*
f12	−0.06	−0.20	0.08	−0.50	−0.04	−0.01	0.45	−0.54	0.03	0.22	−0.03	1	*	*	*
f13	−0.80	−0.63	−0.89	0.62	−0.30	−0.67	−0.86	0.87	−0.79	0.67	0.77	−0.26	1	*	*
f14	−0.88	−0.72	−0.91	0.77	−0.59	−0.83	−0.94	0.69	−0.77	0.82	0.94	−0.21	0.90	1	*
f15	−0.82	−0.80	−0.83	0.03	−0.23	−0.73	−0.40	0.47	−0.92	0.68	0.63	−0.10	0.73	0.58	1

6. Discussion and Conclusions

The primary finding in the SAVRa results was that the ratings show an arch-shaped variation trajectory from QE1 to QE8. This trend was also observed in the CAPE-V rating results. In the SAVRa ratings, the rapid increase of the vocal effort, the vocal discomfort level, and the severity of the soft phonation quality indicated a voice adjustment period. Over this period, the participants' vocal folds were abruptly exposed to a heavy vocal loading, and thus the subjects' feelings of vocal fatigue were strong over this period. After this period, the degrees of the participants' perceived vocal fatigue remained constant at a high level, or increased moderately from QE2 to QE7. The vocal loading intensity for each VLT session was identical. The participants gradually adapted to the vocal loading intensity, thus the increasing rate slowed down after this period. After the S1, the accumulation effect of the vocal loading led to a slow and persistent increase of the participants' perceived vocal fatigue in the late sessions. This indicates that, given constant vocal stimuli for different sessions, the participants' perceived vocal fatigue increased over time (or vocal distance dose). The notable decrease of the SAVRa scores from QE7 to QE8 reflects the effect of vocal rest on participants' vocal fatigue feelings. This indicates that the participants felt much better about their vocal functionalities after the 15-min rest session, but the rest was not sufficient to completely recover to the original status at QE1. A longer rest session was thus presumed to enhance the vocal recovery process. The findings in the CAPE-V rating results show that the overall severity, roughness, and strain ratings have the same arch-shaped variation trend with the SAVRa results. This indicates that vocal fatigue degraded the participants' voice performance by increasing roughness and strain.

The data for the fatigue-indicative symptoms obeyed different trends than the SAVRa results. Previous studies showed that these symptoms were frequently observed on vocally fatigued participants. However, a quantitative relationship between the number of occurrences of these symptoms and the degree of vocal fatigue could not be established. Individual discrepancies in the counts of these symptoms showed varied sensitivities to vocal fatigue. Some participants coughed frequently during the VLT, while others did not cough at all. Swallowing was much more frequently observed than other symptoms for all participants. This finding further validated the results of previous studies on the effect of hydration on vocal fatigue [44,48], i.e., superficial vocal fold hydration (swallowing or drinking) could help relieve vocal dysfunction and improve vocal efficiency.

Fifteen voice metrics (features) were studied to track voice quality variation across VLT sessions. The statistical analysis results in Figure 7 did not include the rest session. The $f0$, SPL_MIC, duty ratio, shimmer_MIC, and shimmer_NSA rapidly increased in early sessions, and remained constant afterwards. The variation of $f0$ in Figure 7 was consistent with the results of previous studies, which found that participants' $f0$ increased with vocal fatigue [49,50]. The shimmer_MIC and shimmer_NSA showed an increase after the VLT session. This finding contradicts Laukkanen's one-day vocal fatigue study results [51], but it is consistent with Gelfer's 60-min vocal fatigue study results [49]. This might be caused by the different phonation durations.

One limitation of the present study was that the voice type was not considered as a parameter in the voice use quantification. For example, breathy voice obviously had a different vocal loading intensity from pressed voice when the $f0$, SPL, duty ratio, and duration were identical for these two voice types. The impact stress between vocal folds for these two voice types were different. The feelings of vocal fatigue that the breathy and pressed voice brought to participants were therefore different. An improved method of calculating D_d that considers voice quality is therefore needed to make the voice use quantification more accurate. Another limitation was that calculation of the D_d from the NSA may be not very accurate because of the rather large uncertainty in the SPL (± 5 dB) estimates from the NSA data [40]. The accuracy of calculating D_d would thus be influenced. This issue limits the use of the dose-based voice use quantification method in long-term voice monitoring. The monitoring of neck surface acceleration is preferable to minimize the influence of extraneous noise and potentially reduce discomfort in occupational settings. A method for directly deriving the magnitude of the vocal fold vibration from the skin acceleration level is therefore needed. The last limitation is that normal swallowing on a daily basis was not measured, and thus the fatigue-indicative symptom analysis lacked a baseline to refer to. This baseline could be established in future work.

Author Contributions: Conceptualization, Z.L., N.Y.-K.L.-J. and L.M. (Luc Mongeau); methodology, Z.L. and L.M. (Luc Mongeau); software, Z.L.; validation, Z.L., N.Y.-K.L.-J. and L.M. (Luc Mongeau); formal analysis, Z.L.; investigation, Z.L.; resources, L.M. (Lisa Martignetti), N.Y.-K.L.-J. and L.M. (Luc Mongeau); data curation, Z.L., L.F. and L.M. (Lisa Martignetti); writing—original draft preparation, Z.L.; writing—review and editing, Z.L., L.F., L.M. (Lisa Martignetti), N.Y.-K.L.-J. and L.M. (Luc Mongeau); visualization, Z.L.; supervision, N.Y.-K.L.-J. and L.M. (Luc Mongeau); project administration, L.M. (Luc Mongeau); funding acquisition, N.Y.-K.L.-J. and L.M. (Luc Mongeau). All authors have read and agreed to the published version of the manuscript.

Funding: This research was funded by the National Institutes of Health (Grant R01 DC-005788) and the Canadian Institutes of Health Research (388583).

Acknowledgments: The financial support of of the National Science and Engineering Research Council of Canada is gratefully acknowledged.

Conflicts of Interest: The authors declare no conflict of interest.

Abbreviations

The following abbreviations are used in this manuscript:

CAPE-V	Consensus Auditory-Perceptual Evaluation of Voice
SAVRa	Self-Administered Voice Rating
GRABAS	Gradem Roughness, Breathiness, Asthenia, Strain
NSA	Neck Surface Accelerometer
SLP	Speech Language Pathologist
MFDR	Maximum Flow Declination Rate
MFCC	Mel-Frequency Spectral Coefficients
VLT	Vocal Loading Task
EGG	Electroglottograph
SPL	Sound Pressure Level
CIRMMT	Centre for Interdisciplinary Research in Music Media and Technology
QE	Quality Evaluation
IPSV	Inability to Produce Soft Voice
CPP	Cepstral Peak Prominence
HRF	Harmonic Richness Factor

References

1. Welham, N.V.; Maclagan, M.A. Vocal Fatigue: Current Knowledge and Future Directions. *J. Voice* **2003**, *17*, 21–30. [CrossRef]
2. Thomas, G.; de Jong, F.; Kooijman, P.G.C.; Donders, A.R.T.; Cremers, C.W. Voice complaints, risk factors for voice problems and history of voice problems in relation to puberty in female student teachers. *Folia Phoniatr. Logop.* **2006**, *58*, 305–322. [CrossRef]
3. Solomon, N.P. Vocal fatigue and its relation to vocal hyperfunction. *Int. J. -Speech-Lang. Pathol.* **2008**, *10*, 254–266. [CrossRef]
4. Remacle, A.; Morsomme, D.; Berrué, E.; Finck, C. Vocal Impact of a Prolonged Reading Task in Dysphonic Versus Normophonic Female Teachers. *J. Voice* **2012**, *26*, 820.e1–820.e13. [CrossRef]
5. Remacle, A.; Morsomme, D.; Finck, C. Comparison of Vocal Loading Parameters in Kindergarten and Elementary School Teachers. *J. Speech Lang. Hear. Res.* **2014**, *57*, 406–415. [CrossRef]
6. Kreiman, J.; Gerratt, B.R. Sources of listener disagreement in voice quality assessment. *J. Acoust. Soc. Am.* **2000**, *108*, 1867–1876. [CrossRef] [PubMed]
7. Kreiman, J.; Gerratt, B.R.; Ito, M. When and why listeners disagree in voice quality assessment tasks. *J. Acoust. Soc. Am.* **2007**, *122*, 2354–2364. [CrossRef] [PubMed]
8. Pabon, J.P.H. Objective acoustic voice-quality parameters in the computer phonetogram. *J. Voice* **1991**, *5*, 203–216. [CrossRef]

9. Roy, N.; Barkmeier-Kraemer, J.; Eadie, T.; Sivasankar, M.P.; Mehta, D.; Paul, D.; Hillman, R. Evidence-Based Clinical Voice Assessment: A Systematic Review. *Am. J. -Speech-Lang. Pathol.* **2013**, *22*, 212–226. [CrossRef]
10. Awan, S.N.; Roy, N. Toward the development of an objective index of dysphonia severity: A four-factor acoustic model. *Clin. Linguist. Phon.* **2006**, *20*, 35–49. [CrossRef] [PubMed]
11. Godino-Llorente, J.I.; Gómez-Vilda, P.; Cruz-Roldán, F.; Blanco-Velasco, M.; Fraile, R. Pathological Likelihood Index as a Measurement of the Degree of Voice Normality and Perceived Hoarseness. *J. Voice* **2010**, *24*, 667–677. [CrossRef] [PubMed]
12. Halberstam, B. Acoustic and Perceptual Parameters Relating to Connected Speech Are More Reliable Measures of Hoarseness than Parameters Relating to Sustained Vowels. *Orl Otorhinolaryngol. Relat. Spec.* **2004**, *66*, 70–73. [CrossRef] [PubMed]
13. Holmberg, E.B.; Hillman, R.E.; Perkell, J.S. Glottal airflow and transglottal air pressure measurements for male and female speakers in soft, normal, and loud voice. *J. Acoust. Soc. Am.* **1988**, *84*, 511–529. [CrossRef] [PubMed]
14. Holmberg, E.B.; Hillman, R.E.; Perkell, J.S.; Guiod, P.C.; Goldman, S.L. Comparisons Among Aerodynamic, Electroglottographic, and Acoustic Spectral Measures of Female Voice. *J. Speech Lang. Hear. Res.* **1995**, *38*, 1212–1223. [CrossRef]
15. Anita Mcallister, Johan Sundberg, S.R.H. Acoustic measurements and perceptual evaluation of hoarseness in children's voices. *Logop. Phoniatr. Vocology* **1998**, *23*, 27–38. [CrossRef]
16. Heman-Ackah, Y.D.; Michael, D.D.; Baroody, M.M.; Ostrowski, R.; Hillenbrand, J.; Heuer, R.J.; Horman, M.; Sataloff, R.T. Cepstral Peak Prominence: A More Reliable Measure of Dysphonia. *Ann. Otol. Rhinol. Laryngol.* **2003**, *112*, 324–333. [CrossRef]
17. Godino-Llorente, J.I.; Gomez-Vilda, P.; Blanco-Velasco, M. Dimensionality Reduction of a Pathological Voice Quality Assessment System Based on Gaussian Mixture Models and Short-Term Cepstral Parameters. *IEEE Trans. Biomed. Eng.* **2006**, *53*, 1943–1953. [CrossRef]
18. Fang, S.H.; Tsao, Y.; Hsiao, M.J.; Chen, J.Y.; Lai, Y.H.; Lin, F.C.; Wang, C.T. Detection of Pathological Voice Using Cepstrum Vectors: A Deep Learning Approach. *J. Voice* **2018**. [CrossRef]
19. Klatt, D.H.; Klatt, L.C. Analysis, synthesis, and perception of voice quality variations among female and male talkers. *J. Acoust. Soc. Am.* **1990**, *87*, 820–857. [CrossRef]
20. Kitch, J.A.; Oates, J. The perceptual features of vocal fatigue as self-reported by a group of actors and singers. *J. Voice* **1994**, *8*, 207–214. [CrossRef]
21. Kitch, J.A.; Oates, J.; Greenwood, K. Performance effects on the voices of 10 choral tenors: Acoustic and perceptual findings. *J. Voice* **1996**, *10*, 217–227. [CrossRef]
22. Welham, N.V.; Maclagan, M.A. Vocal fatigue in young trained singers across a solo performance: A preliminary study. *Logop. Phoniatr. Vocology* **2004**, *29*, 3–12. [CrossRef] [PubMed]
23. Hunter, E.J. General Statistics of the NCVS Self-Administered Vocal Rating (SAVRa). *Natl. Cent. Voice Speech Online Tech. Memo* **2008**, *11*, 1–10.
24. Hunter, E.J.; Titze, I.R. Quantifying Vocal Fatigue Recovery: Dynamic Vocal Recovery Trajectories after a Vocal Loading Exercise. *Ann. Otol. Rhinol. Laryngol.* **2009**, *118*, 449–460. [CrossRef]
25. Nanjundeswaran, C.; Jacobson, B.H.; Gartner-Schmidt, J.; Abbott, K.V. Vocal Fatigue Index (VFI): Development and Validation. *J. Voice* **2015**, *29*, 433–440. [CrossRef]
26. Halpern, A.E.; Spielman, J.L.; Hunter, E.J.; Titze, I.R. The inability to produce soft voice (IPSV): A tool to detect vocal change in school teachers. *Logop. Phoniatr. Vocology* **2009**, *34*, 117–127. [CrossRef]
27. Titze, I.R.; Svec, J.G.; Popolo, P.S. Vocal Dose Measures: Quantifying Accumulated Vibration Exposure in Vocal Fold Tissues. *J. Speech Lang. Hear. Res.* **2003**, *46*, 919–932.[CrossRef]
28. Titze, I.R.; Hunter, E.J. Comparison of Vocal Vibration-Dose Measures for Potential-Damage Risk Criteria. *J. Speech Lang. Hear. Res.* **2015**, *58*, 1425–1439. [CrossRef]
29. Švec, J.G.; Popolo, P.S.; Titze, I.R. Measurement of vocal doses in speech: experimental procedure and signal processing. *Logop. Phoniatr. Vocol.* **2003**, *28*, 181–192. [CrossRef]
30. Carroll, T.; Nix, J.; Hunter, E.; Emerich, K.; Titze, I.; Abaza, M. Objective Measurement of Vocal Fatigue in Classical Singers: A Vocal Dosimetry Pilot Study. *Otolaryngol. Neck Surg.* **2006**, *135*, 595–602. [CrossRef]
31. Echternach, M.; Nusseck, M.; Dippold, S.; Spahn, C.; Richter, B. Fundamental frequency, sound pressure level and vocal dose of a vocal loading test in comparison to a real teaching situation. *Eur. Arch. -Oto-Rhino-Laryngol.* **2014**, *271*, 3263–3268. [CrossRef] [PubMed]

32. Bottalico, P.; Astolfi, A. Investigations into vocal doses and parameters pertaining to primary school teachers in classrooms. *J. Acoust. Soc. Am.* **2012**, *131*, 2817–2827. [CrossRef] [PubMed]
33. Morrow, S.L.; Connor, N.P. Voice Amplification as a Means of Reducing Vocal Load for Elementary Music Teachers. *J. Voice* **2011**, *25*, 441–446. [CrossRef] [PubMed]
34. Titze, I.R.; Sundberg, J. Vocal intensity in speakers and singers. *J. Acoust. Soc. Am.* **1992**, *91*, 2936–2946. [CrossRef]
35. Hunter, E.J.; Banks, R.E. Gender Differences in the Reporting of Vocal Fatigue in Teachers as Quantified by the Vocal Fatigue Index. *Ann. Otol. Rhinol. Laryngol.* **2017**, *126*, 813–818. [CrossRef]
36. Hunter, E.J.; Tanner, K.; Smith, M.E. Gender differences affecting vocal health of women in vocally demanding careers. *Logop. Phoniatr. Vocology* **2011**, *36*, 128–136. [CrossRef]
37. Rowling, J.K. Harry Potter and the Sorcerer's Stone. 2001. Available online: http://www2.sdfi.edu.cn/netclass/jiaoan/englit/download/Harry%20Potter%20and%20the%20Sorcerer's%20Stone.pdf (accessed on 4 February 2020).
38. Lei, Z.; Kennedy, E.; Fasanella, L.; Li-Jessen, N.Y.K.; Mongeau, L. Discrimination between Modal, Breathy and Pressed Voice for Single Vowels Using Neck-Surface Vibration Signals. *Appl. Sci.* **2019**, *9*, 1505. [CrossRef]
39. Mehta, D.D.; Zañartu, M.; Feng, S.W.; Cheyne, H.A.; Hillman, R.E. Mobile Voice Health Monitoring Using a Wearable Accelerometer Sensor and a Smartphone Platform. *IEEE Trans. Biomed. Eng.* **2012**, *59*, 3090–3096. [CrossRef]
40. Švec, J.G.; Titze, I.R.; Popolo, P.S. Estimation of sound pressure levels of voiced speech from skin vibration of the neck. *J. Acoust. Soc. Am.* **2005**, *117*, 1386–1394. [CrossRef]
41. Zanartu, M. Acoustic Coupling in Phonation and Its Effect On Inverse Filtering of Oral Airflow and Neck Surface Acceleration. Ph.D. Thesis, Purdue University, West Lafayette, IN, USA, 2010.
42. Zraick, R.; Kempster, G.; Connor, N.; Thibeault, S.; Klaben, B.; Bursac, Z.; Thrush, C.; Glaze, L. Establishing validity of the consensus auditory-perceptual evaluation of voice (CAPE-V). *Am. J. -Speech-Lang. Pathol.* **2011**, *20*, 14–22. [CrossRef]
43. Rabiner, L.; Schafer, R. *Digital Processing of Speech Signals*; Prentice-Hall Signal Processing Series; Prentice-Hall: Englewood, NJ, USA, 1978.
44. Yiu, E.M.L.; Chan, R.M. Effect of Hydration and Vocal Rest on the Vocal Fatigue in Amateur Karaoke Singers. *J. Voice* **2003**, *17*, 216–227. [CrossRef]
45. Solomon, N.P.; Glaze, L.E.; Arnold, R.R.; van Mersbergen, M. Effects of a Vocally Fatiguing Task and Systemic Hydration on Men's Voices. *J. Voice* **2003**, *17*, 31–46. [CrossRef]
46. Sluijter, A.M.C.; van Heuven, V.J. Spectral balance as an acoustic correlate of linguistic stress. *J. Acoust. Soc. Am.* **1996**, *100*, 2471–2485. [CrossRef] [PubMed]
47. Childers, D.G.; Lee, C.K. Vocal quality factors: Analysis, synthesis, and perception. *J. Acoust. Soc. Am.* **1991**, *90*, 2394–2410. [CrossRef]
48. Sivasankar, M.; Leydon, C. The role of hydration in vocal fold physiology. *Curr. Opin. Otolaryngol. Head Neck Surg.* **2010**, *18*, 171–175. [CrossRef]
49. Gelfer, M.P.; Andrews, M.L.; Schmidt, C.P. Effects of prolonged loud reading on selected measures of vocal function in trained and untrained singers. *J. Voice* **1991**, *5*, 158–167. [CrossRef]
50. Hunter, E.J.; Titze, I.R. Variations in Intensity, Fundamental Frequency, and Voicing for Teachers in Occupational Versus Non-Occupational Settings. *J. Speech Lang. Hear. Res.* **2010**, *53*, 862–875. [CrossRef]
51. Laukkanen, A.M.; Ilomäki, I.; Leppänen, K.; Vilkman, E. Acoustic Measures and Self-reports of Vocal Fatigue by Female Teachers. *J. Voice* **2008**, *22*, 283–289. [CrossRef]

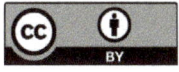

© 2020 by the authors. Licensee MDPI, Basel, Switzerland. This article is an open access article distributed under the terms and conditions of the Creative Commons Attribution (CC BY) license (http://creativecommons.org/licenses/by/4.0/).

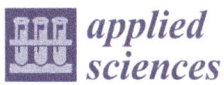

Article

Classification Maps in Studies on the Retirement Threshold

Agnieszka Bielińska [1], Dorota Bielińska-Wąż [2,*] and Piotr Wąż [3]

1 Department of Quality of Life Research, Medical University of Gdańsk, 80-210 Gdańsk, Poland
2 Department of Radiological Informatics and Statistics, Medical University of Gdańsk, 80-210 Gdańsk, Poland
3 Department of Nuclear Medicine, Medical University of Gdańsk, 80-210 Gdańsk, Poland
* Correspondence: djwaz@gumed.edu.pl

Received: 20 January 2020; Accepted: 8 February 2020; Published: 14 February 2020

Abstract: The aim of this work is to present new classification maps in health informatics and to show that they are useful in data analysis. A statistical method, correspondence analysis, has been applied for obtaining these maps. This approach has been applied to studies on expectations and worries related to the retirement threshold. For this purpose two questionnaires formulated by ourselves have been constructed. Groups of individuals and their answers to particular questions are represented by points in the classification maps. The distribution of these points reflects psychological attitudes of the considered population. In particular, we compared structures of the maps searching for factors such as gender, marital status, kind of work, economic situation, and intellectual activity related to the attendance the University of the Third Age, which are essential at the retirement threshold. Generally, in Polish society, retirement is evaluated as a positive experience and the majority of retirees do not want to return to their professional work. This result is independent of the kind of work and of the gender.

Keywords: medical informatics; statistical computing; data analysis; retirement threshold

---

1. Introduction

Classification studies are a valuable source of information in various areas of science. The problem of classification is related to the problem of similarity of objects. Objects arranged in simple, one-dimensional sets may be classified in a unique way according to one, properly chosen, aspect of similarity. The problem becomes more complicated if we consider multidimensional sets, i.e., objects characterized by several different aspects. The degree of similarity depends on the selected aspects, on the number of aspects considered and on the mathematical measure establishing the relations between different properties.

One of class of objects considered by us is biological sequences. Both graphical and numerical classification of these objects is possible using methods based on *Graphical Representations* [1,2]. Within these methods, one can create a large number of different types of numerical characteristics (descriptors) of the plots representing the sequences. One kind of descriptors we propose are the distribution moments related to different statistical distributions describing the DNA sequences. We have shown that using these descriptors a pair of the sequences that differ by only one base can be distinguished. The coordinates of the descriptors representing these sequences are different in the classification maps [1]. The distribution moments we have also introduced as new descriptors of another class of objects—the molecular spectra [3,4]. The applications of the theory of molecular similarity are broad. Except for the studies of the properties of the systems explicitly considered in our works, the new descriptors may have broad range of interdisciplinary applications. For example, they may be applied in computational pharmacology and toxicology [5]. Our new descriptors have also found their application in the classification of the solutions in the chaotic systems [6], or in the classification of the stellar spectra [7,8]. Another kind of descriptor we propose are values used in the classical dynamics such as coordinates of center of mass or the moments of inertia. Examples of the classification studies using these descriptors may be found in the theory of molecular similarity [9] or in bioinformatics [10].

A class of objects considered in this work are groups of individuals. The studies are focused on the *retirement threshold*. A graphical representation of the results known as the *Correspondence Analysis* (CA) proves to be very useful in this kind of study [11]. Recently, CA was applied for studies on a variety of problems, for example, on high school dropouts [12], and also in archeology [13], in food science [14], etc. In the CA the information about the whole system is stored on maps in which objects under consideration are represented by points located in a specific way. The classification of the objects is here performed by studying distances between the points and, in particular, by identifying clusters of the points. Objects corresponding to the points which form a cluster are similar in some way.

Progress of medicine and lower fertility rate caused significant changes in the structure of modern societies. The number of seniors in developed countries is growing dynamically. In Poland in 2010 the percentage of people aged 65 and over was 19%. According to Eurostat forecasts, in 2030 the ratio of elderly people to the population aged 15–64 will be 36%, and in 2050—56% [15].

Due to acceleration of aging process, it seems reasonable to study the quality of life of older people. An important role in shaping the quality of life of seniors plays the retirement threshold, which is described in literature as symbolic moment—starting a new chapter in life. It involves many negative changes such as loss of professional status, deterioration of the economic situation, as well as reduction in the number of social interactions. On the other hand, pensioners have much free time for family life and hobby. Therefore, despite losing one of the most important roles in life, one can set new goals and develop non-professional passions. The change of social role from employee to retiree is a natural process, but such a big change in life may lead to negative psychological effects [16–19]. Changes in different aspects of life due to the retirement threshold have been studied in many countries. For example, changes in the sleep duration were studied in the United States [20] and Finland [21]; changes in the physical activity were studied in Canada [22], Belgium [23], and Finland [24–26]; and changes in the body mass index were studied in the United States [27] and Finland [28]. A variety of changes in the quality of life in different domains have been observed, for example, in the subjective wellbeing [29], in the use of time, activity patterns, in health and wellbeing [30], in the health-related quality of life [31], in the enjoyment of everyday activities [32], and in mobility [33]. The observed changes at the retirement threshold are not unique. Different factors, e.g., sex, social background, and education level, may determine whether they are positive or negative. Education is one of the most important factors determining worry-free retirement [34]. Recently, the Universities of the Third Age (U3A) became popular in many countries, and their positive influence has been broadly discussed [35–39]. The International Association of Universities of the Third Age (AU3A) is a global international organization. The AU3A network includes institutions from Asia, both Americas, Europe, and Australia. The attendance of U3A grows exponentially in the global scale. In China alone the number of universities for senior citizens has grown from 19,000 in 2002 to 70,000 in 2017. The corresponding numbers of students of U3A in China is even more impressive: from 1.0 million to 8 million.

In the present work, we study the influence of factors, such as gender, kind of work, marital status, intellectual activity related to the attendance the University of the Third Age, economic situation, on the expectations and on the worries related to the retirement threshold from the Polish perspective. Some pilot studies on the changes of the quality of life related to the retirement threshold using the World Health Organization Quality of Life-BREF (WHOQOL-BREF) questionnaire, and this graphical representation of the results we have already published [40–45]. The WHOQOL-BREF questionnaire is a standard tool in the quality of life research and many versions of this questionnaire have been created in different countries, for example, the Polish version [46], the Bangla version [47], the Spanish version [48], or the Finnish version [49]. This questionnaire is composed of 26 questions. Two questions are related to *Overall Quality of Life and General Health*. The remaining 24 questions concern four domains: *Physical Health*, *Psychological*, *Social Relationships*, and *Environment*. Using this questionnaire, we have shown that CA classification maps are a convenient tool for the studies on the role of different factors in changing the quality of life after the retirement threshold, such as gender [42] and marital status [43] in four domains, job position in *Physical Health* and *Psychological* domains [44], or in *Social Relationships* and *Environment* domains [45]. In most of cases, these factors play an important role. The considered factors are particularly important in the *Psychological* and in the *Social Relationships* domains. The influence of different factors, such as age, education, marital status, and job position on the *Overall Quality of Life and General Health* has also been studied by us using this graphical approach and WHOQOL-BREF questionnaire [40,41].

2. Materials and Methods

In the present work, the points forming clusters in CA maps correspond to subgroups of all individuals and to their answers to the questions. We used two our own questionnaires: *Questionnaire for an Employed or a Self-Employed Person* and *Questionnaire for a Retiree* (see Appendix A).

The studies have been performed in the period from February 2017 to May 2017 in Bydgoszcz, the eighth largest city in Poland (~350,000 inhabitants). We considered 449 individuals (older than 50): 160 employees (100 females and 60 males) and 289 retirees (186 females and 103 males).

We split the group of the retirees to two subgroups: students of U3A denoted in the figures as *retirees2* and non-students of U3A denoted as *retirees1* (Appendix A, question No. 9R). We also split all the subgroups (*employees, retirees1, retirees2*) according to the marital status. We consider two subgroups: *married* and *others* (Appendix A, question No. 7ER). In subgroup *others* are those individuals who are single, separated, divorced, or widowed.

Groups of individuals and their answers to particular questions (e.g., answer No. 1: *A1*) are represented by points in the classification maps. In this way, we can classify different subgroups, i.e., we can find subgroups of these individuals who answer in a similar way to some specific questions considered in the questionnaires.

The clusters of points are defined by the angles between vectors and the lengths of these vectors. The initial points of all vectors are located at the central point (CP) of the map, i.e., at the crossing point of the dotted lines marked in the maps. The terminal points of the vectors are denoted in the figures by empty squares (groups of individuals) and by full circles (answers). The squares and the circles belong to one cluster if the angles between the vectors (CP-square and CP-circle) are small. The longer are the vectors, the stronger is the positive association. Angles close to 90 degrees indicate no relationship. It the angles are close to 180 degrees, then they indicate a negative association. The longer are the vectors, the stronger is the negative association.

The final results have been generated using the R statistics language [50].

3. Results and Discussion

Figures 1–4 show the results (maps) obtained using CA.

Figure 1 shows maps related to the answers to questions about emptiness after the retirement (Appendix A, questions No. 21E and 18R). The structure of the maps for *males* and for *females* (top panels) are different. For *females* (top right panel), the angles between the vectors CP-*employees* and CP-*A4*, between CP-*retirees2* and CP-*A2* are small. Consequently, we can extract two clusters:

- *employees—A4*,
- *retirees2—A2*.

The lengths of all of the vectors CP-*employees*, CP-*A4*, CP-*retirees2*, and CP-*A2* are large. Then, the two associations are strong.

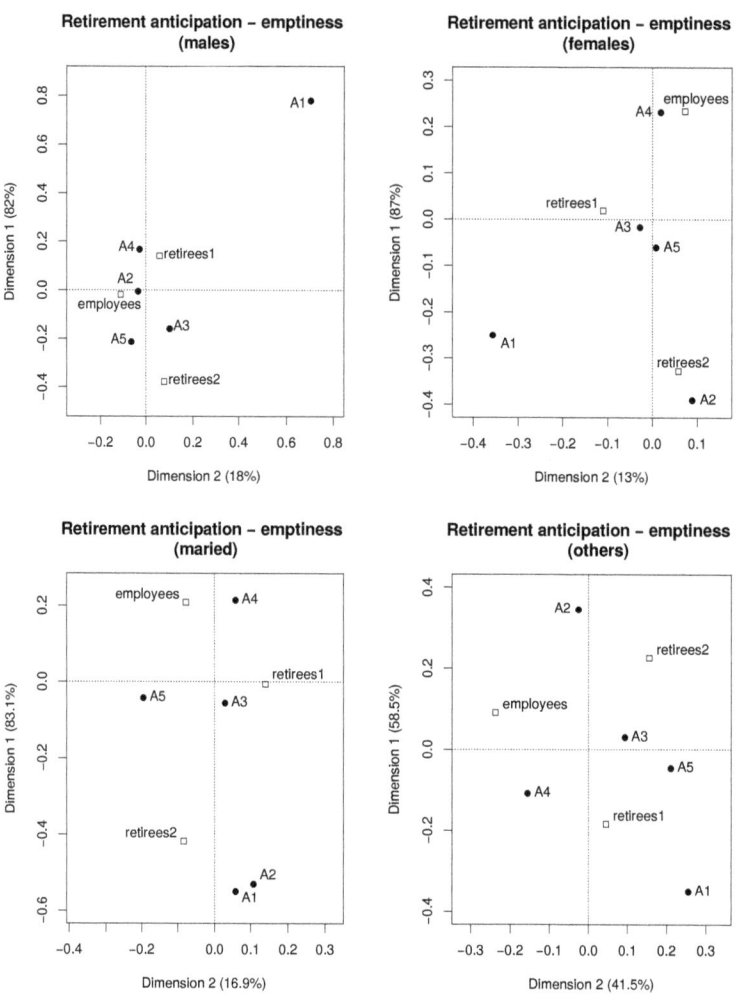

Figure 1. Classification maps (questions No. 21E and 18R).

For *males* (top left panel), the angles are nearly 180 degrees between vectors CP-*retirees2* and CP-*A4*, between CP-*retirees1* and CP-*A5*. Therefore, in this case, we have negative associations:

- retirees2—A4;
- retirees1—A5.

If the spread between the number of answers to different questions is large then the least common answers usually correspond to the negative associations. The least common answer about emptiness after retirement given by *retirees2* is A4 "I was not afraid". The least common answer about emptiness after retirement given by *retirees1* is A5 "I was not afraid at all". Depending on the lengths of the corresponding vectors, the strengths of the association may vary. In this case, the negative association for *males* is weak since the lengths of these vectors are smaller than for *females*. The point representing *employees (males)* is located close to the central point, so there are no strong associations of this group with any of the answers, while the most frequent answer for the *employees (females)* is A4 "I am not afraid" (cluster *employees—A4*).

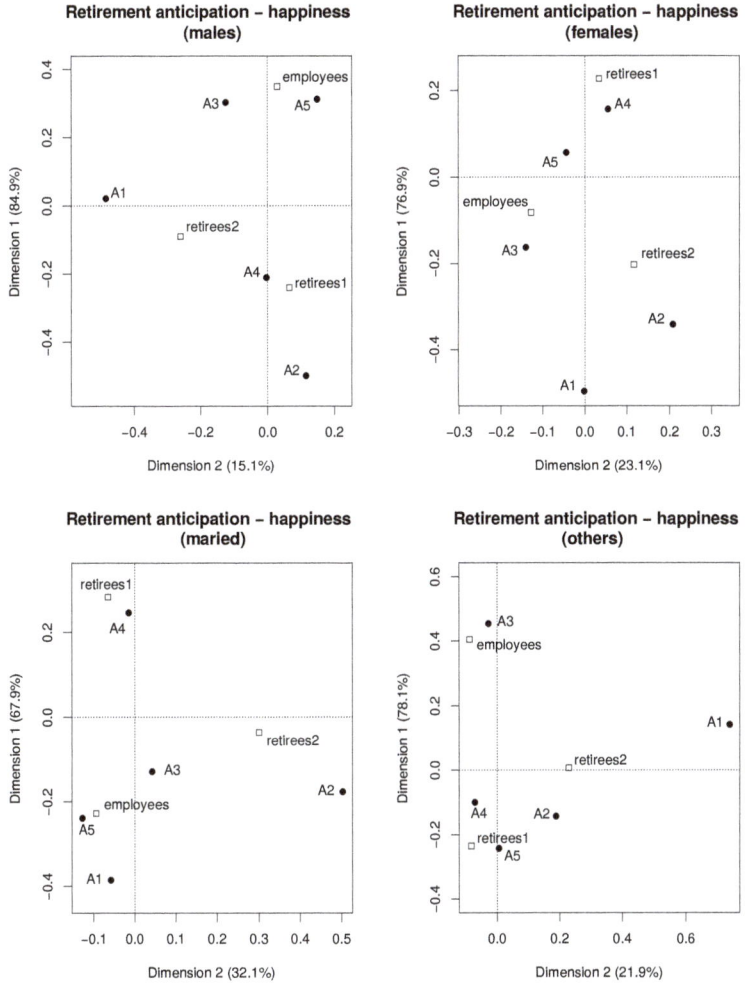

Figure 2. Classification maps (questions No. 15E and 15R).

Transition to retirement is a key moment when an individual must redefine his or her social roles, which is not always successful. Women more often define their social role as a family member: housewife and mother. After the end of their professional activity they find themselves in the role of grandmothers, participating in the family life of their children [51]. According to opinion polls in Polish society men are less involved in family life and performing household duties so after they terminate professional life they would stay without any activities and many of them may feel emptiness [52].

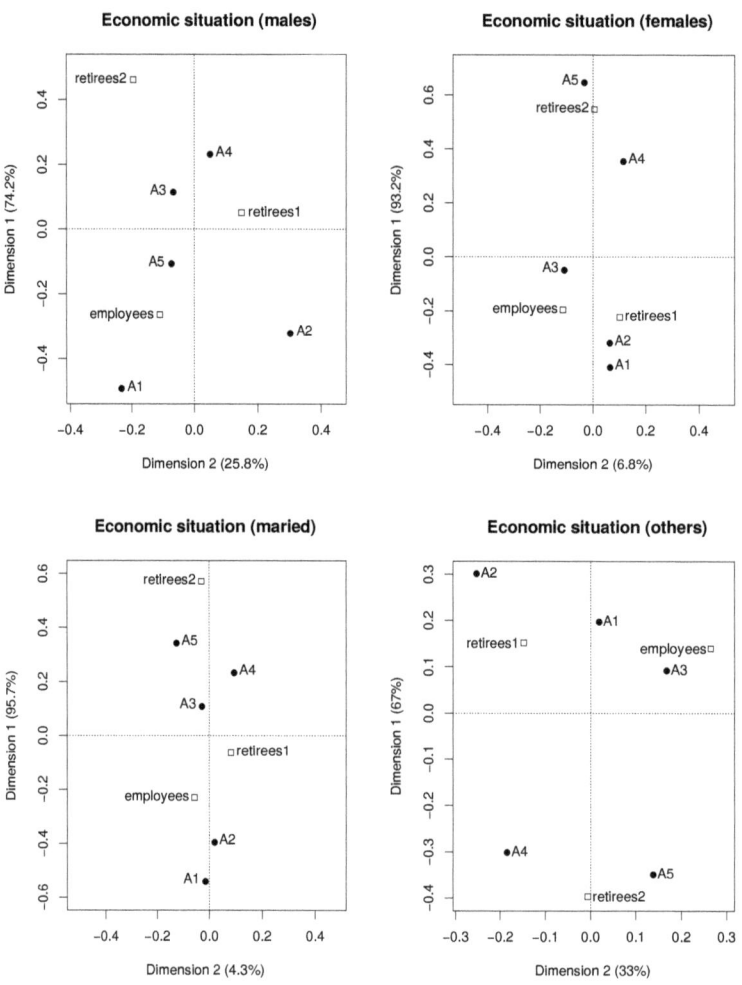

Figure 3. Classification maps (questions No. 19E and 20R).

If we consider the marital status, we observe negative associations for *married* (Figure 1, bottom left panel):

- employees—A1,
- employees—A2,
- retirees2—A4,
- retirees1—A5.

The angles between the vectors CP-*employees* and CP-*A1*, between CP-*employees* and CP-*A2*, between CP-*retirees2* and CP-*A4*, and between CP-*retirees1* and CP-*A5* are close to 180 degrees. The least common answers for *employees (married)* about emptiness after the retirement are A1 "Yes, I am very much afraid" and A2 "Yes, I am slightly afraid". The least common answer to this question of *retirees2 (married)* is A4 "I was not afraid". The least common answer to this question of *retirees1 (married)* is A5 "I was not afraid at all". As the lengths of CP-*A5* and CP-*retirees1* are smaller comparing to other vectors, the association for *retirees1* is the weakest.

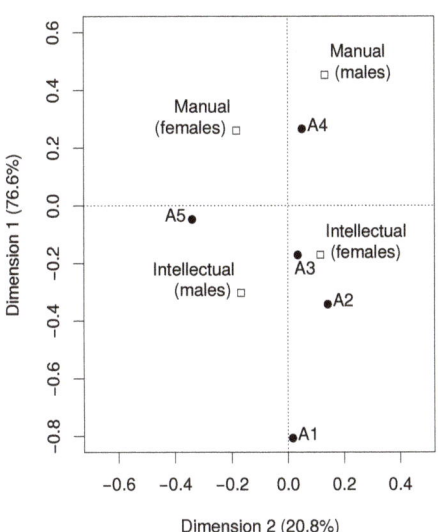

Figure 4. Classification map (question No. 25R).

For *others* (Figure 1, bottom right panel), the structure of the map is different than for *married*. We observe different negative associations:

- *employees—A5*,
- *retirees2—A4*,
- *retirees1—A2*.

Analogously, as for *married*, the least common answer to this question of *retirees2 (others)* is A4 "I was not afraid". The marital status is not an important factor determining the kind of answer to this question for *retirees2*. For *retirees1 (others)* the least common answer is A2, whereas for married is A5. For *employees (others)* the least common answer is A5, whereas for *employees (married)* the least common answers are A1 and A2. For *employees* and *retirees1*, the marital status changes the results of the classification.

Similar studies can be performed for other aspects, for example, satisfaction with retirement (Appendix A, questions No. 15E and 15R). The results are shown in Figure 2: *males* (Figure 2, top left panel), *females* (Figure 2, top right panel), *married* (Figure 2, bottom left panel), and *others* (Figure 2, bottom right panel). The answer A1 corresponds to "Very unhappy", whereas A5 corresponds to "Very happy". We observe different clusters for *males* and *females*, so gender is an important factor influencing the kind of answer to this question. In particular, for *males* we observe the following clusters:

- *retirees1—A2*,
- *employees—A5*.

For *females* the clusters are:

- *retirees1—A4*,
- *retirees2—A2*.

The most frequent answer of *females* attending the U3A (*retirees2*) is the same as *retirees1 (males)*, i.e., A2. There are also several negative associations for *males*:

- employees—A4,
- retirees1—A3.

The least common answer for *retirees1 (males)* is A3. For *females* the negative associations are:

- retirees2—A5,
- retirees1—A1.

The least common answer for *retirees1 (females)* is A1. A5 is located close to the central point so the association for *retirees2 (females)* is weak.

If we consider the marital status, for this question, we also observe different clusters for *married* and for *others*. The marital status is an important factor influencing the results of the classification in this case. In particular, for *married* we observe the clusters (Figure 2, bottom left panel):

- employees—A5,
- retirees1—A4,

and for *others* (Figure 2, bottom right panel)

- employees—A3,
- retirees1—A5,
- retirees2—A1.

The associations *retirees1—A5* and *retirees2—A1* are weak for *others*. The most frequent answer for *employees (married)* is A5 "Very happy", while for *employees (others)* the least common answer is A5 (negative association).

Figure 3 is concerned about the question on the adequate amount of money after retirement (Appendix A, questions No. 19E and 20R). Analogously to Figures 1 and 2, the top panels refer to *males* and to *females* and the bottom ones to *married* and to *others*. A1 corresponds to the answer "Not at all", and A5 to "Quite enough". For *males* (top left panel) the clusters are the following:

- employees—A5,
- retirees2—A3,

and for *females* (Figure 3, top right panel)

- retirees1—A1,
- retirees1—A2,
- retirees2—A5.

The negative associations for *males* are:

- employees—A4,
- retirees2—A2,

and for *females*

- employees—A4,
- retirees2—A1,
- retirees1—A5.

Employees and retirees estimate in a different way the economic situation during the retirement. Some differences are also between *males* and *females*. Considering the marital status, the clusters are also different. In particular, the group *employees (married)* clusters with A1, whereas *employees (others)* clusters with A3.

The summary is contained in the question about the return to the professional work (Appendix A, question No. 25R). The results are shown in Figure 4. The groups are split according to the kind of work—*Manual labor* and *Intellectual labor* (Appendix A, question No. 4ER)—and according to the gender. Finally, four subgroups are considered and denoted in the figure as *Manual (females)*, *Manual (males)*, *Intellectual (females)*, and *Intellectual (males)*. The answer A1 is "Yes, full-time", and the answer A5 is "Absolutely not". We observe the cluster

- *Manual (males)*—A4.

  The negative associations are as follows:

- *Manual (females)*—A2,
- *Manual (males)*—A1,
- *Intellectual (males)*—A4.

The most frequent answer of *Manual (males)* is A4 "No". The associations of *Intellectual (females)* with A3 and A2 are weak. None of the groups clusters with A1 "Yes, full-time". Our analysis shows that in Poland in 2017, reaching the retirement threshold is rather a positive experience.

In line with social expectations, the retirement age was reduced to 60 for females and 65 for males in October 2017.

4. Conclusions

Summarizing, we described a non-standard approach to deriving information about objects met in the medical sciences based on an analysis of classification maps. We demonstrate that the graphical representation of the considered data (of the answers to some questions in the case of groups of individuals) is useful in health informatics, i.e., a lot of information is stored on one map. Searching for the so-called *clusters of points*, we can classify the objects. In this way, one can discover new properties of the considered objects. In the case of groups of individuals, we search for factors such as gender, marital status, kind of work, intellectual activity related to the attendance the University of the Third Age, economic situation, and determining the psychological attitudes of the considered population. For the creation of the classification maps, a statistical method, *Correspondence Analysis*, is used. New applications of the method are proposed: studies on expectations and worries related to the *retirement threshold*. Using standard methods, some considerable part of information may be lost. In particular, the commonly used Pearson's coefficients measure the strength of the linear correlation between the variables. If the correlation is strong but nonlinear, for example, quadratic or exponential, then the standard methods, contrary to the CA, may show that there is no correlation or that the correlation is weak. Similar classification maps we are also going to apply in other medical informatics areas in forthcoming papers related to the studies on the quality of life and to bioinformatics.

Author Contributions: Conceptualization, A.B., D.B.-W., and P.W.; methodology, A.B., D.B.-W., and P.W.; software, P.W., formal analysis, D.B.-W.; data curation, A.B.; writing—original draft preparation, D.B.-W. and A.B.; visualization, P.W. All authors have read and agreed to the published version of the manuscript.

Funding: This research received no external funding.

Conflicts of Interest: The authors declare no conflicts of interest.

Appendix A

Appendix A.1. Questionnaire for an Employed or a Self-Employed Person

I. Personal information

1ER. Gender:

| A1. Male | A2. Female |

2ER. Age (years):

3ER. Education:

| A1. Elementary school | A2. Vocational education | A3. High school | A4. University education | A5. Doctor's degree |

4ER. Kind of work:

| A1. Manual labor | A2. Intellectual labor |

5ER. Business position:

| A1. Staff | A2. Supervisor/manager | A3. Director/president | A4. Business owner |

6ER. In how many years do you plan to retire?

7ER. Marital status

| A1. Single | A2. Married | A3. Separated | A4. Divorced | A5. Widowed |

8ER. Are you chronically ill?

| A1. Yes | A2. No |

If yes, which disease you suffer from?

II. Questions about your current satisfaction level

9E. Are you satisfied with your job?

| A1. Very dissatisfied | A2. Dissatisfied | A3. Neither satisfied nor dissatisfied | A4. Satisfied | A5. Very satisfied |

10E. Does your job make your life meaningful?

| A1. Not at all | A2. Slightly | A3. Moderately | A4. Very much | A5. Essentially |

11E. How do you rate the interpersonal relations in your work?

| A1. Very bad | A2. Bad | A3. Neither bad nor good | A4. Good | A5. Very good |

12E. Are you satisfied with your salary?

| A1. Very dissatisfied | A2. Dissatisfied | A3. Neither satisfied nor dissatisfied | A4. Satisfied | A5. Very satisfied |

13E. Do you feel that you have enough energy to perform your work?

| A1. Not at all | A2. Slightly enough | A3. Moderately enough | A4. Nearly enough | A5. Quite enough |

14E. Are you satisfied with your social life?

| A1. Very dissatisfied | A2. Dissatisfied | A3. Neither satisfied nor dissatisfied | A4. Satisfied | A5. Very satisfied |

III. Retirement-related questions

15E. Are you happy that in several years/months you will retire?

| A1. Very unhappy | A2. Unhappy | A3. Neither happy nor unhappy | A4. Happy | A5. Very happy |

16E. Do you think that after the retirement you will have enough energy to implement your aims?

| A1. Not at all | A2. Slightly enough | A3. Moderately enough | A4. Nearly enough | A5. Quite enough |

17E. Are you afraid that after the retirement you may not be self-sufficient?

| A1. Yes, I am very much afraid | A2. Yes, I am slightly afraid | A3. I do not think of it | A4. I am not afraid | A5. I am not afraid at all |

18E. Are you afraid that after the retirement you will feel lonely?

| A1. Yes, I am very much afraid | A2. Yes, I am slightly afraid | A3. I do not know yet | A4. I am not afraid | A5. I am not afraid at all |

19E. Do you expect to have enough retirement income to support yourself?

| A1. Not at all | A2. Slightly enough | A3. Moderately enough | A4. Nearly enough | A5. Quite enough |

20E. Do you think that you will be satisfied having a lot of free time during retirement?

| A1. Very dissatisfied | A2. Dissatisfied | A3. Neither satisfied nor dissatisfied | A4. Satisfied | A5. Very satisfied |

21E. Are you afraid of emptiness after the retirement, because you will not be so active as before?

| A1. Yes, I am very much afraid | A2. Yes, I am slightly afraid | A3. I do not think of it | A4. I am not afraid | A5. I am not afraid at all |

22E. Are you afraid that during the next several years your health is going to deteriorate?

| A1. Yes, I am very much afraid | A2. Yes, I am slightly afraid | A3. I do not think of it | A4. I am not afraid | A5. I am not afraid at all |

Appendix A.2. Questionnaire for a Retiree

I. Personal information

1ER, 2ER, ... 8ER (see Appendix A.1)
9R. Do you attend classes at the University of the Third Age?

| A1. Yes | A2. No |

II. Professional work-related questions

10R. Were you satisfied with your job?

| A1. Very dissatisfied | A2. Dissatisfied | A3. Neither satisfied nor dissatisfied | A4. Satisfied | A5. Very satisfied |

11R. Did your job make your life meaningful?

| A1. Not at all | A2. Slightly | A3. Moderately | A4. Very much | A5. Essentially |

12R. How did you rate the interpersonal relations in your work?

| A1. Very bad | A2. Bad | A3. Neither bad nor good | A4. Good | A5. Very good |

13R. Were you satisfied with your salary?

| A1. Very dissatisfied | A2. Dissatisfied | A3. Neither satisfied nor dissatisfied | A4. Satisfied | A5. Very satisfied |

III. Just before retirement-questions

14R. Did you have enough energy to perform your work?

| A1. Not at all | A2. Slightly enough | A3. Moderately enough | A4. Nearly enough | A5. Quite enough |

15R. Were you happy that in several years/months you would retire?

| A1. Very unhappy | A2. Unhappy | A3. Neither happy nor unhappy | A4. Happy | A5. Very happy |

16R. Were you afraid that you would have not enough retirement income to support yourself?

| A1. Yes, I was very much afraid | A2. Yes, I was slightly afraid | A3. I did not think of it | A4. I was not afraid | A5. I was not afraid at all |

17R. Were you satisfied that after the retirement you would have a lot of free time?

| A1. Very dissatisfied | A2. Dissatisfied | A3. Neither satisfied nor dissatisfied | A4. Satisfied | A5. Very satisfied |

18R. Were you afraid of emptiness after the retirement, because you would not be so active as before?

| A1. Yes, I was very much afraid | A2. Yes, I was slightly afraid | A3. I did not think of it | A4. I was not afraid | A5. I was not afraid at all |

IV. Questions about your current satisfaction level

19R. Do you think that after the retirement your health deteriorated?

| A1. Yes, it did very much | A2. Yes, it did a little | A3. It is the same | A4. It is not worse | A5. On the contrary, I feel better |

20R. Do you have enough retirement income to support yourself?

| A1. Not at all | A2. Slightly enough | A3. Moderately enough | A4. Nearly enough | A5. Quite enough |

21R. Are you afraid that due to your bad health you will not manage with your housework?

| A1. Yes, I am very much afraid | A2. Yes, I am slightly afraid | A3. I do not think of it | A4. I am not afraid | A5. I am not afraid at all |

22R. Do you feel lonely?

| A1. Yes, very much | A2. Yes, a little | A3. Neither yes nor no | A4. No | A5. Absolutely not |

23R. Are you satisfied with your social life?

| A1. Very dissatisfied | A2. Dissatisfied | A3. Neither satisfied nor dissatisfied | A4. Satisfied | A5. Very satisfied |

24R. Are you satisfied with relations with your children and grandchildren (emotional relations, frequency of visits)?

| A1. Very dissatisfied | A2. Dissatisfied | A3. Neither satisfied nor dissatisfied | A4. Satisfied | A5. Very satisfied |

25R. Would you like to return to your professional work?

| A1. Yes, full-time | A2. Yes, part-time | A3. I do not think of it | A4. No | A5. Absolutely not |

References

1. Bielińska-Wąż, D. Graphical and numerical representations of DNA sequences: Statistical aspects of similarity. *J. Math. Chem.* **2011**, *49*, 2345–2407. [CrossRef]
2. Randić, M.; Novič, M.; Plavšić, D. Milestones in graphical bioinformatics. *Int. J. Quant. Chem.* **2013**, *113*, 2413–2446. [CrossRef]
3. Bielińska-Wąż, D.; Wąż, P.; Basak, S.C. Similarity studies using statistical and genetical methods. *J. Math. Chem.* **2007**, *42*, 1003–1013. [CrossRef]
4. Bielińska-Wąż, D.; Wąż, P. Correlations in Spectral Statistics. *J. Math. Chem.* **2008**, *43*, 1287–1300. [CrossRef]
5. Bielińska-Wąż, D.; Wąż, P.; Jagiełło, K.; Puzyn, T. Spectral Density Distribution Moments as Novel Descriptors for QSAR/QSPR. *Struct. Chem.* **2014**, *25*, 29–35. [CrossRef]
6. Wąż, P.; Bielińska-Wąż, D. Asymmetry Coefficients as Indicators of Chaos. *Acta Phys. Pol. A* **2009**, *116*, 987–991. [CrossRef]
7. Wąż, P.; Bielińska-Wąż, D.; Pleskacz, A.; Strobel, A. Identification of Stellar Spectra Using Methods of Statistical Spectroscopy. *Acta Phys. Polon. B* **2008**, *39*, 1993–2001.
8. Wąż, P.; Bielińska-Wąż, D.; Strobel, A.; Pleskacz, A. Statistical indicators of astrophysical parameters. *Acta Astronom.* **2010**, *60*, 283–293.
9. Wąż, P.; Bielińska-Wąż, D. Moments of Inertia of Spectra and Distribution Moments as Molecular Descriptors. *MATCH Commun. Math. Comput. Chem.* **2013**, *70*, 851–865.
10. Wąż, P.; Bielińska-Wąż, D.; Nandy, A. Descriptors of 2D-dynamic graphs as a classification tool of DNA sequences. *J. Math. Chem.* **2014**, *52*, 132–140. [CrossRef]
11. Beh, E.J.; Lombardo, R. *Correspondence Analysis: Theory, Practice and New Strategies*; John Wiley & Sons: Oxford, UK, 2014.
12. Ziemer, K.S.; Pires, B.; Lancaster, V.; Keller, S.; Orr, M.; Shipp, S. A New Lens on High School Dropout: Use of Correspondence Analysis and the Statewide Longitudinal Data System. *Am. Stat.* **2018**, *72*, 191–198. [CrossRef]
13. Beh, E.J.; Lombardo, R.; Alberti, G. Correspondence analysis and the Freeman-Tukey statistic: A study of archaeological data. *Comput. Stat. Data Anal.* **2018**, *128*, 73–86. [CrossRef]
14. Frost, S.C.; Blackman, J.W.; Ebeler, S.E.; Heymann, H. Analysis of temporal dominance of sensation data using correspondence analysis on Merlot wine with differing maceration and cap management regimes. *Food Qual. Prefer.* **2018**, *64*, 245–252. [CrossRef]
15. Parnowski, T. Medyczne i psychologiczne problemy wieku podeszłego. *Probl. Rodz.* **1996**, *5*, 41–50. (In Polish)
16. Skarborn, M.; Nicki, R. Worry in pre- and post-retirement persons. *Int. J. Aging Hum. Dev.* **2000**, *50* 61–71. [CrossRef]
17. Hershey, D.A.; Henkens, K.; van Dalen, H.P. What drives retirement income worries in Europe? A multilevel analysis. *Eur. J. Ageing* **2010**, *7*, 301–311. [CrossRef]
18. Gutierrez, H.C.; Hershey, D.A. Impact of Retirement Worry on Information Processing. *J. Neurosci. Psychol. Econ.* **2013**, *6*, 264–277. [CrossRef]
19. Kail, B. The Mental and Physical Health Consequences of Changes in Private Insurance Before and After Early Retirement. *J. Gerontol. B Psychol. Sci. Soc. Sci.* **2016**, *71*, 358–368. [CrossRef]
20. Hagen, E.W.; Barnet, J.H.; Hale, L.; Peppard, P.E. Changes in Sleep Duration and Sleep Timing Associated with Retirement Transitions. *Sleep* **2016**, *39*, 665–673. [CrossRef]
21. Myllyntausta, S.; Salo, P.; Kronholm, E.; Aalto, V.; Kivimaki, M.; Vahtera, J.; Stenholm, S. Changes in Sleep Duration During Transition to Statutory Retirement: A Longitudinal Cohort Study. *Sleep* **2017**, *40*. [CrossRef]
22. Regan, K.; Intzandt, B.; Swatridge, K.; Myers, A.; Roy, E.; Middleton, L.E. Changes in Physical Activity and Function with Transition to Retirement Living: A Pilot Study. *Can. J. Aging* **2016**, *35*, 526–532. [CrossRef] [PubMed]
23. Van Dyck, D.; Cardon, G.; De Bourdeaudhuij, I. Longitudinal changes in physical activity and sedentary time in adults around retirement age: What is the moderating role of retirement status, gender and educational level? *BMC Public Health* **2016**, *16*, 1125. [CrossRef] [PubMed]
24. Manty, M.; Kouvonen, A.; Lallukka, T.; Lahti, J.; Lahelma, E.; Rahkonen, O. Pre-retirement physical working conditions and changes in physical health functioning during retirement transition process. *Scand. J. Work Environ. Health* **2016**, *42* 405–412. [CrossRef] [PubMed]

25. Stenholm, S.; Pulakka, A.; Kawachi, I.; Oksanen, T.; Halonen, J.I.; Aalto, V.; Kivimaki, M.; Vahtera, J. Changes in physical activity during transition to retirement: A cohort study. *Int. J. Behav. Nutr. Phys. Act.* **2016**, *13*, 51. [CrossRef]
26. Holstila, A.; Manty, M.; Rahkonen, O.; Lahelma, E.; Lahti, J. Statutory retirement and changes in self-reported leisure-time physical activity: A follow-up study with three time-points. *BMC Public Health* **2017**, *17*, 528. [CrossRef]
27. Gueorguieva, R.; Sindelar, J.L.; Wu, R.; Gallo, W.T. Differential changes in body mass index after retirement by occupation: Hierarchical models. *Int. J. Public Health* **2011**, *56* 111–116. [CrossRef]
28. Stenholm, S.; Solovieva, S.; Viikari-Juntura, E.; Aalto, V.; Kivimaki, M.; Vahtera, J. Change in body mass index during transition to statutory retirement: An occupational cohort study. *Int. J. Behav. Nutr. Phys. Act.* **2007**, *14*, 85. [CrossRef]
29. Barrett, G.F.; Kecmanovic, M. Changes in subjective well-being with retirement: Assessing savings adequacy. *Appl. Econ.* **2013**, *45*, 4883–4893. [CrossRef]
30. Maher, C.A.; Burton, N.W.; van Uffelen, J.G.Z.; Brown, W.J.; Sprod, J.A.; Olds, T.S. Changes in use of time, activity patterns, and health and wellbeing across retirement: Design and methods of the life after work study. *BMC Public Health* **2013**, *13* 952. [CrossRef]
31. Vercambre, M.N.; Okereke, O.I.; Kawachi, I.; Grodstein, F.; Kang, J.H. Self-Reported Change in Quality of Life with Retirement and Later Cognitive Decline: Prospective Data from the Nurses' Health Study. *J. Alzheimers Dis.* **2016**, *52*, 887–897. [CrossRef]
32. Olds, T.S.; Sprod, J.; Ferrar, K.; Burton, N.; Brown, W.; van Uffelen, J.; Maher, C. Everybody's working for the weekend: Changes in enjoyment of everyday activities across the retirement threshold. *Age Ageing* **2016**, *45*, 850–855. [CrossRef]
33. Berg, J. Mobility changes during the first years of retirement. *Qual. Ageing Older Adults* **2016**, *17* 131–140. [CrossRef]
34. Cho, H.; Suh, W.; Lee, J.; Jang, Y.; Kim, M. A worry-free retirement in Korea: Effectiveness of retirement coaching education. *Educ. Gerontol.* **2016**, *42*, 785–794. [CrossRef]
35. Jun, S.K.; Evans, K. The learning cultures of Third Age participants: Institutional management and participants' experience in U3A in the UK and SU in Korea. *KEDI J. Educ. Policy* **2007**, *4*, 53–72.
36. Hebestreit, L. The role of the University of the Third Age in meeting needs of adult learners in Victoria, Australia. *Aust. J. Adult Learn.* **2008**, *48*, 547–565.
37. Sonati, J.G.; Modeneze, D.M.; Vilarta, R.; Maciel É.S.; Boccaletto, E.M.A.; da Silva, C.C. Body composition and quality of life (QoL) of the elderly offered by the "University Third Age" (UTA) in Brazil. *Arch. Gerontol. Geriatr.* **2011**, *52*, e31–e35. [CrossRef]
38. Mackowicz, J.; Wnek-Gozdek, J. "It's never too late to learn"—How does the Polish U3A change the quality of life for seniors? *Educ. Gerontol.* **2016**, *42*, 186–197. [CrossRef]
39. Nascimento, M.D.; Giannouli E. Active aging through the University of the Third Age: The Brazilian model. *Educ. Gerontol.* **2019**, *45*, 11–21. [CrossRef]
40. Bielińska, A.; Majkowicz, M.; Wąż, P.; Bielińska-Wąż, D. Overall Quality of Life and General Health—Changes Related to the Retirement Threshold. In Proceedings of the eTELEMED 2018, The Tenth International Conference on eHealth, Telemedicine, and Social Medicine, Rome, Italy, 25–29 March 2018; XPS IARIA Press: Copenhagen, Denmark, 2018; pp. 1–5.
41. Bielińska, A.; Majkowicz, M.; Bielińska-Wąż, D.; Wąż, P. Influence of the Education Level on Health of Elderly People. In Proceedings of the eTELEMED 2018, The Tenth International Conference on eHealth, Telemedicine, and Social Medicine, Rome, Italy, 25–29 March 2018; XPS IARIA Press: Copenhagen, Denmark, 2018; pp. 6–11.
42. Bielińska, A.; Majkowicz, M.; Bielińska-Wąż, D.; Wąż, P. Classification Studies in Various Areas of Science. In *Numerical Methods and Applications*; NMA 2018, Lecture Notes in Computer Science; Nikolov, G., Kolkovska, N., Georgiev, K.; Eds.; Springer: Cham, Switzerland, 2019; Volume 11189, pp. 326–333.
43. Bielińska, A.; Majkowicz, M.; Wąż, P.; Bielińska-Wąż D. Mathematical Modeling: Interdisciplinary Similarity Studies. In *Numerical Methods and Applications*; NMA 2018, Lecture Notes in Computer Science; Nikolov, G., Kolkovska, N., Georgiev, K.; Eds.; Springer: Cham, Switzerland, 2019; Volume 11189, pp. 334–341.
44. Bielińska, A.; Majkowicz, M.; Bielińska-Wąż, D.; Wąż, P. A New Method in Bioinformatics—Interdisciplinary Similarity Studies. *AIP Conf. Proc.* **2019**, *2116*, 450013.

45. Bielińska, A.; Majkowicz, M.; Wąż, P.; Bielińska-Wąż, D. A New Computational Method: Interdisciplinary Classification Analysis. *AIP Conf. Proc.* **2019**, *2116*, 450014.
46. Jaracz, K.; Kalfoss, M.; Bączyk, G. Quality of life in Polish respondents: Psychometric properties of the Polish WHOQOL—Bref. *Scand. J. Caring Sci.* **2006**, *20*, 251–260. [CrossRef] [PubMed]
47. Tsutsumi, A.; Izutsu, T.; Kato, S.; Islam, A.; Yamada, H.S.; Kato, H.; Wakai, S. Reliability and validity of the Bangla version of WHOQOL-BREF in an adult population in Dhaka, Bangladesh. *Psychiatry Clin. Neurosci.* **2006**, *60*, 493–498. [CrossRef] [PubMed]
48. Benitez-Borrego, S.; Guardia-Olmos, J.; Urzua-Morales, A. Factorial structural analysis of the Spanish version of WHOQOL-BREF: An exploratory structural equation model study. *Qual. Life Res.* **2014**, *23*, 2205–2212. [CrossRef] [PubMed]
49. Siljander, E.; Luoma, M.L.; Merilainen-Porras, S. Validity and reliability of Finnish version of WHOQOL-Bref on adult population in Finland. *IJHD* **2015**, *2*, 52–68. [CrossRef]
50. R Core Team. *R: A Language and Environment for Statistical Computing*; R Foundation for Statistical Computing: Vienna, Austria, 2018.
51. Kim, J.E.; Moen, P. Is Retirement Good or Bad for Subjective Well-Being? *Curr. Dir. Psychol. Sci.* **2001**, *10*, 83–86. [CrossRef]
52. Bożewicz, M. Kobiety i Mężczyźni w Domu. *CBOS, Komunikat z Badań* **2018**, *127*. Available online: https://www.cbos.pl/SPISKOM.POL/2018/K_127_18.PDF (accessed on 1 December 2019). (In Polish)

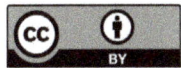

© 2020 by the authors. Licensee MDPI, Basel, Switzerland. This article is an open access article distributed under the terms and conditions of the Creative Commons Attribution (CC BY) license (http://creativecommons.org/licenses/by/4.0/).

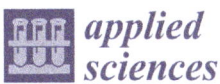

Article

Castration-Resistant Prostate Cancer Outcome Prediction Using Phased Long Short-Term Memory with Irregularly Sampled Serial Data

Jihwan Park [1,2], Mi Jung Rho [2], Hyong Woo Moon [3] and Ji Youl Lee [3,*]

[1] Department of Biomedicine & Health Sciences, College of Medicine, The Catholic University of Korea, Seoul 06591, Korea; bosoagalaxy@gmail.com
[2] Catholic Cancer Research Institute, College of Medicine, The Catholic University of Korea, Seoul 06591, Korea; romy1018@naver.com
[3] Department of Urology, Seoul St. Mary's Hospital, College of Medicine, the Catholic University of Korea, Seoul 06591, Korea; aspasias@catholic.ac.kr
* Correspondence: uroljy@catholic.ac.kr

Received: 11 January 2020; Accepted: 12 March 2020; Published: 15 March 2020

Abstract: It is particularly desirable to predict castration-resistant prostate cancer (CRPC) in prostate cancer (PCa) patients, and this study aims to predict patients' likely outcomes to support physicians' decision-making. Serial data is collected from 1592 PCa patients, and a phased long short-term memory (phased-LSTM) model with a special module called a "time-gate" is used to process the irregularly sampled data sets. A synthetic minority oversampling technique is used to overcome the data imbalance between two patient groups: those with and without CRPC treatment. The phased-LSTM model is able to predict the CRPC outcome with an accuracy of 88.6% (precision-recall: 91.6%) using 120 days of data or 94.8% (precision-recall: 96.9%) using 360 days of data. The validation loss converged slowly with 120 days of data and quickly with 360 days of data. In both cases, the prediction model takes four epochs to build. The overall CPRC outcome prediction model using irregularly sampled serial medical data is accurate and can be used to support physicians' decision-making, which saves time compared to cumbersome serial data reviews. This study can be extended to realize clinically meaningful prediction models.

Keywords: prostate cancer; castration-resistant prostate cancer; deep learning; phased long short-term memory

1. Introduction

Prostate cancer (PCa) is one of the most common male cancers. There are more than 3.3 million men suffering from PCa in the USA [1], and its incidence is increasing in Korea [2]. Recently, a national project in Korea has been developing artificial intelligence medical software for several diseases including PCa [3].

Androgen deprivation therapy (ADT) is commonly used to treat PCa patients. However, this fails patients that are classified as having castration-resistant prostate cancer (CRPC). According to the National Cancer Institute (NCI) of the National Institute of Health (NIH), CRPC is a "prostate cancer that keeps growing even when the amount of testosterone in the body is reduced to very low levels. Many early-stage prostate cancers need normal levels of testosterone to grow, but castration-resistant prostate cancers do not." It is important to administer appropriate treatments at the right time. When a patient has appropriate treatment, it will reduce the time and pain from the treatment such as chemotherapy. However, it is a complicated problem to make a treatment decision from cumbersome medical data, which has many irregularly sampled features. To overcome this situation, a CRPC prediction model can support physicians' decision-making and will help to identify appropriate treatments for PCa patients.

At present, PCa outcomes are usually predicted using nomograms [4–7]. Recently, researchers have begun to explore the use of deep learning methods, which show some promise [8–11], but the majority of these techniques rely on image segmentation and classification [12,13]. Data from longitudinal electronic health records (EHRs) that are irregularly sampled, such as PCa data, does not fit well with deep learning prediction models. Therefore, in this study, we adopt a phased long short-term memory (phased-LTSM) method with the aim of developing a model that can predict the outcome of PCa patients from asynchronously sampled data for various variables using deep learning [14]. In particular, we will develop a model that can identify CPRC patients.

2. Materials and Methods

2.1. Materials

Data from 1592 patients who had undergone prostatectomy were used to predict the use of CRPC medication. The data consisted of clinical stage information, laboratory data, and treatment events. In total, 8 patients received CRPC medication and 1584 patients did not. We used the receipt of CPRC medication as the binary classification condition. These medications included docetaxel, cabazitaxel, abiraterone, enzalutamide, and radium-223 (see Table 1).

Table 1. Demographics of prostate cancer patients.

Category	Non-Castration-Resistant Prostate Cancer (CRPC) Medication	CRPC Medication	p-Value (chi-Squared Test)
Number of cases (n = 1592 cases)	1584	8	
Age at diagnosis (%)			0.253
<40	1 (0.1)	0 (0.0)	
40–44	3 (0.2)	0 (0.0)	
45–49	16 (1.0)	0 (0.0)	
50–54	54 (3.4)	0 (0.0)	
55–59	165 (10.4)	2 (25.0)	
60–64	303 (19.1)	1 (12.5)	
65–69	461 (29.1)	0 (0.0)	
70–74	429 (27.1)	2 (25.0)	
75–80	146 (9.2)	3 (37.5)	
80–84	6 (0.4)	0 (0.0)	
Mean	63.64	66.5	
T-stage (%)			0.008
T1	1 (0.1)	0 (0.0)	
T1a	7 (0.4)	0 (0.0)	
T1c	3 (0.2)	0 (0.0)	
T2	100 (6.3)	0 (0.0)	
T2a	141 (8.9)	0 (0.0)	
T2b	56 (3.5)	0 (0.0)	
T2c	746 (47.1)	0 (0.0)	
T3	4 (0.3)	0 (0.0)	
T3a	312 (19.7)	3 (37.5)	
T3b	195 (12.3)	4 (50.0)	
T3c	1 (0.1)	0 (0.0)	
T4	14 (0.9)	1 (12.5)	
Tx	4 (0.3)	0 (0.0)	
N stage (%)			0.305
N0	379 (23.9)	3 (37.5)	
N1	68 (4.3)	1 (12.5)	
Nx	1137 (71.8)	4 (50.0)	
M-stage (%)			0.422
M0	304 (19.2)	3 (37.5)	
M1	3 (0.2)	0 (0.0)	
Mx	1277 (80.6)	5 (62.5)	

CRPC patients are treated with specific treatments including chemotherapy, such as docetaxel [15], cabazitaxel [16], abiraterone [17], enzalutamide [18], and radium-223 [19]. These CRPC treatments are delivered in many different combinations alongside ADT medications such as leuprorelin, bicalutamide, goserelin, and degarelix.

We preprocessed the serial data into three-dimensional (3D) vectors to use as the input for the deep learning model. Seven features were used: two laboratory data, prostate specific antigen (PSA) and PSA doubling time (DT), the use of radiation therapy (RT), and four ADT medications—leuprorelin, bicalutamide, goserelin, and degarelix. The timesteps were the days when the features were observed. However, not all of the features are observed at every interval and each observation has irregularly sampled follow-up data (see Figure 1). Because PSA is commonly examined lab data through all of the patient's follow up periods, PSA is the most important factor. PSADT shows the characteristic of PSA kinetics.

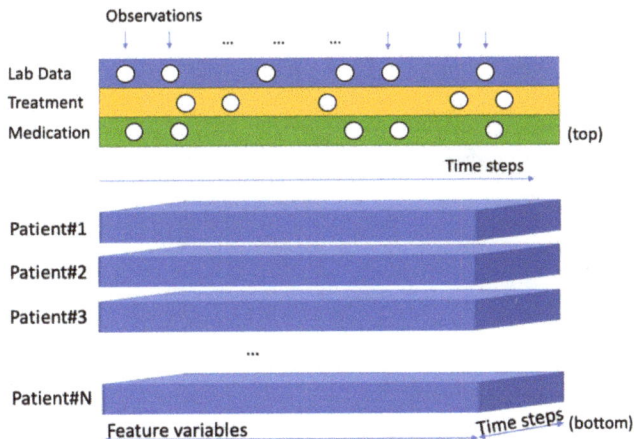

Figure 1. Irregularly collected events observations (top) 3D format input for serial data model (bottom).

2.2. Ethics

This study procedures were carried out in accordance with the Declaration of Helsinki and were approved by the Institutional Review Board of the Catholic University (IRB number: KC18SNDI0512). Identifying information was removed from the electronic health record (EHR) data, which was then formatted. Unless locally managed mapping information was exposed, specific patients could not be identified.

2.3. Methods

We used a 3D fixed time format to input serial data into the model. For the serial data modeling, a recurrent neural network (RNN) managed the data using a circular network model. Simple RNNs have a vanishing gradient problem, which cannot generate proper gradient values from repeated activation functions. The gradient value is an operator that directs the RNN's learning. The activation function calculates the gradient value for each iteration and will produce a value close to 0 after circular network executions. In contrast, long short-term memory (LSTM) uses a gating method to adjust the signal, which eliminates the vanishing gradient problem (see Figure 2). The input vector adjusts the value based on the tanh activation function. The forget vector adjust part of the previous input value to the current input. The output vector adjusts the output values using the previous input and current adjusted input. After all of these gating methods, the final output is used as the next input for the tanh and sigmoid layers.

Typically, the clinical event observations were not collected regularly. This irregular sampling meant that the intervals between consecutive events were not evenly spaced. LSTM cannot learn effectively from such data.

Phased-LSTM selectively updates the status to account for irregular sampling times through an additional time gate [14]. At each time step, the time gate switches on and off to update the state and the hidden output state. These updates only happen for the open phase. Otherwise, the previous values will be used. The time gate addresses the LSTM problems caused by irregularly sampled data (see Figure 3).

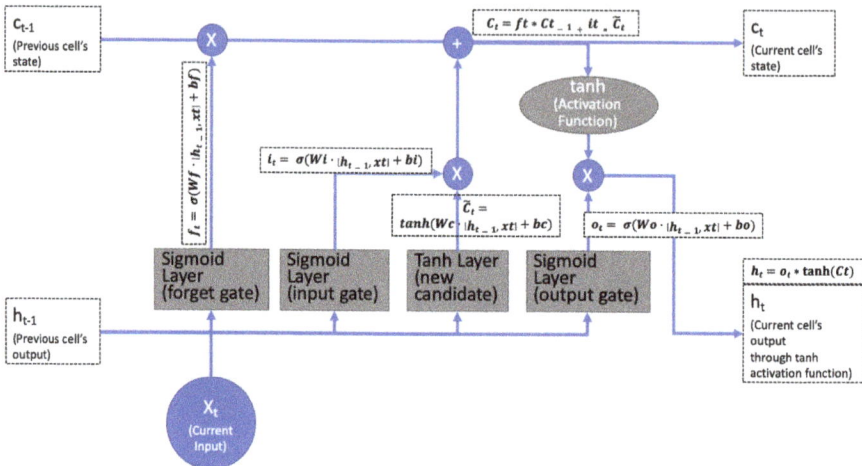

Figure 2. Standard long short-term memory (LSTM) using three gates (forget, input, and output) to eliminate the vanishing gradient problem.

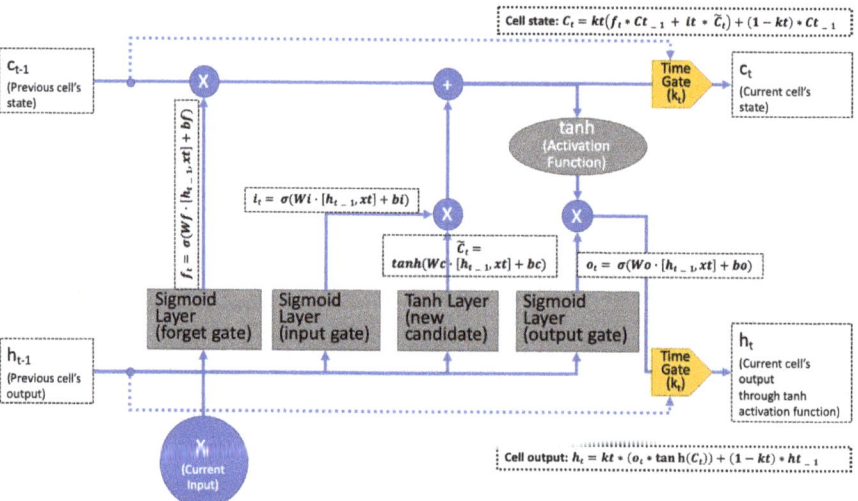

Figure 3. Phased LSTM using rectified linear units as the time-gate kt that propagates the gradient well.

There are two patterns of serial medical data: in the first, more than two features are sampled simultaneously and, in the second, some parts of the features are missing and others are not. To manage both patterns, missing imputation must be applied. The phased-LSTM's time gate addresses these patterns based on three phases (see Figure 4).

The time gate of phased-LSTM k_t has three phases: phase 1, "openness-rise" 0 to 1, phase 2, "openness-drop" 1 to 0, and phase 3, "closed" a leak at a rate α [14].

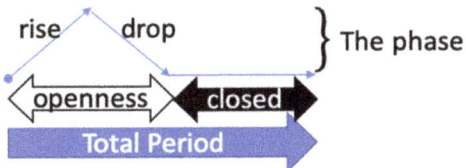

Figure 4. Phased LSTM time gate: phase visualization [14].

The time gate k_t is described by

$$\phi_t = \frac{(t-s) \bmod \tau}{\tau} \qquad (1)$$

and

$$k_t \begin{cases} \frac{2\phi_t}{r_{on}}, & if\ \phi_t < \frac{1}{2} r_{on} \\ 2 - \frac{2\phi_t}{r_{on}}, & if\ \frac{1}{2} r_{on} < \phi_t < r_{on} \\ \alpha \phi_t, & otherwise \end{cases} \qquad (2)$$

In this case, ϕ_t is an auxiliary variable that represents the phase of the cycle (Equation (1)), t is the time point, s is the phase shift, τ is the period that controls the real-time period, and r_{on} is the ratio of the open period to the total period τ [14].

Phased-LSTM's time gate k_t is a kind of rectified linear unit that can propagate gradient information effectively [14] (Equation (2)). Thus, k_t has three parameters: τ, s, and r_{on}. These parameters were used during the phased-LSTM model learning. During the open-phase, the rise or drop period in Figure 4 known as propagates new cell states or α-weighted gradient information. Ultimately, k_t is able to propagate irregularly sampled data selectively. In other words, it deals with complicated time series medical data effectively. Neil et al. presented this algorithm, which outperforms previous LSTM algorithms [14].

We used a chi-squared test to find the characteristic of patients' data. The chi-squared result showed the information of group differences, which represent how each of the groups performed in the study [20].

Due to the imbalance in the ratio of CRPC and non-CRPC patients, we used the synthetic minority oversampling technique (SMOTE) algorithm [21]. The SMOTE generates sample data that is similar to a prior set. This method is frequently used for imbalanced data analysis [22–25]. Based on the SMOTE oversampling algorithm, we generated a 50:50 ratio of CRPC data using the prior data.

We used k-fold cross validation to verify that the result of model training was not overfitted. The k-fold cross validation splits the data set into a k number of sets and validates the model with shuffled different sets [26]. We used 10-folds to verify the model.

The phased-LSTM prediction model was built using TensorFlow [27]. The model consists of a a phased-LSTM layer and used a SoftMax [28] dense layer to generate a binary result: CRPC or non-CRPC treated. It also used the Adam [29] optimizer and sparse_categorical_crossentropy loss function [12].

We used linear interpolation to build serial input data for the phased-LSTM model with an appropriate shape. Linear interpolation is one of the most common algorithms used to build connected serial data from data that has been irregularly recorded.

3. Results

The majority of age distribution resided between 55 and 80 years. The mean of age is 63.64 and 66.5 years for each Non-CRPC medication and CRPC medication group. The majority of T-stage data distribution resided between T2 and T3. Most of N-stage and M-stage data resided at a 0 or X stage, which means the absence of metastasis. Though it is highly imbalanced, the data distribution showed a similar shape from two groups.

Figure 5 shows the prior data shape, oversampling result, and scaling result for 120 and 360 days of serial data. We used SMOTE to generate CRPC-treated data similar to the prior CRPC cases. Lastly, we obtained balanced data (1575:1576, CRPC: non-CRPC treated) compared to the prior data that was highly imbalanced (8:1584, CRPC: non-CRPC treated).

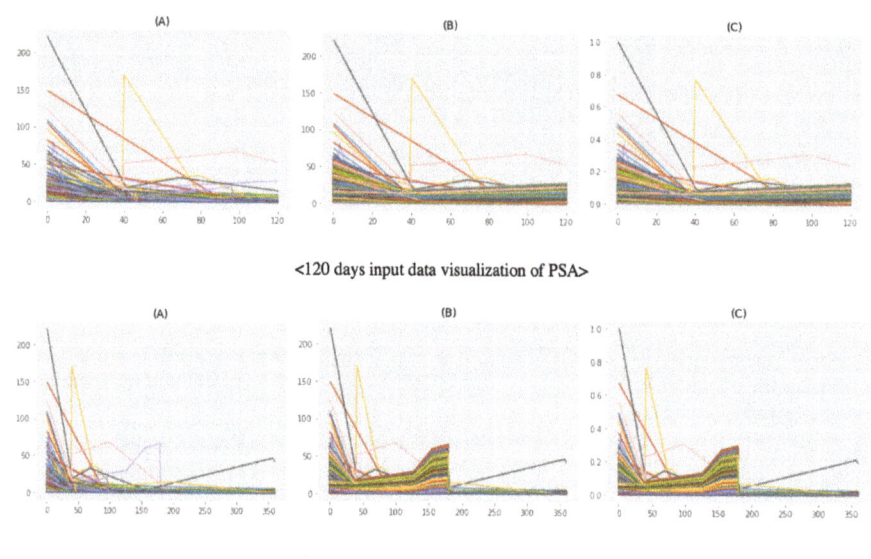

Figure 5. Shape of the input data for prostate specific antigens: (**A**) prior data, (**B**) oversampling result from prior data, and (**C**) scaling result from oversampling data.

We used two sets of serial data: 120 days and 360 days. Each set had a plus-one timestep. For instance, in the 120-day case, there were 121 (120 + 1) time steps including the start time point. The 120-day set contained 3152 cases, 121 timesteps, and seven features. The 360-day set contained 3152 cases, 361 timesteps, and seven features. The model parameter number for the model was 70,016, which was trained by the deep learning model.

Both sets used four epochs (blue lines), which is the number of training iterations. To prevent building the overfitted model, we manually determined four epochs by testing 10 epochs (see Table 2). Although the training time was short, the 120-day set has a recall precision of 91.6% and the 360-day set had a recall precision of 96.9%. The validation loss (red lines) of the 120-day set converged slowly, while that of the 360-day set converged quickly (see Figure 6). Ultimately, the Receiver Operating Characteristic/Area Under the Curve (ROCAUC) accuracy result of the 120-day model is 88.6% and the 360-day model is 94.8% (see Figure 7).

Because the loss of the model continued decreasing and the accuracy of the model continued increasing after four epochs, we did 10-fold cross-validation to verify 10 epochs' training results did not overfit (see Table 3). We have 97.81% and 97.68% average accuracy of the model's evaluations every 120 days and 360 days.

Table 2. Determining epochs to build model.

Category	Running Result: 10 Epochs to Determine Early Stop			Category	Running Result: Determine 4 Epochs for Preventing Overfitting		
	Epoch (10)	Loss	Accuracy		Epoch (4)	Loss	Accuracy
120-day model	1	0.6892	0.5743	120-day model	1	0.6889	0.5168
	2	0.6722	0.5549		2	0.6705	0.6954
	3	0.5841	0.7257		3	0.5720	0.7756
	4	0.4445	0.8073		4	0.3924	0.8391
	5	0.2879	0.8957				
	6	0.1943	0.9379				
	7	0.1496	0.9560				
	8	0.1428	0.9615				
	9	0.1341	0.9637				
	10	0.1140	0.9701				
360-day model	1	0.6848	0.5698	360-day model	1	0.6882	0.4932
	2	0.5190	0.7969		2	0.5423	0.8196
	3	0.2708	0.9021		3	0.3228	0.8930
	4	0.2302	0.9180		4	0.2388	0.9288
	5	0.1519	0.9569				
	6	0.1065	0.9719				
	7	0.1060	0.9742				
	8	0.0861	0.9764				
	9	0.0749	0.9837				
	10	0.0942	0.9782				

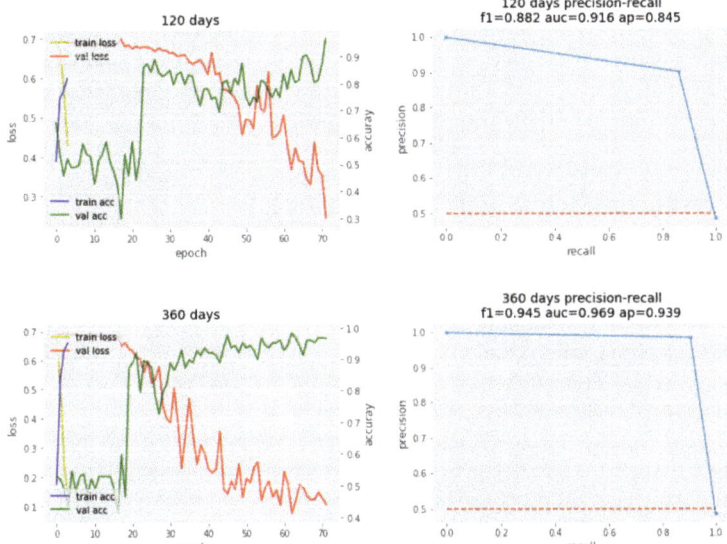

Figure 6. Phased LSTM training/validation (left) and precision-recall plots (right).

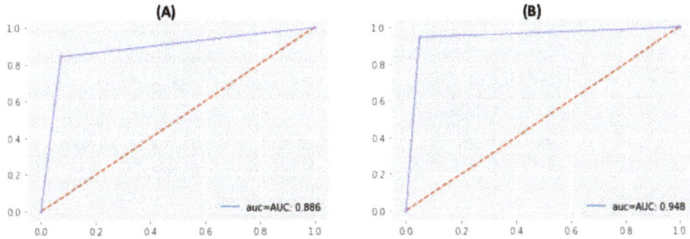

Figure 7. Accuracy Result (ROCAUC): (**A**) 120-day model's accuracy is 88.6%, (**B**) 360-day model's accuracy is 94.8%.

Table 3. 10-fold cross validation of the model.

10-Fold Cross Validation	120-Day Model		360-Day Model	
	Loss	Accuracy	Loss	Accuracy
1	0.1067	0.9778	0.2015	0.9937
2	0.0596	0.9810	0.0548	0.9873
3	0.0750	0.9778	0.1027	0.9714
4	0.1263	0.9587	0.1008	0.9778
5	0.2235	0.9841	0.0897	0.9746
6	0.1063	0.9714	0.1090	0.9746
7	0.1342	0.9905	0.0859	0.9683
8	0.2189	0.9937	0.0930	0.9746
9	0.0863	0.9810	0.1290	0.9651
10	0.1190	0.9651	0.0744	0.9810
Average	0.1256	0.9781	0.1041	0.9768

4. Discussion

In this study, we built a model to predict CPRC-treated patients. From this, we were able to draw the following conclusions.

Serial medical data is an important factor in predicting the likely outcome of patients with PCa. For example, predicting the likelihood of CRPC helps medical professionals to make appropriate decisions at the right time. Some previous studies have predicted time or variables related to CRPC. For example, Elishmereni et al. used a mathematical algorithm to predict the time until biochemical failure of ADT using data from 83 hormone sensitive prostate cancer patients [30]. Although this study only used data from 83 patients, it had a prediction accuracy of 90%. In this study, we used data from 1592 patients to predict CRPC, which is a large number of patients for building a prediction model. Another study by Humphreys et al. tried to find a relationship between age at diagnosis and CRPC. They found that those aged between 55 and 75 years have the shortest survival time [31]. We did not use age as an input variable since there was no significant difference (chi-squared test p-value of 0.253) between the groups with and without CRPC treatment (see Table 1). In another study, Angulo et al. used DNA hypermethylation profiles to predict CRPC. They found 61 genes related to CRPC [32]. However, DNA sequencing is not commonly used for PCa patients and it incurs extra expenses for the patient. We used typical follow-up data from PCa patients. A model based on commonly collected data make it more applicable in real out-patient scenarios.

We built a CRPC prediction model, which can support physicians' decision making and allows them to review more patients in a short period of time. When medical staff do not have enough time to track the status of each patient in need of significant interventions, human errors are more likely to occur and opportunities for treatment may be missed until the condition becomes serious. If prediction support is available, such as the likelihood of a PCa patient developing CPRC, patients in need of treatment can be identified quickly. Therefore, patients will receive the right treatment at the right time.

We used the state-of-the-art deep learning method to handle serial medical data. Because it is difficult to predict a patient's outcome with serial data that is collected irregularly, including medications, treatments, and laboratory test results such as blood tests. Typical deep learning methods such as RNN and LSTM can be used to analyze serial data. However, they must be improved in order to handle irregularly-sampled serial datasets. To overcome this, we adopted recently developed deep learning technology. The phased-LSTM [14] deep learning method builds a fast and accurate prediction model using serial medical data. The predictions show high precision recall scores, which means that they are highly accurate.

The results of this study can be extended to other areas such as emergency room or intensive care units, which receive a significant amount of serial data from patients. In addition, follow-up data from many patient care organizations can be used with this method to make accurate predictions that support clinicians' decision-making.

Although we produced meaningful results, this study still has some limitations. We used data from 1592 patients taken from one hospital. Because we were not permitted to use data from other hospitals for this study, we only used one hospital's data for this study. Though the data was from only one hospital, 10 years of follow-up data of 1592 patients is a big enough number to build a prediction model. Because there were many missing values for other features such as family history, genotype, and lifestyle, we built a model without those features.

In addition, we used imbalanced PCa treatment data with only a small number of CRPC-treated patients. Extremely imbalanced data is not enough to verify the model. For instance, when validation data have only a few CRPC patients out of hundreds of PCa patients, it does not make sense to verify the model's accuracy. Chawla et al. proposed SMOTE and presented results with imbalanced data sets, which has 10923 examples in the majority class and 260 examples in the minority class originally [21]. We used the SMOTE method to build oversampling data. Lastly, we got well balanced data, which has a similar shape to the prior data based on SMOTE.

In future studies, we will obtain more CRPC-treated cases in order to improve the model. However, our study is an example of how irregularly sampled serial medical data can be used to build a decision support prediction model.

Ultimately, this study shows how the state-of-the-art phased-LSTM deep learning method can be used to make meaningful prediction models based on serial medical data. This can help clinicians who want to know their patients' likely outcomes from irregularly sampled follow up data.

Author Contributions: J.P. wrote the article and helped to develop the CRPC prediction model. M.J.R. supported in writing the article and in developing the CRPC prediction model. H.W.M. gave medical advice for the development of the CRPC prediction model. J.Y.L. supervised the research and tested the CRPC prediction model. All four authors substantially contributed their expertise. All authors have read and agreed to the published version of the manuscript.

Funding: The Institute for Information & Communications Technology Promotion (IITP) and grant funded by the Korea government (MSIT) (2018-2-00861, Intelligent SW Technology Development for Medical Data Analysis) funded this research. The Smart Healthcare Research Grant through the Daewoong Foundation (DF-201907-0000001) also supported this research.

Conflicts of Interest: The authors declare no conflict of interest.

References

1. Siegel, R.; Miller, K.; Jemal, A. Cancer statistics, 2018. *CA Cancer J. Clin.* **2018**, *68*, 7–30. [CrossRef]
2. Jung, K.-W.; Won, Y.-J.; Kong, H.-J.; Lee, E.S. Cancer statistics in korea: Incidence, mortality, survival, and prevalence in 2016. *Cancer Res. Treat.* **2019**, *51*, 417–430. [CrossRef] [PubMed]
3. Park, J.; Rho, M.J.; Park, Y.H.; Jung, C.K.; Chong, Y.; Kim, C.-S.; Go, H.; Jeon, S.S.; Kang, M.; Lee, H.J. Promise clip project: A retrospective, multicenter study for prostate cancer that integrates clinical, imaging and pathology data. *Appl. Sci.* **2019**, *9*, 2982. [CrossRef]
4. Koh, H.; Kattan, M.W.; Scardino, P.T.; Suyama, K.; Maru, N.; Slawin, K.; Wheeler, T.M.; Ohori, M. A nomogram to predict seminal vesicle invasion by the extent and location of cancer in systematic biopsy results. *J. Urol.* **2003**, *170*, 1203–1208. [CrossRef] [PubMed]
5. Omlin, A.; Pezaro, C.; Mukherji, D.; Cassidy, A.M.; Sandhu, S.; Bianchini, D.; Olmos, D.; Ferraldeschi, R.; Maier, G.; Thompson, E. Improved survival in a cohort of trial participants with metastatic castration-resistant prostate cancer demonstrates the need for updated prognostic nomograms. *Eur. Urol.* **2013**, *64*, 300–306. [CrossRef] [PubMed]
6. Hirasawa, Y.; Nakashima, J.; Sugihara, T.; Takizawa, I.; Gondo, T.; Nakagami, Y.; Horiguchi, Y.; Ohno, Y.; Namiki, K.; Ohori, M. Development of a nomogram for predicting severe neutropenia associated with docetaxel-based chemotherapy in patients with castration-resistant prostate cancer. *Clin. Genitourin. Cancer* **2017**, *15*, 176–181. [CrossRef]
7. Mun, S.; Park, J.; Dritschilo, A.; Collins, S.; Suy, S.; Choi, I.; Rho, M. The prostate clinical outlook (pco) classifier application for predicting biochemical recurrences in patients treated by stereotactic body radiation therapy (sbrt). *Appl. Sci.* **2018**, *8*, 1620. [CrossRef]

8. Fakoor, R.; Ladhak, F.; Nazi, A.; Huber, M. Using deep learning to enhance cancer diagnosis and classification. In Proceedings of the International Conference on Machine Learning, Atlanta, GA, USA, 17–19 June 2013.
9. Liu, S.; Zheng, H.; Feng, Y.; Li, W. Prostate cancer diagnosis using deep learning with 3d multiparametric MRI. *arXiv* **2017**, arXiv:1703.04078.
10. Litjens, G.; Sánchez, C.I.; Timofeeva, N.; Hermsen, M.; Nagtegaal, I.; Kovacs, I.; Hulsbergen-Van De Kaa, C.; Bult, P.; Van Ginneken, B.; Van Der Laak, J. Deep learning as a tool for increased accuracy and efficiency of histopathological diagnosis. *Sci. Rep.* **2016**, *6*, 26286. [CrossRef]
11. Wang, X.; Yang, W.; Weinreb, J.; Han, J.; Li, Q.; Kong, X.; Yan, Y.; Ke, Z.; Luo, B.; Liu, T. Searching for prostate cancer by fully automated magnetic resonance imaging classification: Deep learning versus non-deep learning. *Sci. Rep.* **2017**, *7*, 15415. [CrossRef]
12. He, B.; Xiao, D.; Hu, Q.; Jia, F. Automatic magnetic resonance image prostate segmentation based on adaptive feature learning probability boosting tree initialization and cnn-asm refinement. *IEEE Access* **2017**, *6*, 2005–2015. [CrossRef]
13. Bhattacharjee, S.; Park, H.-G.; Kim, C.-H.; Prakash, D.; Madusanka, N.; So, J.-H.; Cho, N.-H.; Choi, H.-K. Quantitative analysis of benign and malignant tumors in histopathology: Predicting prostate cancer grading using svm. *Appl. Sci.* **2019**, *9*, 2969. [CrossRef]
14. Neil, D.; Pfeiffer, M.; Liu, S.-C. Phased lstm: Accelerating recurrent network training for long or event-based sequences Advances in neural information processing systems. *arXiv* **2016**, arXiv:1610.09513.
15. Bianchini, D.; Lorente, D.; Rodriguez-Vida, A.; Omlin, A.; Pezaro, C.; Ferraldeschi, R.; Zivi, A.; Attard, G.; Chowdhury, S.; De Bono, J.S. Antitumour activity of enzalutamide (mdv3100) in patients with metastatic castration-resistant prostate cancer (crpc) pre-treated with docetaxel and abiraterone. *Eur. J. Cancer* **2014**, *50*, 78–84. [CrossRef]
16. Miyoshi, Y.; Sakamoto, S.; Kawahara, T.; Uemura, K.; Yokomizo, Y.; Uemura, H. Correlation between automated bone scan index change after cabazitaxel and survival among men with castration-resistant prostate cancer. *Urol. Int.* **2019**, *103*, 279–284. [CrossRef]
17. Attard, G.; Reid, A.H.; A'Hern, R.; Parker, C.; Oommen, N.B.; Folkerd, E.; Messiou, C.; Molife, L.R.; Maier, G.; Thompson, E. Selective inhibition of cyp17 with abiraterone acetate is highly active in the treatment of castration-resistant prostate cancer. *J. Clin. Oncol.* **2009**, *27*, 3742. [CrossRef]
18. Penson, D.F.; Armstrong, A.J.; Concepcion, R.; Agarwal, N.; Olsson, C.; Karsh, L.; Dunshee, C.; Wang, F.; Wu, K.; Krivoshik, A. Enzalutamide versus bicalutamide in castration-resistant prostate cancer: The strive trial. *J. Clin. Oncol.* **2016**, *34*, 2098–2106. [CrossRef]
19. Parker, C.; Heinrich, D.; OSullivan, J.; Fossa, S.; Chodacki, A.; Demkow, T.; Cross, A.; Bolstad, B.; Garcia-Vargas, J.; Sartor, O. Overall survival benefit of radium-223 chloride (alpharadin) in the treatment of patients with symptomatic bone metastases in castration-resistant prostate cancer (crpc): A phase iii randomized trial (alsympca). *Eur. J. Cancer* **2011**, *47*, 3. [CrossRef]
20. McHugh, M.L. The chi-square test of independence. *Biochem. Med. Biochem. Med.* **2013**, *23*, 143–149. [CrossRef]
21. Chawla, N.V.; Bowyer, K.W.; Hall, L.O.; Kegelmeyer, W.P. Smote: Synthetic minority over-sampling technique. *J. Artif. Intell. Res.* **2002**, *16*, 321–357. [CrossRef]
22. Wang, J.; Xu, M.; Wang, H.; Zhang, J. Classification of imbalanced data by using the smote algorithm and locally linear embedding. In Proceedings of the 2006 8th international Conference on Signal Processing, Guilin, China, 16–20 November 2006.
23. Jeatrakul, P.; Wong, K.W.; Fung, C.C. Classification of imbalanced data by combining the complementary neural network and smote algorithm. In Proceedings of the International Conference on Neural Information Processing, Sydney, Australia, 22–25 November 2010; pp. 152–159.
24. Ditzler, G.; Polikar, R.; Chawla, N. An incremental learning algorithm for non-stationary environments and class imbalance. In Proceedings of the 2010 20th International Conference on Pattern Recognition, Istanbul, Turkey, 23–26 August 2010; pp. 2997–3000.
25. Torgo, L.; Ribeiro, R.P.; Pfahringer, B.; Branco, P. Smote for regression. In Proceedings of the Portuguese Conference on Artificial Intelligence, Azores, Portugal, 9–12 September 2013; pp. 378–389.
26. Boyce, M.S.; Vernier, P.R.; Nielsen, S.E.; Schmiegelow, F.K. Evaluating resource selection functions. *Ecol. Model.* **2002**, *157*, 281–300. [CrossRef]

27. Jia, Y.; Martín, A.; Ashish, A.; Paul, B.; Eugene, B.; Zhifeng, C.; Craig, C.; Greg, S.C.; Andy, D.; Jeffrey, D.; et al. Tensorflow: Large-Scale Machine Learning on Heterogeneous Systems. 2015. Available online: http://tensorflow.org/ (accessed on 1 October 2019).
28. Goodfellow, I.; Bengio, Y.; Courville, A. *Deep Learning*; MIT Press: Cambridge, MA, USA, 2016.
29. Kingma, D.P.; Ba, J. Adam: A method for stochastic optimization. *arXiv* **2014**, arXiv:1412.6980.
30. Elishmereni, M.; Kheifetz, Y.; Shukrun, I.; Bevan, G.H.; Nandy, D.; McKenzie, K.M.; Kohli, M.; Agur, Z. Predicting time to castration resistance in hormone sensitive prostate cancer by a personalization algorithm based on a mechanistic model integrating patient data. *Prostate* **2016**, *76*, 48–57. [CrossRef] [PubMed]
31. Humphreys, M.R.; Fernandes, K.A.; Sridhar, S.S. Impact of age at diagnosis on outcomes in men with castrate-resistant prostate cancer (crpc). *J. Cancer* **2013**, *4*, 304. [CrossRef]
32. Angulo, J.C.; Andrés, G.; Ashour, N.; Sánchez-Chapado, M.; López, J.I.; Ropero, S. Development of castration resistant prostate cancer can be predicted by a DNA hypermethylation profile. *J. Urol.* **2016**, *195*, 619–626. [CrossRef]

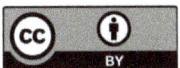

© 2020 by the authors. Licensee MDPI, Basel, Switzerland. This article is an open access article distributed under the terms and conditions of the Creative Commons Attribution (CC BY) license (http://creativecommons.org/licenses/by/4.0/).

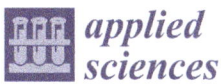

Article

A Comparison of Deep Learning Methods for ICD Coding of Clinical Records

Elias Moons [1,*], Aditya Khanna [1,2], Abbas Akkasi [1] and Marie-Francine Moens [1]

1. Department of Computer Science, KU Leuven, 3000 Leuven, Belgium; adityakhanna@iitb.ac.in (A.K.); abbas.akkasi@kuleuven.be (A.A.); sien.moens@cs.kuleuven.be (M.-F.M.)
2. Department of Electrical Engineering, IIT Bombay, Maharashtra 400076, India
* Correspondence: elias.moons@cs.kuleuven.be

Received: 29 June 2020; Accepted: 28 July 2020; Published: 30 July 2020

Abstract: In this survey, we discuss the task of automatically classifying medical documents into the taxonomy of the International Classification of Diseases (ICD), by the use of deep neural networks. The literature in this domain covers different techniques. We will assess and compare the performance of those techniques in various settings and investigate which combination leverages the best results. Furthermore, we introduce an hierarchical component that exploits the knowledge of the ICD taxonomy. All methods and their combinations are evaluated on two publicly available datasets that represent ICD-9 and ICD-10 coding, respectively. The evaluation leads to a discussion of the advantages and disadvantages of the models.

Keywords: ICD coding; hierarchical classification; electronic healthcare

1. Introduction

The International Classification of Diseases (ICD), which is endorsed by the World Health Organization, is the diagnostic classification standard for clinical and research purposes in the medical field. ICD defines the universe of diseases, disorders, injuries, and other related health conditions, listed in a comprehensive, hierarchical fashion. ICD coding allows for easy storage, retrieval, and analysis of health information for evidenced-based decision-making; sharing and comparing health information between hospitals, regions, settings, and countries; and data comparisons in the same location across different time periods (https://www.who.int/classifications/icd/en/). ICD has been revised periodically to incorporate changes in the medical field. Today, there have been 11 revisions of the ICD taxonomy, where ICD-9 and ICD-10 are the most studied when it comes to their automated assignment to medical documents. In this paper, we compare state-of-the-art neural network approaches to classification of medical reports written in natural language (in this case English) according to ICD categories.

ICD coding of medical reports has been a research topic for many years [1]. Hospitals need to label their patient visits with ICD codes to be in accordance with the law and to gain subsidies from the government or refunds from insurance companies. When the documents are in free text format, this process is still done manually. Automating (a part of) this process would greatly reduce the administrative work.

In this paper, we compare the performance of several deep learning based approaches for ICD-9 and ICD-10 coding. The codes of ICD-9 consist of, at most, five numbers. The first three numbers represent a high level disease category, a fourth number narrows this down to specific diseases, and a fifth number differentiates between specific disease variants. This leads to a hierarchical taxonomy with four layers underneath a root node. The first layer ($L1$) consists of groups of 3-numbered categories, the next three layers ($L2$ through $L4$) correspond to the first 3, 4, or 5 numbers of the ICD code as is displayed in the upper part of Figure 1. In the lower part of this figure, a concrete example of the coding is shown.

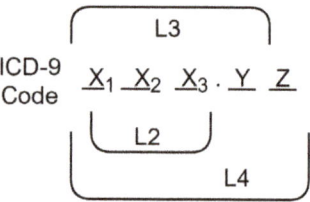

240-279: Endocrine, nutritional and metabolic diseases   (L1)
250:       Diabetes mellitus   (L2)
250.2:   Diabetes with hyperosmolarity   (L3)
250.21:   Diabetes with hyperosmolarity of type 1   (L4)

Figure 1. ICD-9 code structure with second through fourth layer representations and diabetes as an example.

In this paper, we survey state-of-the-art deep learning approaches for ICD-9 coding. We especially focus on the representation learning that the methods accomplish.

Experiments with ICD-9 are carried out on the MIMIC-III dataset [2]. This dataset consists of over 50,000 discharge summaries of patient visits in US hospitals. These summaries are in free textual format and labeled with corresponding ICD-9 codes, an example snippet is visible in Figure 2. Most discharge summaries are labeled with multiple categories, leading to a multiclass and multilabel setting for category prediction.

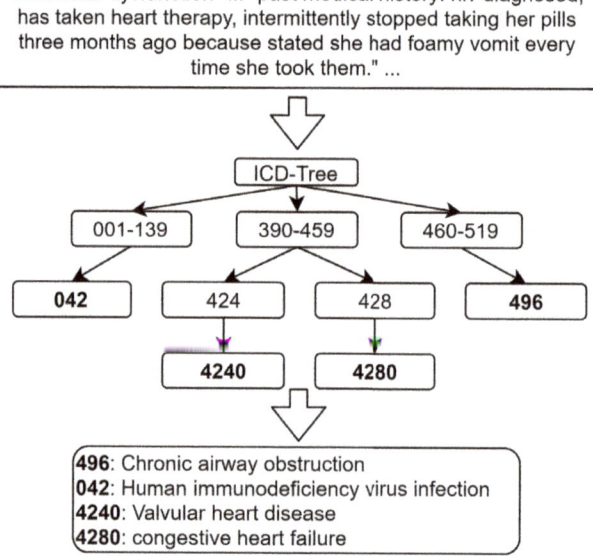

Figure 2. Example snippet of discharge summary from the MIMIC-III dataset with corresponding target International Classification of Diseases (ICD) codes.

Codes from the ICD-10 version are very similar to those of ICD-9. The main difference is that they consist of up to seven characters of which at least the first three are always present, the latter four are optional. The first character is an uppercase alphabetic letter, all other characters are numeric. The first three characters indicate the category of the diagnoses, and the following three characters indicate the etiology, anatomic site, severity, or other clinical details. A seventh character indicates an extension. An example of the ICD-10 structure is visible in Figure 3, it visualizes the same diagnosis as in Figure 1 but for ICD-10 instead of ICD-9.

Experiments with ICD-10 are conducted on the CodiEsp dataset, which is publicly available. This dataset consists of 1000 discharge summaries of patient visits in Spain. The documents are in free text format, which is automatically translated to English from Spanish, and they are manually labeled with ICD-10 codes by healthcare professionals.

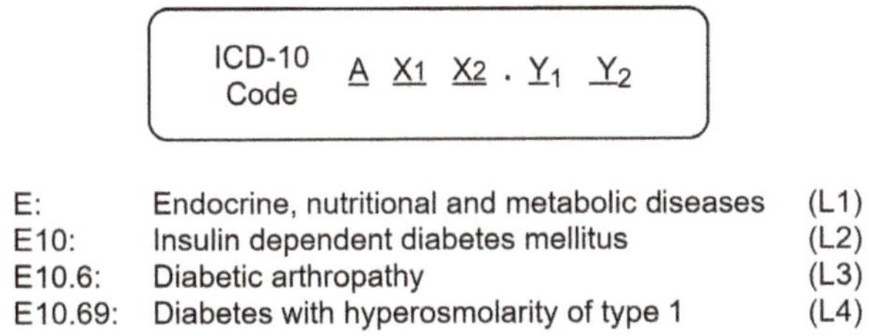

$$\text{ICD-10 Code} \quad \underline{A} \ \underline{X_1} \ \underline{X_2} \cdot \underline{Y_1} \ \underline{Y_2}$$

E:	Endocrine, nutritional and metabolic diseases	(L1)
E10:	Insulin dependent diabetes mellitus	(L2)
E10.6:	Diabetic arthropathy	(L3)
E10.69:	Diabetes with hyperosmolarity of type 1	(L4)

Figure 3. ICD-10 code structure with second through fourth layer representations and diabetes as an example.

The deep learning methods that we discuss in this paper encompass different neural network architectures including convolutional and recurrent neural networks. It is studied how they can be extended with suitable attention mechanisms and loss functions and how the hierarchical structure of the ICD taxonomy can be exploited. ICD-10 coding is especially challenging, as in the benchmark dataset that we use for our experiments the ICD coding model has to deal with very few manually labeled training data.

In our work we want to answer the following research questions. What are the current state-of-the-art neural network approaches for classifying discharge summaries? How do they compare to each other in terms of performance? What combination of techniques gives the best results on a public dataset? We hypothesize the following claims. (1) A combination of self-attention and convolutional layers yields the best classification results. (2) In a setting with less training samples per category, attention on description vectors of the target categories improves the results. (3) Using the hierarchical taxonomy explicitly in the model improves classification on a small dataset. The most important contribution of our work is an extensive evaluation and comparison of state-of-the-art deep learning models for ICD-9 and ICD-10 coding which currently does not exist in the literature.

The remainder of this paper is organized as follows. In Section 2, related work relevant for the conducted research will be discussed. Section 3 will elaborate on the datasets used in the experiments and how this data is preprocessed. The compared deep learning methods are described in Section 4. These methods are evaluated on the datasets in different settings and all findings are reported in Section 5. The most important findings will be discussed in Section 6. Finally, we conclude with some recommendations for future research.

2. Related Work

The most prominent and more recent advancements in categorizing medical reports with standard codes will be described in this section.

2.1. Traditional Models for ICD Coding

Larkey and Croft [3] are the first to apply machine learning techniques to ICD coding. Different techniques including a k-nearest neighbor classifier, relevance feedback, and a Bayesian classifier are applied to the texts of inpatient discharge summaries. The authors found that an ensemble of models yields the best results. At that time, and still later, one has experimented with rule-based pattern matching techniques, which are often expressed as regular expressions (see, e.g., in [4]). Farkas et al. [5] have proposed a hybrid system that partially relied on handcrafted rules and partially on machine learning. For the latter, the authors compare a decision tree learner with a multinomial logistic regression algorithm. The system is evaluated on the data from the CMC Challenge on Classifying Clinical Free Text Using Natural Language Processing, support vector machines (SVMs) were also a popular approach for assigning codes to clinical free text (see, e.g., in [6] who evaluate a SVM using n-gram word features on the MIMIC-II dataset). A systematic overview of earlier systems for automated clinical coding is found in [7]. The authors of [8] show that datasets of different sizes and different numbers of distinct codes demand different training mechanisms. For small datasets, it is important to select relevant features. The authors have evaluated ICD coding performance on a dataset consisting of more than 70,000 textual Electronic Medical Records (EMRs) from the University of Kentucky (UKY) Medical Center tagged with ICD-9 codes. Integrating feature selection on both structured and unstructured data is researched by the authors of [9] and has proven to aid the classification process. Two approaches are evaluated in this setting: early and late integration of structured and unstructured data, the latter yielding the better results. Documents are tagged with ICD-9 and ICD-10 medical codes.

2.2. Deep Learning Models for ICD Coding

More recently, and following a general trend in text classification, deep learning techniques have become popular for ICD coding. These methods learn relevant features from the raw data and thus skip the feature engineering step of traditional machine learning methods. Deep learning proved its value in computer vision tasks [10], and rapidly has conquered the field of text and language processing. Deep learning techniques also have been successfully applied to Electronic Health Records (EHR) [11]. In the 2019 CLEF eHealth evaluation lab, deep learning techniques had become mainstream models for ICD coding [12].

A deep learning model that encompasses an attention mechanism is tested by the authors of [13] on the MIMIC-III dataset. In this work, a Long Short-Term Memory network (LSTM) is used for both character and word level representations. A soft attention layer here helps in making predictions for the top 50 most frequent ICD codes in the dataset. Duarte et al. [14] propose bidirectional GRUs for ICD-10 coding of the free text of death certificates and associated autopsy reports. Xie et al. [15] have developed a tree-of-sequences LSTM architecture with an attention mechanism to simultaneously capture the hierarchical relationships among codes. The model is tested on the MIMIC-III dataset. Huang et al. [16] have shown that deep learning-based methods outperform other conventional machine learning methods such as a SVM for predicting the top 10 ICD-9 codes on the MIMIC-III dataset, a finding confirmed by Li et al. [17], who have confirmed that ICD-9 coding on the MIMIC-II and MIMIC-III datasets outperforms a classical hierarchy-based SVM and a flat SVM. This latter work also shows that convolutional neural networks (CNNs) are successful in text classification given their capability to learn global features that abstract larger stretches of content in the documents. Xu et al. [18] have implemented modality-specific machine learning models including unstructured text, semistructured text, and structured tabular data, and then have used an ensemble method to integrate all modality-specific models to generate the ICD codes. Unstructured and semistructured text is handled by a deep neural network, while tabular data are converted to binary features which are input as features in a decision tree learning algorithm [19]. The text classification problem can also be modeled as a joint label-word embedding problem [20]. An attention framework is proposed that measures the compatibility of embeddings between text sequences and labels. This technique is evaluated on both the MIMIC-II and MIMIC-III datasets but achieves inferior results to the neural models presented further in this paper. Zeng et al. [21] transfer MeSH domain knowledge to improve automatic ICD-9 coding but improvements compared to baselines are limited. Baumel et al. [22] have introduced the Hierarchical Attention bidirectional Gated Recurrent Unit model (HA-GRU). By identifying relevant sentences for each label, documents are tagged with corresponding ICD codes. Results are reported both on the MIMIC-II and MIMIC-III datasets. Mullenbach et al. [23] present the Convolutional Attention for Multilabel classification (CAML) model that combines the strengths of convolutional networks and attention mechanisms. They propose adding regularization on the long descriptions of the target ICD codes, especially to improve classification results on less represented categories in the dataset. This approach is further extended with the idea of multiple convolutional channels in [24] with max pooling across all channels. The authors also shift the attention from the last prediction layer, as in [23], to the attention layer. Mullenbach et al. [23,24] achieve state-of-the art results for ICD-9 coding on the MIMIC-III dataset. As an addition to these models, in this paper a hierarchical variant of each of them is constructed and evaluated.

Recently, language models have become popular in natural language processing. The use of Bidirectional Encoder Representations from Transformers (BERT) models, which uses a transformer architecture with multi-head attention, and especially BioBERT has improved the overall recall values at the expense of precision compared to CNN and LSTM models when applied in the ICD-10 coding task at CLEF eHealth in 2019 [25], a finding which we have confirmed in our experiments. Therefore, we do not report on experiments with this architecture in this survey.

Finally, Campbell et al. [26] survey the literature on the benefits, limitations, implementation, and impact of computer-assisted clinical coding on clinical coding professionals. They conclude that human coders could be greatly helped by current technologies and are likely to become clinical coding editors in an effort to raise the quality of the overall clinical coding process. Shickel et al. [11] review deep learning models for EHR systems by examining architectures, technical aspects, and clinical applications. Their paper discusses shortcomings of the current techniques and future research directions among which the authors cite ICD coding of free clinical text as one of the future challenges.

2.3. Hierarchical Models for Classification

In this paper, we foresee several mechanisms to exploit the hierarchical taxonomy of ICD codes in a deep learning setting, in other words we exploit the known dependencies between classes. Although this is a rather novel topic, hierarchical relationships between classes have been studied in traditional machine learning models. Deschacht et al. [27] have modeled first-order hierarchical dependencies between classes as features in a conditional random field and applied this model to text classification. Babbar et al. [28] study error generalization bounds of multiclass, hierarchical classifiers using the DMOZ hierarchy and the International Patent Classification by simplifying the taxonomy and selectively pruning some of its nodes with the help of a meta-classifier. The features retained in this meta-classifier are derived from the error generalization bounds. Furthermore, hierarchical loss functions have been used in non-deep learning approaches. Gopal et al. [29] exploit the hierarchical or graphical dependencies among class labels in large-margin classifiers, such as a SVM, and in logistic regression classifiers by adding a suitable regularization term to their hinge-loss and logistic loss function, respectively. This regularization enforces the parameters of a child classifier to be similar to the parameters of its parent using a Euclidean distance function, in other words, encouraging parameters which are nearby in the hierarchy to be similar to each other. This helps classes to leverage information from nearby classes while estimating model parameters. Cai and Hofmann [30] integrate knowledge of the class hierarchy into a structured SVM. Their method also considers the parent–child relationship as a feature. All parameters are learned jointly by optimizing a common objective function corresponding to a regularized upper bound on the empirical loss. During training it is enforced that the score of a training example with a correct labeling should be larger than or equal to the score of a training example of an incorrect labeling plus some loss or cost. It is assumed that assignment of confusing classes that are "nearby" in the taxonomy is less costly or severe than predicting a class that is "far away" from the correct class. This is realized by scaling the penalties for margin violation. A similar idea is modeled in a deep learning model for audio event detection [31]. These authors propose the hierarchy-aware loss function modeled as a triplet or quadruplet loss function that favors confusing classes that are close in the taxonomy, over ones that are far away from the correct class. In [32], an hierarchical SVM is shown to outperform that of a flat SVM. Results are reported on the MIMIC-II dataset. In a deep neural network setting, recent publications on hierarchical text classification outside the medical field make use of label distribution learning [18], an hierarchical softmax activation function [33], and hierarchical multilabel classification networks [34].

Recent research shows the value of hierarchical dependencies using hierarchical attention mechanisms [22] and hierarchical penalties [34], which are also integrated in the training of the models surveyed in this paper.

If the target output space of categories follows a hierarchy of labels—as is also the case in ICD coding—the trained models efficiently use this hierarchy for category assignment or prediction [32,35,36]. During categorization the models apply a top-down or a bottom-up approach at the classification stage. In a top-down approach parent, categories are assigned first and only children of assigned parents are considered as category candidates. In a bottom-up approach, only leaf nodes in the hierarchy are assigned which entail that parent nodes are assigned.

In the context of category occurrences in hierarchical target spaces, a power-law distribution is described in [37]. Later, the authors of [38] have addressed this phenomenon quantitatively deriving a relationship in terms of space complexity for those kind of distributions. They have proved that hierarchical classifiers have lower space complexity than their flat variants if the hierarchical target space satisfies certain conditions based on, e.g., maximum branching factor and the depth of the hierarchy. The hierarchical variants discussed in this survey are of different shape than those discussed in these works, layer-based instead of node-based, and do not suffice the necessary conditions for these relationships to apply.

2.4. Models Relevant for This Survey

The experiments reported in Section 5 are carried out starting with and expanding the models described in [23,24]. These models are evaluated against common baselines, partly inspired by other models e.g., the GRU form [22]. For all models, the state-of-the-art, and the baselines, a hierarchical version is constructed using the principles explained in [34]. This hierarchical version duplicates the original model for each layer in the corresponding ICD taxonomy (ICD-9 or ICD-10). These are then trained in parallel. Furthermore, the weights in these networks are influenced by the weights of neighboring layers via the addition of a hierarchical loss function. This loss function penalizes hierarchical inconsistencies that arise when training the model. This leads to a clear comparison between all tested models among themselves as well as with their hierarchical variants.

3. Materials

3.1. ICD-9 Datasets

The publicly available MIMIC-III dataset [2] is used for ICD-9 code predictions. MIMIC-III is an openly accessible clinical care database. For this research, following the trends of previous related work, the patient stay records from the database are used. Every hospital admission has a corresponding unique HADM-ID. In the MIMIC-III database, some patients have also an added Addendum to their stay. Based on earlier studies, records of only those patients who have discharge summaries linked are selected. The addendum is concatenated to the patient's discharge summary. Analogous to the work in [24], out of the the original database, three sub-datasets are extracted. These datasets are used for the experiments and allow for evaluation in different settings. The sub-datasets are the following.

- **Dis-50** consists of a selection of the discharge summaries from the MIMIC-III dataset (11,369 out of 52,726) for the classification of Top-50 ICD-9 codes. We use the publicly available split [23] for training (8066), testing (1729), and development (1574) of the models.
- **Dis** describes the full label setting where all Diagnostic (6918) and Procedural (2011) ICD-9 codes are used. This leads to a total of 8929 Unique codes on the 52,726 discharge summaries. We again use the publicly available split for training (47,723), testing (3372), and development (1631) of the models.
- **Full** extends the **Dis** dataset with other notes regarding the patient (radiology notes, nursing notes, etc.) in addition to the discharge summaries. This dataset, contains almost thrice the number of tokens for training. We use the same test, train, development split as used in the **Dis** dataset.

3.2. ICD-10 Dataset

The **CodiEsp** corpus [39] consists of 1000 clinical cases, tagged with various ICD-10 codes by health specialists. This dataset is released in the context of the CodiEsp track for CLEF ehealth 2020. The dataset corresponding to the subtask of classifying diagnostic ICD codes is used. The original text fragments are in Spanish but an automatically translated version in English is also provided by the organizers, this version is used in this research. The publicly available dataset contains a split of 500 training samples, 250 development samples, and 250 test samples. In total, the 1000 documents comprises of 16,504 sentences and 396,988 words, with an average of 396.2 words per clinical case. The biggest hurdle while training with this dataset is the size and consequently the small number of training examples for each category present. Figure 4 gives a sorted view of all categories present in the training dataset and the amount of examples tagged with that specific category.

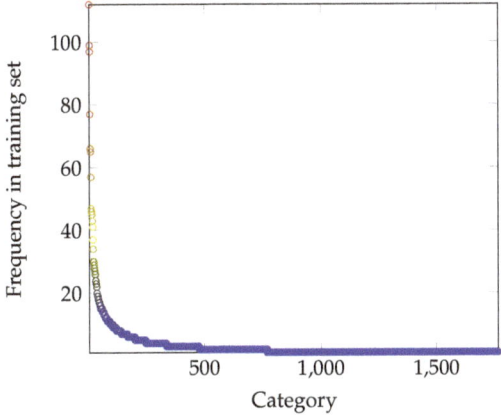

Figure 4. Category frequencies of CodiEsp training dataset.

There are in total 1767 different categories spread out over only 500 training documents. Every document is labeled with on average 11.3 different categories and each category is on average represented by 3.2 training examples. Even the top 50 most frequently occurring categories have only between 15 and 112 corresponding positive training documents. Therefore, tests for this dataset are conducted on these 50 categories. Table 1 gives an overview of statistics for all discussed training datasets. The specifics for the corresponding development and test sets are similar. Displayed statistics for the Dis and the Full dataset are the same since the only difference lies in larger text fragments, resulting in 72,891 unique tokens for the Full dataset compared to 51,917 for Dis. There are no differences concerning the labels.

Table 1. Dataset specifics overview.

Dataset	#Training Docs	#Labels	Avg. #Labels/Doc	Avg. #Training Docs/Label
Dis-50	8067	50	5.7	920
Dis	47,724	8922	15.9	85
Full	47,724	8922	15.9	85
CodiEsp	500	1767	11.3	3.2

3.3. Preprocessing

The preprocessing follows the standard procedure described in [23], i.e., tokens that contain no alphabetic characters are removed and all tokens are put to lowercase. Furthermore tokens that appear in fewer than three training documents are replaced with the "UNK" token. All documents are then truncated to a maximum length of 2500 tokens.

4. Methods

In this section, all tested models will be discussed in detail. First, a simple convolutional and a recurrent baseline commonly used in text classification are described. Then, two recent state-of-the-art models in the field of ICD coding are explained in detail. These models are implemented by the authors following the original papers and are called **DR-CAML** [23] and **MVC-(R)LDA** [24], respectively. We discuss in detail the attention mechanisms and loss functions of these models. Afterwards, as a way of handling the hierarchical dependencies of the ICD-codes, we propose various ways of their integration in all models. This is based on advancements in hierarchical classification as inspired by [34].

All discussed models have for each document i as input a sequence of word vectors x^i as their representation and as output a set of ICD-codes y^i.

4.1. Baselines

The performance of all models will be evaluated and compared against two simple common baselines used for handling sequential input data (text). These models are, respectively, based on convolutional and recurrent neural principles.

4.1.1. Convolutional

The baseline convolutional neural network model, or **CNN**, consists of a 1D temporal convolutional neural layer. This convolutional layer consists of different kernels, which are filters with a specific pattern that are tested against all sequences of the input data with the same length. This is followed by a (max-)pooling layer, to reduce the data size by only remembering the maximum value over a certain range. More formally, for an input x and a given 1D kernel f on element s of the input sequence, the convolutional and pooling operation can be defined as follows.

$$F_1(s) = (x \circledast f)(s) = \sum_{i=0}^{h-1} f(i) \cdot x_{s-i} \qquad (1)$$

$$F_2(s) = max_{i=0}^{l-1} F_1(s-1) \qquad (2)$$

The amount of filters k and l in the convolutional and pooling layer, respectively, as well as their sizes are optimizable parameters of this model. For both layers a stride length, i.e., the amount by which the filter shifts in the sequence, can be defined leading to a trade-off between output size and observability of detailed features.

4.1.2. Recurrent

As the recurrent neural network baseline, two common approaches are considered.

BiGRU

The **GRU**, or Gated Recurrent Unit, is a gating mechanism in recurrent neural networks. It is the mechanism of recurrent neural networks allowing the model to "learn to forget" less important fragments of the data and "learn to remember" the more important fragments with respect to the learning task. More formally, consider an input vector x_t, update gate vector z_t, reset gate vector r_t, and output vector h_t at time t. The respective values can be calculated as follows.

$$z_t = \sigma(W_z \cdot [h_{t-1}, x_t] + b_z) \tag{3}$$

$$r_t = \sigma(W_r \cdot [h_{t-1}, x_t] + b_r) \tag{4}$$

$$h_t^* = tanh(W_h \cdot [t_t \times h_{t-1}, x_t] + b_h) \tag{5}$$

$$h_t = (1 - z_t) \times h_{t-1} + z_t \times h_t^* \tag{6}$$

This leads to weight matrices W_z, W_r, and W_h to train as well as biases b_z, b_r, and b_h, σ stands for the sigmoid activation function. **BiGRU** is the bidirectional variant of such a model that processes the input data front-to-back and back-to-front in parallel.

BiLSTM

An **LSTM**, or Long Short-Term Memory neural network model, is very similar to a GRU but replaces the update gate with a forget gate and an additional output gate. This way it usually has more computational power than a regular GRU, but at the expense of more trainable parameters and more chance of overfitting when the amount of training data is limited [40–42]. Formally, consider again an input vector x_t and a hidden state vector h_t at time t. Activation vectors for the update gate, forget gate, and output gate are, respectively, represented by z_t, f_t, and o_t. These states relate to each other like follows.

$$z_t = \sigma(W_z \cdot [h_{t-1}, x_t] + b_z) \tag{7}$$

$$f_t = \sigma(W_f \cdot [h_{t-1}, x_t] + b_f) \tag{8}$$

$$o_t = \sigma(W_o \cdot [h_{t-1}, x_t] + b_o) \tag{9}$$

$$c_t^* = tanh(W_c \cdot [h_{t-1}, x_t] + b_c) \tag{10}$$

$$c_t = (f_t) \times c_{t-1} + z_t \times c_t^* \tag{11}$$

$$h_t = o_t \times tanh(c_t) \tag{12}$$

This again leads to weight matrices W_z, W_f, W_o, and W_c to train as well as biases b_z, b_f, b_o, and b_c with σ being the sigmoid activation function. **BiLSTM** is the bidirectional variant of a regular LSTM, analogous to BiGRU, which is the bidirectional variant of GRU.

4.2. Advanced Models

This subsection describes the details of recent state-of-the-art models presented in [23,24] in the way they are used for the experiments in Section 5.

4.2.1. DR-CAML

DR-CAML is a CNN-based model adopted for ICD coding [23]. When an ICD code is defined by the WHO, it is accompanied by a label definition expressed in natural language to guide the model towards learning the appropriate parameter values of the model. For this purpose, the model employs a per-label attention mechanism enabling it to learn distinct document representations for each label. It has been shown that for labels for which there are very few training instances available, this approach is advantageous. The idea is that the description of a target code is itself a very good training example for the corresponding code. Similarity between the representation of a given test sample and the representation of the description of a target code gives extra confidence in assigning this label.

In general, after the convolutional layer, DR-CAML employs a per-label attention mechanism to attend to the relevant parts of text for each predicted label. An additional advantage is that the per-label attention mechanism provides the model with the ability of explaining why it decided to assign each code by showing the spans of text relevant for the ICD code.

DR-CAML consists of two modules: one for the representation of the input text, and the other for the embedding of the label's description as is visualized in Figure 5. The CAML module has a CNN at the base layer which takes a sequence of the embeddings of the text tokens as input and consequently represents the document as the matrix H. Then, the per-label attention mechanism applies. Attention in this context means learning which parts of some context (the label description vectors) are relevant for a given input vector.

After calculating the attention vector α using a softmax activation function, it is applied as a product with H. With h_l, the vector parameter for label l, the vector representation for each label is computed as

$$v_l = \sum_{n=1}^{N} \alpha_{l,n} h_n \qquad (13)$$

Given the vector representation of a document and the probability for label l, $\hat{y}_l$ can be obtained as shown in Figure 5.

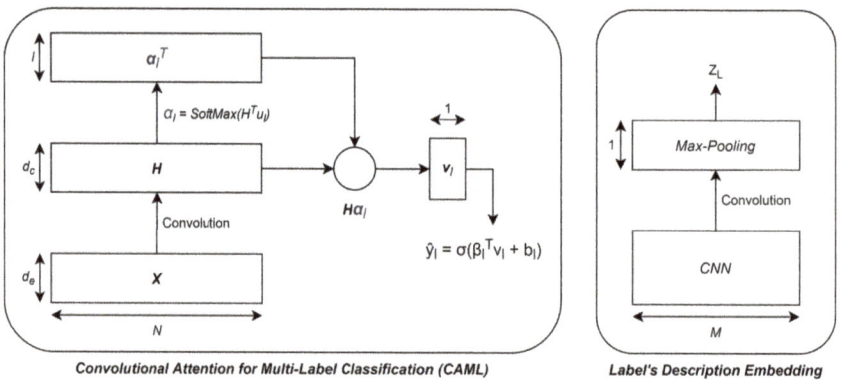

Figure 5. DR-CAML (after [23]).

The CNN modules on the left hand side try to minimize the binary cross entropy loss. The second module is a max-pooling CNN model which produces a max-pooled vector, z_l, by getting the description of code l. Assuming n_y is the number of true labels in train data, the final loss is computed by adding a regularization term to the base loss function. The loss function is explained in more detail in Section 4.2.3.

4.2.2. MVC-(R)LDA

MVC-LDA and **MVC-RLDA** can be seen as extensions of DR-CAML. Similar to that model, they are based on a CNN architecture with a label attention mechanism that considers ICD coding as a multi-task binary classification problem. The added functionality lies in the use of parallel CNNs with different kernel sizes to capture information of different granularity. MVC-LDA, the top module in Figure 6, is a multi-view CNN model stacked on an embedding layer. MVC-RLDA reintroduces the per-label attention mechanism introduced in the previous subsection.

In general, the multi-view CNNs are constructed with four CNNs that have the same number of filters but with different kernel sizes. This convolutional layer is followed by a max-pooling function across all channels to select the most relevant span of text for each filter. A separate attention layer for each label comes next, helping the model to attend to relevant parts of a document for each label. A linear layer with weight vector V_j is implemented for the jth label and CV_j is the attention for the input C and label j. This attention vector CV_j is the output of a dense layer with softmax activation function leading to a relative weighting of the input elements C.

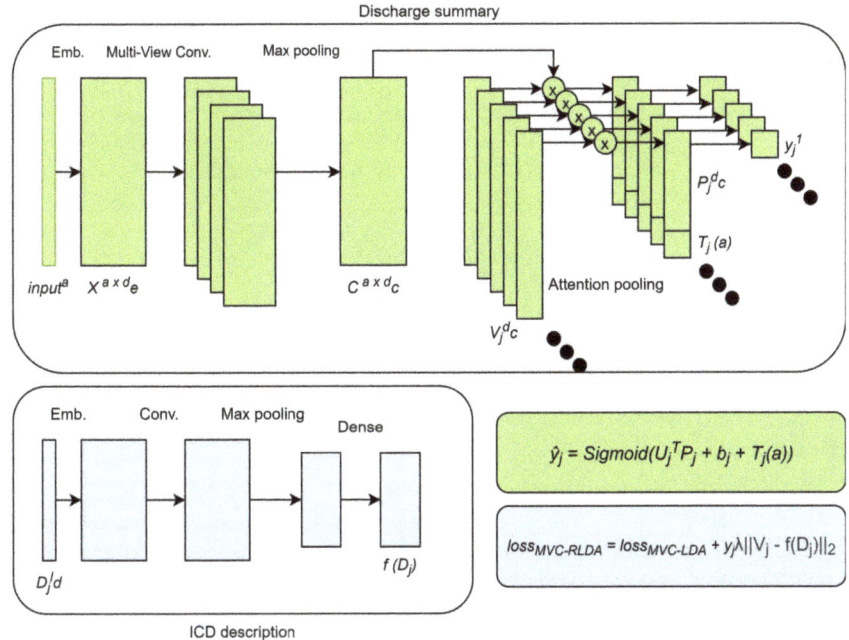

Figure 6. MVC-(R)LDA (after the work in [24]).

Then, the pooled outputs of the attention layer are computed as

$$P_j = C^T(CV_j). \tag{14}$$

At the end, a dense layer is used for each label. The length of an input document is also encoded into the output layers with embedding function

$$T_j(l) = Sigmoid(K_j l + d_j), \tag{15}$$

to decrease the problem of under-coding to some extent. This is done as in [24], which showed a statistically significant Pearson's correlation between the input length and the number of ground truth codes. Therefore, the model can derive an underlying bias that, on average, shorter input documents represent a lower amount of categories.

Parameters a, K_j, and d_j in the length embedding function respectively represent the input length, and the layer's weight and bias, respectively, for a given label j. The prediction y_j for class j is then computed as

$$y_j = Sigmoid(U_j^T P_j + b_j + T_j(a)). \tag{16}$$

Similar to DR-CAML, this model tries to minimize the binary loss function. Adding the label description embedding to MVC-LDA, the lower part of Figure 4 leads to MVC-RLDA whose loss function includes an extra weighted term as a regularizer. It guides the attention weights to avoid overfitting. In addition, this regularization forces the attention for classes with similar descriptions to be closer to each other. The loss function is again explained in more detail in Section 4.2.3.

4.2.3. Loss Function

The loss functions used to train DR-CAML and the multiview models MVD-(R)LDA are calculated in the same way. The general loss function is the binary cross entropy loss $loss_{BCE}$. This loss is extended by regularization on the long description vectors of the target categories, visualized in Figure 6 on the lower right corner.

Given N different training examples x^i. The values of $\hat{y}_l$ and max-pooled vector z_l can be calculated as represented in Figure 5 by getting the description of code l out of all L target codes. In this figure, and the following formulas, β_l is a vector of prediction weights and v_l the vector representation for code l. Assuming n_y is the number of true labels in the training data, the final loss is computed by adding regularization to the base loss function as

$$\hat{y}_l = \sigma(\beta_l^t v_l + b_l) \tag{17}$$

$$loss_{BCE}(X) = -\sum_{i=1}^{N}\sum_{l=1}^{L} y_l \log(\hat{y}_l) + (1-y_l)\log(1-\hat{y}_l) \tag{18}$$

$$loss_{Model}(X) = loss_{BCE} + \lambda \frac{1}{n_y}\sum_{i=1}^{N}\sum_{l=1}^{L} \|z_l - \beta_l\|_2 \tag{19}$$

4.3. Modeling Hierarchical Dependencies

In this section, we investigate the modeling of hierarchical dependencies as extensions of the models described above. A first part integrates the hierarchical dependencies directly into the structure of the model. This leads to **Hierarchical models**, which are layered variants of the already discussed approaches. The second way hierarchical dependencies are explicitly introduced into the model is via the use of a hierarchical loss function to penalize hierarchical inconsistencies across the model's prediction layer.

4.3.1. Hierarchical Models

Hierarchical relationships can be shaped directly into the architecture of any of the described models above. The ICD-9 taxonomy can be modeled as a tree with a general ICD root and 4 levels of depth, as already described in Section 1. This leads to a hierarchical variant of any of the models. In this variant, not 1 but 4 identical models will be trained, one for each of the different layers in the ICD hierarchy (corresponding to the length of the codes).

Such an approach is presented in [34] and is adapted to the target domain of ICD categories. An overview of the approach is given in Figure 7.

The input for each layer is partially dependent on an intermediary representation from the previous layer as well as the original input through concatenation of both. Layers are stacked from most to least specific in from leaf to root node in the taxonomy. Models corresponding to different layers will then rely on different features, or characteristics, to classify the input vectors. This way the deepest, most advanced representations, can be used for classifying the most abstract and broad categories. On the other hand, for the most specific categories, word level features can directly be used to make detailed decisions between classes that are very similar.

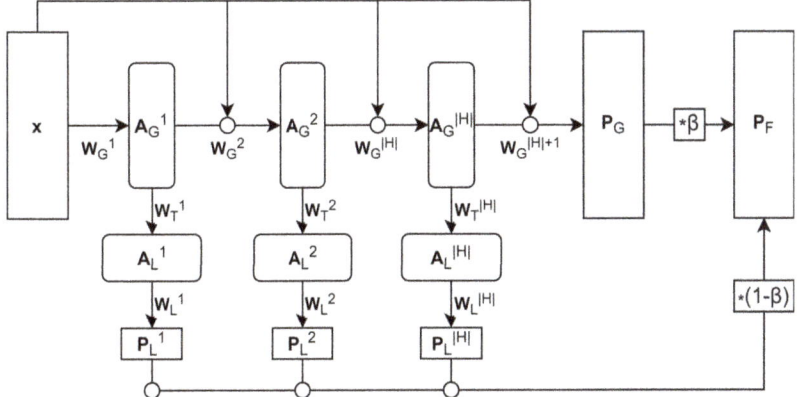

Figure 7. Overview of hierarchical variant of a model, inspired by [34].

4.3.2. Hierarchical Loss Function

To capture the hierarchical relationships in a given model, the loss function of the above models can be extended with an additional term. This leads to the definition of a **Hierarchical loss function** ($loss_H$). This loss function penalizes classifications that contradict the inherent ICD hierarchy. More specifically, when a parent category is not predicted to be true, none of its child categories should be predicted to be true. The hierarchical loss between a child and its parent in the tree is then defined as the difference between their computed probability scores, with 0 as a lower bound. More formally, for the entire loss function $loss_{H\_Model}$ for a category of layer X, combining the regular training loss $loss_{Model}$ described above and the hierarchical loss $loss_H$, is calculated as follows,

$$P(X) = Probability(X == True) \tag{20}$$
$$Par(X) = Probability(Parent(X) == True) \tag{21}$$
$$L(X) = True\ label\ of\ X (0\ or\ 1) \tag{22}$$
$$loss_H(X) = Clip(P(X) - Par(X), 0, 1) \tag{23}$$
$$loss_{H\_Model}(X) = (1 - \lambda) loss_{Model}(X) + \lambda loss_H(X) \tag{24}$$

which leaves a parameter λ to optimize the loss function (parameter λ is optimized over the training set).

5. Results

5.1. MIMIC-III

Results are displayed for five different models. First, results for the two baseline models, **CNN** and **BiGRU**, are shown. Because in most of the experiments, the BiGRU models performed at least on par with their BiLSTM variants, we only report the results of **BiGRU** as a recurrent neural network baseline. The reason for this good performance of GRU models compared to LSTM models most likely resides in the amount of available training data for various target categories. Then, we report on three more advanced models as discussed in the Method section: **DR-CAML**, **MVC-LDA**, and **MVD-RLDA**. Different hyperparameter values are considered and tested on the development set of MIMIC-III the setting giving the highest average performance on the development set is reported in Table 2.

Table 2. Optimal hyperparameter values obtained on the development set of the MIMIC-III dataset.

	CNN	BiGRU	DRCAML	MVC-LDA	MVC-RLDA
# of filters	500	-	50	6,8,10,12	6,8,10,12
Filter Sizes	4	-	10	70	90
λ	-	0.0005	-	-	0.0005
Lr	0.003	0.003	0.0001	0.001	0.001
Batch size	16	16	16	4	4
Seq. length~	2500	2500	2500	10000	10000

For all these models using their optimal hyperparameter settings, the average performance is reported in terms of Micro F1, Macro F1, Micro AUC (ROC), and Precision@X. For models that are only evaluated on the top 50 most frequent categories in the training data, results are displayed in Table 3. This experiment is then repeated over all categories, which leads to the results in Table 4. Last, Table 5 gives the results of training the models on all labels for the Full dataset.

Table 3. Results of flat models on top 50 most frequent categories of the MIMIC-III Dis-50 dataset.

		Micro F1	Macro F1	Micro AUC	P@5
	CNN	63.42	59.74	91.57	62.33
	GRU	63.49	55.72	91.79	61.72
Dis-50	DR-CAML	69.64	64.56	93.90	65.39
	MVC-LDA	69.07	64.17	93.69	65.15
	MVC-RLDA	69.53	64.85	93.77	64.91

Table 4. Results of flat models on all labels of the MIMIC-III Dis dataset.

		Micro F1 Proc	Micro F1 Diag	Micro F1 Both	Micro AUC	P@5
	CNN	51.01	40.80	42.58	84.38	59.48
	GRU	53.88	40.86	43.40	85.36	61.59
Dis	DR-CAML	48.99	59.03	50.47	89.45	68.28
	MVC-LDA	59.75	51.60	53.03	90.02	69.77
	MVC-RLDA	58.84	50.74	52.10	89.77	68.71

Table 5. Results of flat models on all labels of the MIMIC-III Full dataset.

		Micro F1 Proc	Micro F1 Diag	Micro F1 Both	Micro AUC	P@5
	CNN	46.19	41.19	42.18	83.96	57.53
	GRU	46.50	37.74	39.64	83.19	55.00
Full	DR-CAML	57.90	41.40	49.94	89.42	67.16
	MVC-LDA	58.12	50.70	51.97	89.93	68.53
	MVC-RLDA	57.61	49.67	50.97	89.68	67.60

This experiment is repeated for the hierarchical variants of all described models. This time, only results on the top 50 most frequent target categories are reported in Table 6. As hierarchical models introduce a large number of additional intermediate categories, the target space is too large to train these hierarchical variants in a full category setting.

Table 6. Results of hierarchical models obtained on the MIMIC-III Dis-50 dataset.

		Micro F1	Macro F1	Micro AUC	P@5
Dis-50	CNN	61.70	53.79	90.62	59.87
	GRU	62.38	54.88	91.77	60.03
	DR-CAML	67.68	63.74	93.47	63.48
	MVC-LDA	65.21	60.06	92.29	62.41
	MVC-RLDA	65.43	61.22	92.34	61.73

To assess the importance of the different components of the highest performing model on MIMIC-III Dis, an ablation study is conducted. The multi-view and the hierarchical component are added and the regularization on long descriptions of the target ICD-codes is removed while all other components stay the same. The difference in performance is measured and visualized in Figure 8.

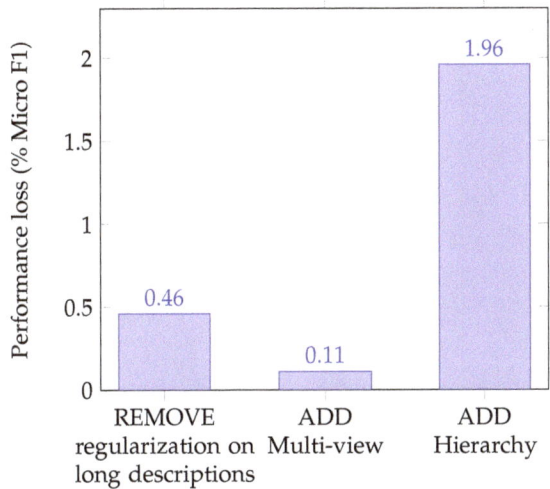

Figure 8. Ablation study on highest performing model (hierarchical MVC-RLDA) for MIMIC-III dataset.

5.2. CodiEsp

Similar experiments are carried out on the CodiEsp dataset, while only using the top 50 most frequent codes. The same hyperparameter settings are used as in Table 2. Results are visualized in Tables 7 and 8. Results for the full target space are not reported, as 90% of the target categories would only have 5 or less positive training examples. Furthermore, this would lead to a target space of 1767 different categories with only 500 training examples in total, which makes training of a decent model unfeasible.

Table 7. Results of flat models on top 50 codes obtained on the CodiEsp dataset.

		Micro F1	Macro F1	Micro AUC	P@5
CodiEsp	CNN	12.52	6.17	49.35	7.96
	GRU	11.54	11.03	50.54	7.68
	DR-CAML	9.58	8.24	48.63	7.96
	MVC-LDA	10.84	6.23	49.26	4.17
	MVC-RLDA	11.52	6.67	48.01	3.70

Table 8. Results of hierarchical models for top 50 codes obtained on the CodiEsp dataset.

		Micro F1	Macro F1	Micro AUC	P@5
	CNN	12.44	6.18	53.08	2.84
	GRU	11.87	11.50	50.14	7.68
CodiEsp	DR-CAML	10.35	3.97	53.61	5.59
	MVC-LDA	13.00	2.79	60.76	11.94
	MVC-RLDA	13.92	4.21	56.38	8.72

To assess the importance of the different components of the highest performing model on CodiEsp, an ablation study is conducted. The multi-view, the hierarchical component, and the regularization on long descriptions of the target ICD-codes are each removed while all other components stay the same. The difference in performance is measured and visualized in Figure 9.

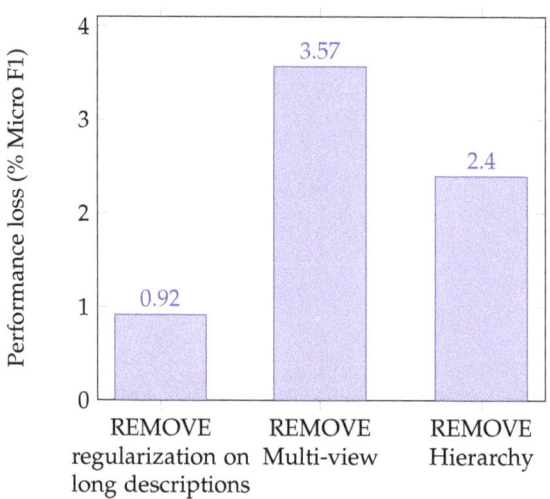

Figure 9. Ablation study on highest performing model (hierarchical MVC-RLDA) for CodiEsp dataset.

6. Discussion

A comparison between the results displayed in Tables 3 and 4 shines a light on the value of the multiview component. The micro F1 scores of the five models are in similar relationship to each other in both tables, except for the two multiview models. They outperform CAML in the full label setting of the MIMIC-III Dis dataset, where they show very similar behavior to CAML in a top-50 category setting, where for each of the categories a decent amount of training samples is available. When the target space increases and more categories have fewer training examples, the added granularity of having multiple kernel sizes in the MVC-(R)LDA model pays off. Table 5 shows results for models trained on the Full dataset. The best performing model (MVC-LDA, 58.12%) gets outperformed by the best performing model for all labels on Dis (MVD-LDA, 59,75%). The addition of the information in other medical documents than just discharge summaries thus seems to complicate instead of facilitate the classification process.

Furthermore, comparing Tables 3 and 6, where the influence of the hierarchical parameter can be assessed in a top-50 category setting, reveals a shift in the opposite direction. While in general, the modeling of the hierarchical relationships hurts the classification process for all categories, it hinders the multiview models the most. This time, DR-CAML is clearly the best performing model. Adding multiview and simultaneously modeling the hierarchical relationships between the target categories tend to make the model overfit on the training data.

Looking at Tables 7 and 8, it is clear that the lack of a sufficient amount of training data in CodiEsp (about 100 times less than for the Dis dataset) for most categories led to lower performance of all models on this dataset. For the flat variants of the models, a regular CNN even outperforms the more complex models. As the amount of training data is low, the added complexity of the latter models hinders them generalizing well for unseen data. Comparing the results in both tables also leads to the conclusion that in contrast to the results on MIMIC-III, on average the hierarchical component increases the classification performance based on Micro F1 on CodiEsp. Where the information embedded in the ICD taxonomy is redundant and even counteracting the performance for the larger MIMIC-III dataset, it is leveraged when there is a lack of information in the training data itself, which is the case for CodiEsp.

Last, Figures 8 and 9 display the relative importance of the long description regularization, the multi-view. and the hierarchy for the top performing model on both the Dis and CodiEsp datasets. For the Dis dataset, not using the hierarchy is by far the most important component. The regularization on long descriptions still adds 0.46% and the multi-view almost does not influence the results. For CodiEsp, it shows that the multi-view component has the biggest influence, followed by the hierarchy, whose importance on this smaller dataset is already shown previously.

7. Conclusions

In this paper, we have surveyed the current methods used for classification of clinical reports based on ICD codes using neural networks. We have combined the techniques already present in the literature and assessed the relative importance of all present components. Combining a convolutional framework with self-attention as well as regularizing, the loss function with attention on the long descriptions of target ICD codes proved to be valuable. Furthermore, a hierarchical objective was integrated in all presented models. Its added value lies especially in a setting with low amounts of available training data. Last, extending the dataset with the information present in other medical documents introduced too much noise into the data, hindering the performance of the tested models.

Concerning future research directions, it would be valuable to test the techniques on a ICD-10 or ICD-11 dataset of larger size. This would give better insights into which performance these models could achieve in current hospital settings. On a similar note, tackling the problem of lack of data by finding a way to combine the available training data from different datasets (e.g., MIMIC-III and CodiEsp) and different ontologies (e.g., ICD-9, ICD-10, and MeSH) could further improve the classification performance of all models. Last, it would be interesting to investigate the use of hierarchical descriptions as an addition to the loss function, giving another use for the information inherently present in the ICD taxonomy.

Author Contributions: Conceptualization, E.M. and M.-F.M.; Methodology, E.M. and M.-F.M.; Software, E.M., A.A. and A.K.; Validation, E.M., A.A. and A.K.; Formal Analysis, E.M. and M.-F.M.; Investigation, E.M.; Resources, A.K.; Data Curation, A.K.; Writing-Original Draft Preparation, E.M. and M.-F.M.;Writing-Review Editing, E.M., A.A., A.K. and M.-F.M.; Visualization, E.M.; Supervision, M.-F.M.; Project Administration, A.A. and M.-F.M.; Funding Acquisition, M.-F.M. All authors have read and agreed to the published version of the manuscript.

Funding: This research was funded by the VLAIO SBO project, grant number 150056. M.-F.M. is co-funded by the ERC Advanced Grant CALCULUS H2020-ERC-2017-ADG 788506.

Conflicts of Interest: Authors declare no conflict of interest.

References

1. Larkey, L.; Croft, W.B. *Automatic Assignment of ICD9 Codes To Discharge Summaries*; Technical Report; University of Massachusetts: Amherst, MA, USA, 1995.
2. Johnson, A.E.W.; Pollard, T.J.; Shen, L.; Lehman, L.w.H.; Feng, M.; Ghassemi, M.; Moody, B.; Szolovits, P.; Anthony Celi, L.; Mark, R.G. MIMIC-III, a freely accessible critical care database. *Sci. Data* **2016**, *3*, 1–9. [CrossRef] [PubMed]
3. Larkey, L.S.; Croft, W.B. Combining classifiers in text categorization. In Proceedings of the 19th Annual International ACM SIGIR Conference on Research and Development in Information Retrieval, Zurich, Switzerland, 18–22 August 1996; (Special Issue of the SIGIRForum); pp. 289–297.
4. Goldstein, I.; Arzumtsyan, A.; Özlem, U. Three approaches to automatic assignment of ICD-9-CM codes to radiology reports. In *Proceedings of the AMIA Annual Symposium*; American Medical Informatics Association: Washington, DC, USA, 2007; pp. 279–283.
5. Farkas, R.; Szarvas, G. Automatic construction of rule-based ICD-9-CM coding systems. *BMC Bioinform.* **2008**, *9* (Suppl. 3), S10. [CrossRef] [PubMed]
6. Marafino, B.J.; Davies, J.M.; Bardach, N.S.; Dean, M.L.; Dudley, R.A. N-gram support vector machines for scalable procedure and diagnosis classification, with applications to clinical free text data from the intensive care unit. *J. Am. Med. Inform. Assoc.* **2014**, *21*, 871–875. [CrossRef] [PubMed]
7. Stanfill, M.; Williams, M.; Fenton, S.; Jenders, R.; Hersh, W. A systematic literature review of automated clinical coding and classification systems. *J. Am. Med. Inform. Assoc. JAMIA* **2010**, *17*, 646–651. [CrossRef] [PubMed]
8. Kavuluru, R.; Rios, A.; Lu, Y. An empirical evaluation of supervised learning approaches in assigning diagnosis codes to electronic medical records. *Artif. Intell. Med.* **2015**, *65*, 155–166. [CrossRef]
9. Scheurwegs, E.; Cule, B.; Luyckx, K.; Luyten, L.; Daelemans, W. Selecting relevant features from the electronic health record for clinical code prediction. *J. Biomed. Inform.* **2017**, *74*, 92–103. [CrossRef]
10. Leo, M.; Furnari, A.; Medioni, G.G.; Trivedi, M.M.; Farinella, G.M. Deep Learning for Assistive Computer Vision. In Proceedings of the Computer Vision—ECCV 2018 Workshops—Part VI, Munich, Germany, 8–14 September 2018; pp. 3–14.
11. Shickel, B.; Tighe, P.; Bihorac, A.; Rashidi, P. Deep EHR: A survey of recent advances in deep learning techniques for electronic health record (EHR) analysis. *IEEE J. Biomed. Health Inform.* **2018**, *22*, 1589–1604. [CrossRef]
12. Kelly, L.; Suominen, H.; Goeuriot, L.; Neves, M.; Kanoulas, E.; Li, D.; Azzopardi, L.; Spijker, R.; Zuccon, G.; Scells, H.; et al. Overview of the CLEF eHealth Evaluation Lab 2019. In *International Conference of the Cross-Language Evaluation Forum for European Languages*; Springer: Cham, Switzerland, 2019; pp. 322–339.
13. Shi, H.; Xie, P.; Hu, Z.; Zhang, M.; Xing, E.P. Towards automated ICD coding using deep learning. *arXiv* **2017**, arXiv:1711.04075.
14. Duarte, F.; Martins, B.; Pinto, C.S.; Silva, M.J. Deep neural models for ICD-10 coding of death certificates and autopsy reports in free-text. *J. Biomed. Inform.* **2018**, *80*, 64–77. [CrossRef]
15. Xie, P.; Xing, E. A neural architecture for automated ICD coding. In *Proceedings of the 56th Annual Meeting of the Association for Computational Linguistics (Volume 1: Long Papers)*; ACL: Melbourne, Australia, 2018.
16. Huang, J.; Osorio, C.; Sy, L.W. An empirical evaluation of deep learning for ICD-9 code assignment using MIMIC-III clinical notes. *Comput. Methods Prog. Biomed.* **2019**, *177*, 141–153. [CrossRef]
17. Li, M.; Fei, Z.; Zeng, M.; Wu, F.; Li, Y.; Pan, Y.; Wang, J. Automated ICD-9 coding via a deep learning approach. *IEEE/ACM Trans. Comput. Biol. Bioinform.* **2019**, *16*, 1193–1202. [CrossRef] [PubMed]
18. Xu, K.; Lam, M.; Pang, J.; Gao, X.; Band, C.; Mathur, P.; Papay, F.; Khanna, A.K.; Cywinski, J.B.; Maheshwari, K.; et al. Multimodal machine learning for automated ICD coding. In *Proceedings of the 4th Machine Learning for Healthcare Conference*; Doshi-Velez, F., Fackler, J., Jung, K., Kale, D., Ranganath, R., Wallace, B., Wiens, J., Eds.; PMLR: Ann Arbor, MI, USA, 2019; Volume 106, pp. 197–215.
19. Quinlan, J.R. Induction of decision trees. *Mach. Learn.* **1986**, *1*, 81–106. [CrossRef]
20. Wang, G.; Li, C.; Wang, W.; Zhang, Y.; Shen, D.; Zhang, X.; Henao, R.; Carin, L. Joint embedding of words and labels for text classification. In *Proceedings of the 56th Annual Meeting of the Association for Computational Linguistics (Volume 1: Long Papers)*; ACL: Melbourne, Australia, 2018.

21. Zeng, M.; Li, M.; Fei, Z.; Yu, Y.; Pan, Y.; Wang, J. Automatic ICD-9 coding via deep transfer learning. *Neurocomputing* **2018**, *324*, 43–50. [CrossRef]
22. Baumel, T.; Nassour-Kassis, J.; Elhadad, M.; Elhadad, N. Multi-Label Classification of Patient Notes: A Case Study on ICD Code Assignment. In Proceedings of the Workshops at the Thirty-Second AAAI Conference on Artificial Intelligence, Hilton, NO, USA, 2–7 February 2018.
23. Mullenbach, J.; Wiegreffe, S.; Duke, J.; Sun, J.; Eisenstein, J. Explainable prediction of medical codes from clinical text. In *Proceedings of the 2018 Conference of the North American Chapter of the Association for Computational Linguistics: Human Language Technologies, Volume 1 (Long Papers)*; ACL: New Orleans, LA, USA, 2018.
24. Sadoughi, N.; Finley, G.P.; Fone, J.; Murali, V.; Korenevski, M.; Baryshnikov, S.; Axtmann, N.; Miller, M.; Suendermann-Oeft, D. Medical code prediction with multi-view convolution and description-regularized label-dependent attention. *arXiv* **2018**, arXiv:1811.01468.
25. Amin, S.; Neumann, G.; Dunfield, K.; Vechkaeva, A.; Chapman, K.A.; Wixted, M.K. MLT-DFKI at CLEF eHealth 2019: Multi-label classification of ICD-10 codes with BERT. In Proceedings of the Working Notes of CLEF 2019—Conference and Labs of the Evaluation, Forum, Lugano, Switzerland, 9–12 September 2019.
26. Campbell, S.; Giadresco, K. Computer-assisted clinical coding: A narrative review of the literature on its benefits, limitations, implementation and impact on clinical coding professionals. *Health Inf. Manag. J.* **2019**, *49*, 183335831985130. [CrossRef] [PubMed]
27. Deschacht, K.; Moens, M. Efficient hierarchical entity classifier using conditional random fields. In Proceedings of the 2nd Workshop on Ontology Learning and Population: Bridging the Gap between Text and Knowledge@COLING/ACL 2006, Sydney, Australia, 22 July 2006; pp. 33–40.
28. Babbar, R.; Partalas, I.; Gaussier, É.; Amini, M. On flat versus hierarchical classification in large-scale taxonomies. In Proceedings of the Advances in Neural Information Processing Systems 26: Proccedings of the 27th Annual Conference on Neural Information Processing Systems 2013, Lake Tahoe, NV, USA, 5–8 December 2013; pp. 1824–1832.
29. Gopal, S.; Yang, Y. *Recursive Regularization for Large-Scale Classification with Hierarchical and Graphical Dependencies*; Association for Computing Machinery: New York, NY, USA, 2013.
30. Cai, L.; Hofmann, T. Hierarchical document categorization with support vector machines. In Proceedings of the Thirteenth ACM International Conference on Information and Knowledge Management, Washington, DC, USA, 8–13 November 2004.
31. Jati, A.; Kumar, N.; Chen, R.; Georgiou, P. Hierarchy-aware loss function on a tree structured label space for audio event detection. In Proceedings of the ICASSP 2019–2019 IEEE International Conference on Acoustics, Speech and Signal Processing (ICASSP), Brighton, UK, 12–17 May 2019; pp. 6–10.
32. Perotte, A.; Pivovarov, R.; Natarajan, K.; Weiskopf, N.; Wood, F.; Elhadad, N. Diagnosis code assignment: Models and evaluation metrics. *J. Am. Med. Inform. Assoc.* **2014**, *21*, 231–237. [CrossRef]
33. Mohammed, A.A.; Umaashankar, V. Effectiveness of hierarchical softmax in large scale classification tasks. In Proceedings of the 2018 International Conference on Advances in Computing, Communications and Informatics (ICACCI), Bangalore, India, 19–22 September 2018; pp. 1090–1094.
34. Wehrmann, J.; Cerri, R.; Barros, R. Hierarchical multi-label classification networks. In Proceedings of the Thirty-Fifth International Conference on Machine Learning, Stockholm, Sweden, 10–15 July 2018; pp. 5075–5084.
35. Silla, C.N.; Freitas, A.A. A survey of hierarchical classification across different application domains. *Data Min. Knowl. Discov.* **2011**, *22*, 31–72. [CrossRef]
36. Kowsari, K.; Brown, D.E.; Heidarysafa, M.; Meimandi, K.J.; Gerber, M.S.; Barnes, L.E. HDLTex: Hierarchical Deep Learning for Text Classification. In Proceedings of the 2017 16th IEEE International Conference on Machine Learning and Applications, Cancun, Mexico, 18–21 December 2017.
37. Yang, Y.; Zhang, J.; Kisiel, B. A scalability analysis of classifiers in text categorization. In Proceedings of the 26th Annual International ACM SIGIR Conference on Research and Development in Informaion Retrieval, Toronto, ON, Canada, 28 July–1 August 2003; pp. 96–103.
38. Babbar, R.; Metzig, C.; Partalas, I.; Gaussier, E.; Amini, M.R. On power law distributions in large-scale taxonomies. *ACM Sigkdd Explor. Newsl.* **2014**, *16*, 47–56. [CrossRef]

39. Miranda-Escalada, A.; Gonzalez-Agirre, A.; Krallinger, M. CodiEsp Corpus: Spanish Clinical Cases Coded in ICD10 (CIE10)—eHealth CLEF2020. Available online: https://zenodo.org/record/3758054#.XxXGgy17E6h (accessed on 29 July 2020).
40. Chung, J.; Gulcehre, C.; Cho, K.; Bengio, Y. Empirical evaluation of gated recurrent neural networks on sequence modeling. *arXiv* **2014**, arXiv:1412.3555.
41. Yin, W.; Kann, K.; Yu, M.; Schütze, H. Comparative study of CNN and RNN for natural language processing. *arXiv* **2017**, arXiv:1702.01923.
42. Kaiser, Ł.; Sutskever, I. Neural GPUs learn algorithms. *arXiv* **2015**, arXiv:1511.08228.

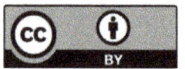

© 2020 by the authors. Licensee MDPI, Basel, Switzerland. This article is an open access article distributed under the terms and conditions of the Creative Commons Attribution (CC BY) license (http://creativecommons.org/licenses/by/4.0/).

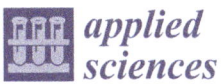

Article

Applying Machine Learning for Healthcare: A Case Study on Cervical Pain Assessment with Motion Capture

Juan de la Torre [1,*], Javier Marin [1], Sergio Ilarri [2,3] and Jose J. Marin [1,4]

1. IDERGO-Research and Development in Ergonomics, Biomechanical Laboratory, I3A-University Institute of Research of Engineering of Aragon, University of Zaragoza, 50018 Zaragoza, Spain; 647473@unizar.es (J.M.); jjmarin@unizar.es (J.J.M.)
2. Computer Science for Complex System Modelling (COSMOS), I3A-University Institute of Research of Engineering of Aragon, University of Zaragoza, 50018 Zaragoza, Spain; silarri@unizar.es
3. Department of Computer Science and Systems Engineering, University of Zaragoza, 50018 Zaragoza, Spain
4. Department of Design and Manufacturing Engineering, University of Zaragoza, 50018 Zaragoza, Spain
* Correspondence: 627471@unizar.es

Received: 9 July 2020; Accepted: 24 August 2020; Published: 27 August 2020

Abstract: Given the exponential availability of data in health centers and the massive sensorization that is expected, there is an increasing need to manage and analyze these data in an effective way. For this purpose, data mining (DM) and machine learning (ML) techniques would be helpful. However, due to the specific characteristics of the field of healthcare, a suitable DM and ML methodology adapted to these particularities is required. The applied methodology must structure the different stages needed for data-driven healthcare, from the acquisition of raw data to decision-making by clinicians, considering the specific requirements of this field. In this paper, we focus on a case study of cervical assessment, where the goal is to predict the potential presence of cervical pain in patients affected with whiplash diseases, which is important for example in insurance-related investigations. By analyzing in detail this case study in a real scenario, we show how taking care of those particularities enables the generation of reliable predictive models in the field of healthcare. Using a database of 302 samples, we have generated several predictive models, including logistic regression, support vector machines, k-nearest neighbors, gradient boosting, decision trees, random forest, and neural network algorithms. The results show that it is possible to reliably predict the presence of cervical pain (accuracy, precision, and recall above 90%). We expect that the procedure proposed to apply ML techniques in the field of healthcare will help technologists, researchers, and clinicians to create more objective systems that provide support to objectify the diagnosis, improve test treatment efficacy, and save resources.

Keywords: data mining; data anonymization; health; cervical injury; neck pain; inertial sensors

1. Introduction

In the field of healthcare, the exponential increase in the data that health centers must produce and manage is significant. The need has arisen to develop procedures that make this process easier and that take advantage of all the data generated [1], detecting unknown and valuable information in health data [2]. Thus, the volume of data generated is such that its processing and analysis by traditional methods is too complex and overwhelming [3]. To tackle this challenge, data mining (DM) can play a key role, as it allows the discovery of patterns and trends in large amounts of complex data and the extraction of hidden information to help in making decisions that can improve the quality of the care processes [4–7]. It is closely linked with the scientific discipline in the field of artificial intelligence called machine learning (ML), which "employs a variety of statistical, probabilistic and optimization techniques that allow computers to learn from past examples and to detect hard-to-discern patterns from large, noisy or complex data sets" [8].

Consequently, ML is generating growing interest in the field of healthcare (e.g., see [9,10]) for relevant special issues related to this topic), mainly derived from its possible applications, such as assessing the effectiveness of treatments, detecting fraud and abuse in health insurance, managing healthcare, making lower-cost medical solutions available to the patients, detecting symptoms and diseases [11], discovering treatment patterns from electronic medical records [12], detecting groups of incidents [13], and identifying medical treatment methods [2,3]. Likewise, ML also presents health benefits: (1) a potential reduction in the time and effort required for diagnosis and treatment, (2) the ability to examine multiple areas simultaneously, (3) a decreased potential for human error, and (4) data that are accessible anytime and anywhere [14]. Besides, DM and ML are key in the path towards personalized medicine, where the goal is to customize treatments to the specifics of each individual [15–18].

However, to take full advantage of the benefits offered by ML in the field of healthcare, several considerations are necessary. Among others, the following aspects can be highlighted:

- The data have to be structured and organized in order to properly process and transform them into suitable variables, which is essential in the development of any pattern recognition software and a highly problem-dependent task [19,20].
- Moreover, the secure treatment and management of data acquires special relevance in the field of healthcare, where the privacy of the patient must be ensured. The management of sensitive data contrasts with other fields of application of ML (fraud detection, stock prediction, etc.), where anonymization treatments may be sometimes not necessary or critical. Therefore, a specific treatment involving the anonymization and categorization of the data must be performed in order to ensure the privacy of the patients [21]. Due to privacy policies, on certain occasions if a suitable anonymization of the data is not performed and/or the required authorizations to access some data are not obtained, the needed health studies cannot be carried out. Therefore, data availability should also be considered as a key factor [21].
- Another difference with other ML applications is the existence of different costs of failures; in the health area, the cost of a false negative (e.g., failing to detect that a patient has a specific disease) is usually much higher than the cost of a false positive (e.g., if a person is initially considered to have a disease that he/she does not really have, additional tests will be performed to rule this out, which may be costly but usually less harmful than failing to diagnose an existing disease).
- It should also be considered that ML hardly ever follows a linear sequence ending at the first attempt; instead, it is rather an iterative feedback process where the stages interact with each other. Furthermore, in the field of healthcare, where the flow of data is continuous and constant, it is reasonable to assume that the model can be designed to be a "learning" model that must be continuously updated to improve its predictions over time. Therefore, the different stages needed to generate a reliable predictive model should be properly structured, from the acquisition of raw data to decision-making, which is essential to achieve the effectiveness of the model [22].

All this motivates the need to define the particularities of the application of ML techniques in the field of healthcare, where different stages in the ML workflow must be correctly defined and structured. The proper application of ML techniques would be beneficial for the clinicians, researchers, developers, and designers involved in the field of health, where the management of information acquires a transcendental role. It would favor the design of new products and services for improving healthcare access [23], creating truly accessible technological solutions [24], and enhance the relationship between health systems and people by providing adequate services at the right time [23].

Based on the above, the aims of this study are the following: (1) to show and develop the particularities of applying ML techniques in the field of healthcare, detailing all the stages that comprise this process, from the acquisition of raw data to the decision-making derived from the predictive model generated; and (2) to demonstrate and show its practical application in a real use case. Specifically, the ML process is applied in a cervical pain assessment study with patients affected by whiplash pathologies derived from traffic accidents or other causes. This case study shows the proposed methodology in action to solve a specific relevant problem. Moreover, the applied procedure can be used as an ML application guide for other similar studies in the field of healthcare. We believe that the combination of the use case study and the machine learning methodology is a relevant contribution of this paper. We do not remain in the theoretical/methodological part only or limit our work to apply different machine learning algorithms and compare the results, as many other works do; instead, we describe the whole machine learning process, highlighting the aspects that are more relevant for our use case but at the same time providing a general framework that could be used in other health-related projects. In this way, we think that the paper could be relevant both as a specific case study and also as a reference and guideline for other similar projects.

The structure of the rest of this paper is as follows. In Section 2, we present the use case scenario studied and the clinical methods used for data collection. In Section 3, we describe the proposed procedure to develop predictive models for healthcare, illustrating each step with our work on the case study. In Section 4, we present an overall discussion of the proposal and the lessons learnt. Finally, in Section 5, we summarize our conclusions, the limitations of the study, and some ideas for future work.

2. Use Case Scenario and Clinical Methods

To illustrate the particularities of using ML techniques in the health area, a case study related to the detection of cervical pain is considered. The goal is to try to estimate automatically the presence of cervical pain, which can help to objectify a diagnosis and to clarify issues in case of insurance litigation. The selection of cervical pathology as a case study in this work is motivated by the fact that musculoskeletal disorders of the cervical spine have a high incidence and prevalence and are considered a public health problem, especially in developed countries [25,26]. Likewise, cervical injuries (usually due to whiplash after a traffic accident) are difficult to diagnose [26] because traumatic cervical spine injuries and their associated symptoms are diverse [25].

A real dataset was collected by evaluating the movement of the cervical spine in 151 patients (60 asymptomatic subjects, 42 with cervical pain resulting from a traffic accident, and 49 with neck discomfort due to other causes). Cervical movement assessment tests were performed by using an MH-sensor motion capture system [27,28] (see Figure 1). The participants performed a sequence of functional cervical Range of Motion (ROM) tests of the following movements: flexion-extension, rotation, and lateralization (Figure 2). The patients were collaborating subjects in order to avoid disturbances produced by non-collaborating subjects immersed in a judicial process with an insurance company [29]. The medical test was performed twice with each patient, giving a total of 302 samples.

Moreover, all the participants, who were either asymptomatic or had cervical pain, were also assessed with a clinical examination to verify that they met the inclusion criteria:

- age between 18 and 65 years;
- not immersed in a judicial process;
- no presence of surgery and/or cervical fracture.

The medical inspection, assessment by scales/clinical tests, and development of the clinical profile of the patients were conducted by clinicians. All the participants received information about the experiment and signed a consent agreement prior to the testing. The study received a favorable verdict from the Bioethics Committee of Aragón in Spain (CEICA) on 25 July 2017.

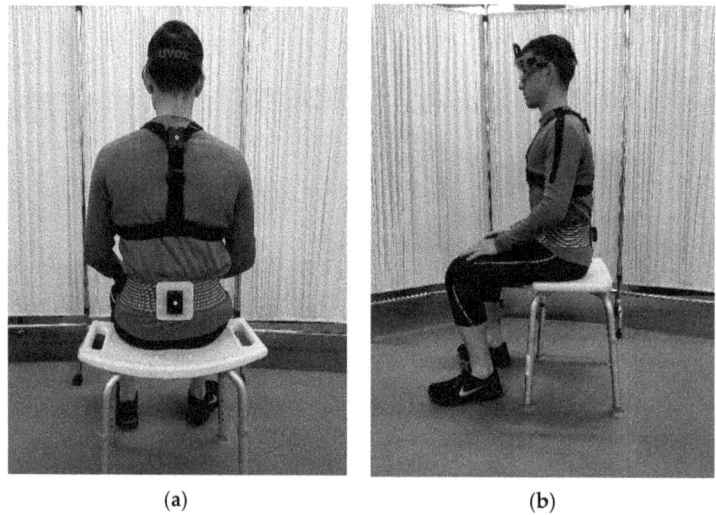

Figure 1. Move Human (MH)-sensor motion capture system, cervical assessment. (**a**) Back view. (**b**) Lateral view.

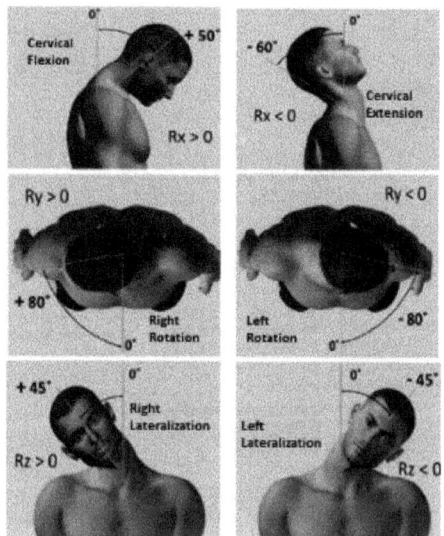

Figure 2. Cervical movements evaluated.

3. Proposed Procedure to Develop Predictive Models in Healthcare

A predictive model to support decision-making in the field of healthcare should be able to make predictions relative to relevant target clinical variables. The final goal is to deploy a system that can help in clinical decision-making (e.g., objectifying diagnoses, testing the efficacy of treatments, saving resources, providing suitable and customized treatments, etc.). The proposed procedure for continuous use in the field of healthcare is summarized and outlined in Figure 3.

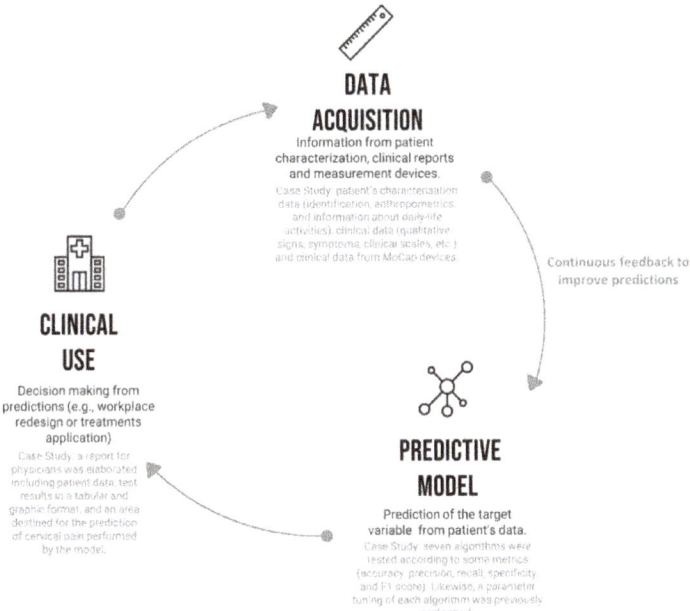

Figure 3. Application of predictive models for clinical decision-making. Icons made by monkik, smashicons and mynamepong.

The complete ML process has been considered, with the particularities of its application in the healthcare area. It is based on seven stages that range from the definition of the target to the clinical use of the system, as shown in Figure 4. Each stage is explained in the following subsections. Besides, this paper is accompanied by electronic Supplementary Material to facilitate the understanding of the different stages of application in the case study considered; specifically, we provide sample data files obtained at the end of different stages of the process (anonymized datasets) and an example report that a health professional could obtain as the output of the process.

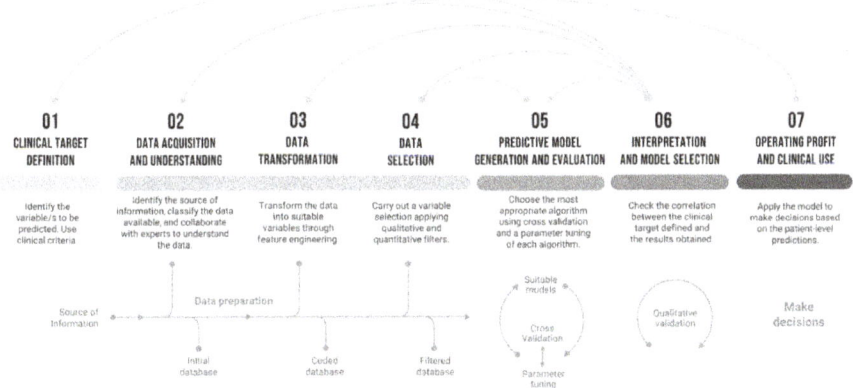

Figure 4. Project management procedure proposed for the application of machine learning in healthcare.

In order to adapt and particularize the usual process of applying ML techniques in the healthcare field and develop the project management procedure, some outstanding studies such as [20,30], as well as the most widespread DM processes, such as knowledge discovery in databases (KDD) [31,32]; sample, explore, modify, model, and assess (SEMMA) [14,32]; and the cross-industry standard process for DM (CRISP-DM) [32–35], have been considered as a reference. Likewise, the project management procedure scheme proposed (shown in Figure 4) has been inspired by different outlines of clinical applications proposed by different authors [4,19,36–38] and adapted and extended according to our own experience and the work performed with clinicians in our case study and other related collaborations, such as the project "Mobile units for functional assessment of the musculoskeletal system" (CEICA reference of the project: OTRI-2019/0108) in collaboration with the hospital MAZ (Mutua de Accidentes de Zaragoza, Zaragoza, Spain), whose goal was to predict the degree of collaboration of patients in insurance litigation.

From the related proposals mentioned above, the CRISP-DM process has been our main inspiration to develop the project management procedure proposed in this paper. This is to be expected because CRISP-DM sets a general common framework that can be adapted to different scenarios. Thus, there are similarities between the six stages in CRISP-DM and our seven-stage proposal. For example, the CRISP-DM stage 6 "deployment" is closely related to our last stage, which is "operating profit and clinical use". As another example, stage 6 of CRISP-DM establishes that the creation of the model is not the end of the project and, similarly, in healthcare the knowledge provided to the clinician through the application of the predictive model is not the end of the process, since the system is continuously acquiring new data to improve the clinical performance. As the main difference between both procedures, we put more emphasis on data management aspects, since this is a key point in healthcare, and consider the whole process from the perspective of its application in a healthcare scenario. While only one stage for data management is considered in the CRISP-DM process (stage 3, "data preparation"), data management is the focus of three stages in our proposal (stage 2 "data acquisition and understanding", stage 3 "data transformation", and stage 4 "data selection").

The works mentioned in this section have inspired our proposal, which extends existing models by including a thorough analysis of all the data management challenges, as well as an illustration of each step through a real practical case study. Although the particularities of applying ML techniques in healthcare are exemplified in a specific case study, the procedure presented is flexible enough to adapt to any healthcare case.

3.1. Stage 1: Clinical Target Definition

In the first stage, the aim of the system is established—that is, the variables with clinical significance that the system should be able to predict are identified. Likewise, the final performance of the model and the statistical measures that will define its performance must also be defined. Measures such as the accuracy, precision, or recall are usual metrics used to assess the performance of a classification model, and metrics such as the Mean Absolute Error (MAE) or Root Mean Squared Error (RMSE), to cite two examples can be used to evaluate the accuracy of a numeric prediction.

In predictive classification in a healthcare domain, it is usual that some metric must be highlighted in such a way that the model must always be generated with the aim to minimize it. This metric is usually the number of false negatives (affecting the recall metric). The reason for this is that, in healthcare, false negatives and false positives have no similar costs, which has always been an issue that clinicians have had to deal with [39]. Moreover, the clinical need must be identified (e.g., to classify a certain type of pathology, to predict a pattern or behavior, etc.). In addition, the sample size and viability of the project must be assessed prior to its realization [34].

Application to our Case Study

In our case study, the aim of the prediction model is to predict the presence of cervical pain (the target variable) in patients who have suffered whiplash or suffer from chronic cervical pathology. In our collected dataset, the cervical pain is a binary variable (the presence or absence of pain) which has been reported by the collaborating subjects, who were real patients undergoing an assessment process in a hospital.

Predicting the presence of cervical pain is of interest especially in the forensic field, as the incidence and prognosis of whiplash injury from motor vehicles is relevant to insurance litigations for pain and suffering [29]. The aim is to determine the presence or absence of pain with enough confidence to be able to aid clinicians to detect possible magnifications of the injury by the affected individuals and thus establish an unbiased compensation for the cervical pain [40]. It can help to identify and objectify pain in patients with a high degree of anxiety and in hypochondriac patients.

Without a loss of generality, the following target metrics have been determined for the purpose of this study, whose required threshold values have been stablished according to the criteria of clinical experts (for this particular case study, they considered that achieving this quality criteria would be enough for the system to be used as a decision-support system in production):

- Accuracy: greater than 85%.
- Precision: greater than 85%.
- Recall: greater than 90%.

The sample size is 302; although this is not a very large dataset, it contains a lot of variables with relevant information to characterize the presence of cervical pain during insurance litigation, which allows predicting the target variable, thus considering the project viable.

3.2. Stage 2: Data Acquisition and Understanding

The second stage implies identifying different sources that will allow access to the data necessary to feed the model, both in the initial phase of model design (initial training), as well as regarding a future continuous feedback when it reaches the operational stage of application in the field of healthcare. Likewise, the typology of these data will also be identified and selected. The level of accuracy that these sources of information can provide and the frequency of data collection (which may be determined by aspects such as the cost of the equipment needed, the availability of collaborating patients, etc.) will be considered in the choice [34].

In the field of healthcare, due to the diverse origins of data, their typology, their consistency, and even their veracity, the process of categorization of the data acquires special relevance for their correct structuring, understanding, and subsequent treatment.

When there are patient's personal data that make the identification of the patient possible, proper anonymization techniques must be applied. Apart from direct identification data (such as the name and last name of the patient, his/her history number, or his/her card ID), other data such as the age, nationality, height, weight, diagnosis, etc., can be used for indirect patient identification. In stage 3 "Data transformation" (see Section 3.3), certain techniques are presented to safeguard the privacy of patients and avoid the loss of useful information for the generation of the model, but these sensitive variables must be identified in this second phase.

Although there are classifications of information and data in the healthcare environment [30], alternative complementary classifications are proposed in this paper for a better understanding and structuring of the data. This has been motivated by the needs of medical staff, as well as by specialists of the medical legal/forensic field collaborating with us in our case study: a greater variety of classifications is of interest in order to include the perspectives of all the parties involved.

Clinical Data and Patient Data

Firstly, two types of data related to patients can be identified when we distinguish between clinical data and other data related to the patient:

- Patient characterization data. They are generally static data (although there may be small fluctuations in certain data values over large time intervals, such as in the case of the weight of the patient). They can be grouped in the following categories:

- Identification data: name, age, gender, educational level, nationality, etc.
- Temporary data: dates of control or highlighted clinical evolution, visits to the hospital, start and end of treatments, etc.
- Anthropometric data: measurements of the size and proportions of the human body, such as the height, weight, percentage of fat and muscle, foot length, abdominal perimeter, etc., that usually require instrumentation to be obtained (scale, tape measure, etc.).
- Daily life activities (DLA) data: data usually reported by the patient related to the habits and activities that he/she usually performs on a daily basis. In some cases, some of these data can be measured using wearables sensors or other devices deployed in smart homes.
- Clinical data: data of a medical nature that may require instrumentation and medical tests for their acquisition.

Data According to the Degree of Objectivity

Another possible classification is to categorize the data according to the degree of objectivity:

- Measures: objective data that do not require assessment by a clinician. These data are not affected by the reproducibility factor. Examples are test or clinical scales, test results, or data collected by medical instrumentation. Data recorded by sensor devices provide objective data on some measurable dimensions of the patient and can be of different types: motion capture (MoCap) sensors, surface electromyography (EMG), stabilometric platforms, dynamometers, etc.
- Assessed data: information that depends on the assessment of the clinician, such as diagnoses and treatments.
- Reported data: subjective information provided by the patient regarding his/her condition (perceived symptoms).

Data According to Clinical Considerations

We also present a classification that groups the collected data according to clinical considerations:

- Clinical profile: data about symptoms and clinical signs of the patient that can lead to a diagnosis by the clinician. We refer to symptoms when they are of subjective nature, reported by the patient, and to signs if they are objective and obtained by the clinician about the pathology. In addition, the signs can be qualitative (binary) or (discrete or continuous) quantitative (e.g., the temperature of a thermometer, image tests, other measurements, etc.).
- Treatment data: data about the treatment that the clinician has prescribed, such as the type of treatment, number of rehabilitation sessions, drugs received, surgery, etc.
- Clinical scales, tests, or surveys: data resulting from scales or validated and protocolized tests whose objective is to obtain objective information about the patient (e.g., the timed up and go test, the Unterberger test, psychological tests, etc.).
- Medical history: data concerning the patient's clinical history, ordered chronologically (e.g., first hospital visit, imaging test for diagnosis, treatment administration after diagnosis, etc.).

Data According to their Data Types

Finally, the different data variables can be grouped according to their types, independently of the specifics of the health area. For example, we could consider:

- Qualitative variables: also called categorical variables, they are variables that are not numerical. They describe data that fit into categories (e.g., educational level, the level of development of a disease, the level of invasiveness of a treatment, etc.).
- Quantitative variables: also called measurement or numerical variables, they represent quantities of different nature. They can be divided into discrete variables that can only take a finite number of values (e.g., the number of rehabilitation sessions, score on a clinical scale, age, etc.),

and continuous variables, which can take values in an infinite/continuous range of possible values (e.g., the temperature of a thermometer, weight, Body Mass Index (BMI), etc.).
- Textual data: data that are directly collected in text format, such as handwritten annotations in medical histories.

In this stage, data profiling [41] and cleaning [42] must be applied to detect potential problems and, if possible, fix them. By categorizing the data, using one of the proposed classifications (or another one that could be useful for a specific use case) independently, or several of them at the same time, the process of the understanding and assimilation of the data available and their scope is facilitated. This step must be carried out to obtain a preliminary database, containing the data collected, that will be called the initial database. For this task, having the support of both a clinical expert and a technologist is recommended. In some cases, when the amount of data to handle is large or coming from different data sources, a data warehouse can be created to integrate all the information and allow the easy and efficient analysis of the data stored [43,44].

During data collection for classification tasks, it is also important to collect enough instances/samples to represent in an appropriate way the different classes that must be predicted. In case there is imbalance regarding the number of samples in the different target classes, this should be identified as part of the data profiling, and some strategies could be applied to deal with this issue [45,46] (e.g., to try to prevent the majority class from dominating the predictions in a harmful way).

Application to Our Case Study

In this case study, the initial database was prepared according to the final goal, which was predicting the presence/absence of cervical pain. The categorization of the data was jointly agreed by physicians and technologists, considering the application of this research in the legal field and the degree of objectivity of the data. According to the four classifications presented, the data from our case study could be classified as shown in Table 1, following the exposed criteria:

Table 1. Possible classifications of the case study data.

1. Clinical Data and Patient Data	2. Data According to the Degree of Objectivity	3. Data According to the Clinical Considerations	4. Data According to Their Data Types
Patient characterization data: - Identification: name, age, gender, educational level, etc. - Temporary: accident date, visits to the hospital, date of the range of motion (ROM) test, etc. - Anthropometric: weight, height, body mas index, foot length, etc. - Daily life activities: physical activity intensity, workplace, etc.	Measures: all the data from the MoCap sensors or Whiplash scale (WDQ).	Clinical profile: - Symptoms: pain periodicity, feeling of instability, limitation of mobility, etc. - Signs: contracture, limitation of mobility, spinal column alterations, etc.	Qualitative variables: educational level, limitation of mobility, contracture, etc.
Clinical data: feeling of instability, surgery, all the data from the MoCap sensors, etc.	Assessed data: contracture, limitation of mobility, Jackson contraction, etc.	Treatment: n/a.	Quantitative variables: - Discrete: WDQ, age, etc. - Continuous: all the data from the MoCap sensors, weight, height, etc.
	Reported data: pain periodicity, feeling of instability, etc.	Clinical scales or tests: WDQ.	Textual data: n/a.
		Medical history: accident date, visits to the hospital, etc.	

The classifications shown in Table 1 illustrate different useful perspectives of the data collected in the case study. Specifically, and considering the final goal of objectively predicting the presence of cervical pain, the classification that best suited the point of view of the health professionals participating in our case study was the following (a combination of the first two classification approaches described):

- Patient characterization data: the data measured and reported, such as the identification information (e.g., ID, age, gender, etc.), anthropometrics (e.g., height, weight, BMI, etc.), and data relative to the activities of daily life (e.g., weekly physical activity and its intensity, workplace, etc.).
- Assessed and reported data: such as the characterization of a cervical accident (e.g., the time since the accident, type of impact of the traffic accident, position of the head, type of effect, etc.), qualitative signs (e.g., column alterations and contractures), clinical scales (e.g., whiplash scale—WDQ), and symptoms (e.g., instability, limitation of mobility, etc.).
- Measured data: such as data from a cervical assessment test with MoCap or from each movement studied, for example the angles reached and the speeds of the movements (e.g., maximum values, minimum values, average values, etc.).

For the purposes of medical legal/forensic assessments, a classification according to the degree of objectivity of the clinical data (assessed and reported) is of interest. Thanks to the understanding of an expert technologist in insurance litigation, it has been possible to identify objective information in the case study, such as the presence of a contracture, column alterations, the WDQ, the characterization of the traffic accident (in case such an event had occurred), etc.

The initial database is presented as Supplementary Material File S1, which collects the dataset that has been considered for the development of the model.

3.3. Stage 3: Data Transformation

Once the data to be considered in the initial database have been selected, certain transformations of the data must be performed in order to handle empty values, perform data transformations to define the required variables and adapt them to the required format, and ensure the anonymization of the data.

The information obtained from the different sources can correspond to variables already defined and structured or to raw data, and it can be presented as numerical, text, curves, images, etc. [47]. Transforming raw data into the format required for the application of specific ML algorithms is a common pre-processing step to be performed, and it could also be useful because the volume of data to be handled could be reduced, and its predictive power could be significantly increased, making it possible to have a significantly lower volume of data to achieve a reliable and stable predictive model [5,19]. To be exploited by traditional DM and ML algorithms, textual data can be transformed into structured variables and different text mining techniques can be applied [48,49]. Besides, depending on the purpose, unsupervised learning approaches can be applied on the texts—for example, for dimensionality reduction (e.g., using the Self-Organizing Map (SOM) method [50]), for clustering documents according to their similarity, or for discovering topics in documents (e.g., probabilistic topic modeling by using Latent Dirichlet Allocation) [51].

This stage of transformation of raw data is known as feature engineering and is performed prior to modelling [52]. In some cases, several data mining techniques can be applied to extract features from raw data. For example, Principal Component Analysis (PCA), like the SOM method mentioned above, is a dimensionality reduction method that is often used to reduce the dimensionality of large data sets; it can be used to tackle the problem of high dimensionality that appears in some projects when the number of variables is excessively high compared to the total number of samples (see Section 3.5) [39]. In the field of healthcare, the following types of transformations can be highlighted:

- Texts that become "positive or negative opinions", concepts, dates, values, etc., through the application of text mining techniques [53,54].

- Images of medical tests that are converted into binary variables related to a pathology or other binary representations.
- Curves or other graphical representations from which information can be extracted as statistical variables, such as the mean, standard deviation, skewness, quartiles, etc.
- Different imputation techniques [18,55–57] that can be applied in order to fill empty values, either by means of interpolation or by using other procedures. Alternatively, some records may need to be discarded (e.g., if several key data values are missing).
- The potential addition or creation of variables based on the knowledge of clinical experts and technologists, either as a combination of existing variables or based on experience acquired in similar studies [30].
- Data anonymization, applied in order to preserve the privacy of patients [58]. The trade-off between privacy and information loss should be considered. A detailed analysis of data anonymization techniques for health data is out of the scope of this work but, for illustration purposes, some examples of transformations that can be applied to guarantee the privacy of sensitive information are:
    - Transformation of continuous variables (e.g., age, size, weight, income, etc.) into ordinal variables by defining suitable ranges. Normalization (e.g., min-max normalization) or standardization (z-score scaling) techniques could also be applied to transform the quantitative variables into variables in the range from 0 to 1.
    - Transformation of qualitative variables (e.g., diagnosis, treatment, education level, etc.), that could be classified, according to a scale, into ordinal variables (e.g., severity of diagnosis, treatment risks, range of studies ("high school", "BS", "MS", "PhD"), etc.). In this way, these variables cannot be associated with a specific patient, thus preserving the patient's privacy.
    - Transformation of qualitative variables (e.g., nationality, physical description, address, etc.), that could not be classified according to a scale into groups (e.g., by continents or country grouping, by groups according to a general description, by postal code, etc.) so that these variables cannot be associated with a specific patient.
    - The previous anonymization techniques are examples of the generalization of attribute values. Other possible techniques and privacy-preservation methodologies include adding noise [59], k-anonymity [60], differential privacy [61], etc.

Another important aspect to mention here is the need for the normalization of quantitative attributes; if we have quantitative variables with very different scales, the variables that can take larger values could end up dominating others when learning a predictive model. This is unsuitable because it mistakenly attributes more importance to those variables just because their usual values are higher than the values of other variables.

After applying the specified transformations, the initial database is transformed to an encoded (modified) database, which includes all the available information in the format of multiple variables.

Application to Our Case Study

In the case of the cervical pain assessment study, this process consisted of transforming the data from the MoCap sensors into variables (i.e., mean, deviation, maximum, minimum, etc., of the range of the movement) and transforming the clinical and characterization data of the patients into variables considering sensitive variables and their anonymization. Some ranges of variables were associated with a numeric coding to improve the anonymization process and the generation of the predictive model. The process was carried out jointly by a clinical expert and a technologist. As in our case study we have transformed all the quantitative variables into discrete variables, no additional normalization was needed. The following are examples of the transformations performed (the numeric coding used is indicated in brackets):

- Age transformation in a three-tier classification: under 30 (0), between 30 and 55 (1), and over 55 (2).
- Transformation of the level of weekly exercise into a classification of three levels as a function of the time required and the intensity of the exercise: slight (0), moderate (1), and intense (2).
- Transformation of the level of studies in a classification of three levels with their assigned numerical coding: basic/high school (0), medium/bachelor (1), and superior/university studies (2).
- Weight transformation in a three-tier classification: less than 60 Kg (0), between 60 and 85 Kg (1), and greater than 85 Kg (2).
- Height transformation in a three-level classification: less than 158 cm (0), between 158 and 185 cm (1), and greater than 185 cm (2).
- Transformation of the body mass index (BMI) into a three-tier classification: under 24 (0), between 24 and 30 (1), and over 30 (2).
- Grouping of the cervical pain periodicity to create a variable of three levels: sporadic (0), discontinuous (1), and frequent (2).

The completeness and quality of the data recorded is also a key aspect in any ML pipeline, and particularly in the health area. In our case study, some variables were initially incomplete, due to the lack of collected data from certain patients (five patients). These incomplete data were related to specific features (e.g., the workplace of the patient, his/her age, the dominant side of his/her body, the date of the traffic accident, etc.), and were later collected by a telephone call.

The encoded database is presented as Supplementary Material File S2, where the variables are obtained after the transformations that are carried out from the initial database are collected and the anonymized variables are highlighted (see Variable_View).

3.4. Stage 4: Data Selection

The next stage is to filter the encoded database obtained in the previous phase and select the most useful variables, applying different filters in a way that will lead to obtaining a filtered database, which will be the basis of the predictive model. Possible successive filters to be used include the following:

1. Filters due to ethical and legal issues: Discard personal or private variables and those that are unimportant for the purpose of the predictive model, such as names, clinical history numbers, telephone numbers, and addresses. The filtered database must be anonymous with respect to existing regulations on the protection of personal data, so a previous anonymization process becomes essential in order to keep as much important data as possible. Notice that during the previous step (data transformation, see Section 3.3), some data are transformed to increase privacy; in this step, privacy might need to be further increased by not selecting some sensitive data in case those data have not been properly transformed previously or in the case of other sensitive data that are irrelevant for predictions.
2. Manual selection: Screening based on the needs set by the target of the prediction, removing outliers or variables with a lot of missing data [5]. It is highly recommended that this filtering be conducted by an expert in the healthcare field.
3. Automated attribute selection: specific software and algorithms can be used for filtering, calculating the gain ratio for each of the variables and rejecting those with low predictive power—for example, using regression techniques.

Application to Our Case Study

In our case study, the encoded database initially included 230 variables in the initial dataset (the "Coded database"), which were reduced to 28 after the following consecutive filtering steps (see Table 2):

1. The removal of variables related to personal and ethical data not anonymized previously and with no predictive power. The variables name, surname, telephone number, address, and email were removed in this filtering.
2. Manual filtering performed by physicians and technologists, corresponding to non-objective or inappropriate variables in the medical legal/forensic field (e.g., the sensation of instability, mobility limitation, pain periodicity, etc.), as well as variables with missing data that could not be completed (e.g., the position of the head and type of effect in case of a traffic accident, intensity of work, etc.). In this filtering, 74 variables were removed according to the criteria indicated.
3. Finally, a filtering was applied based on the gain ratio of the variables. We used the IBM SPSS modeler software [62] (v. 18), discarding 123 variables with low predictive power (we selected those with a gain ratio higher than 0.95 out of 1). Variables such as the average angle, standard deviation, complementary angle, weight, height, etc., were selected. The selection of these 28 variables is consistent with the target variable (the presence or absence of pain) and its associated requirements, since it is a desirable situation for clinicians that these variables are objective, represent the main cervical movements, and correspond to clinical data objectively acquired by the clinicians.

Table 2. Final variables considered in the case study after feature selection.

Patient Characterization Data	Gender		Age		Educational Level	
Clinical data: assessed and reported data	Contracture		Traffic accident		Spinal column alterations	WDQ
Clinical data: data measured with sensors	Mean Speed [°/s] in:		Flex.-Ext.		Rotation	Lateralization
	Max Speed [°/s] in:		Flexion		Right Rotation	Right Lateral
			Extension		Left Rotation	Left Lateral
	Max Angle [°] in:		Flexion		Right Rotation	Right Lateral
			Extension		Left Rotation	Left Lateral
	Total Range [°] in:		Flex.-Ext.		Rotation	Lateralization
	Total Length [°] in:		Flex.-Ext.		Rotation	Lateralization

Table 2 shows the 28 final variables of the filtered database; the detailed information of each variable, with the different associated values for the different data instances, is included as Supplementary Material File S3.

3.5. Stage 5: Predictive Model Generation and Evaluation

In the next stage, a predictive model according to the established objective is designed based on the filtered database obtained in the previous stage. To do this, we must select those algorithms that are considered viable for the specific clinical project, such as decision trees, neural networks, or support vector machines (SVM), among others [63]. If the volume of data is very high, the use of specific support software can facilitate selecting a suitable algorithm by performing iterations before generating the full predictive model. For example, the IBM SPSS modeler classifier node (v. 18) can create several models and then compare them to select the best approach for a particular analysis.

In this stage, the performance of the selected algorithms should be tested to choose the most convenient one to implement in the predictive model. To evaluate their stability and effectiveness, different cross-validation approaches can be considered [19,30,64–66]. The simplest method consists of separating the sample into two sub-samples: one to train the model and another one to test it (holdout method). Other more advanced methods include dividing the sample into k sub-samples (k-fold cross validation), stratifying the sample with the same percentage of each class (stratified k-fold cross validation), or even making as many combinations as the number of data instances (leave-one-out cross validation). Furthermore, a validation set could be used (besides the "test set" and the "training set"), which is a set of examples used to tune the parameters of a classifier [67]. This is useful because the performance of the selected algorithms can be improved through parameter tuning, which consists of varying values of parameters of the algorithms in order to find the most suitable configuration for each of them. Once the suitable parameter configuration for each algorithm is selected, the performance of the different algorithms can be compared.

It must be stressed that the most appropriate prediction method depends on the data. Besides, overfitting (a phenomenon that occurs when the adjustment of the model to the training data is too strong and, as a consequence, finds difficulties in obtaining suitable conclusions about unobserved data) should be avoided, as this would lead to a model that will only be able to make predictions for the data with which it has been trained [52]. There are several techniques to deal with this, such as regularization (smoothing the models), data augmentation (increasing the training data), early stopping, etc. As an example, early stopping implies that the training process of the model must be stopped before overfitting [30,68,69], that is, before the model adjusts too much to the training data (i.e., before the performance of model gets worse on the validation data).

Over-parametrization is a recurrent problem in the application of ML techniques in healthcare, where there are cases where the ratio between variables and data is very high and overfitting effects can occur. The opposite can also happen when the volume of data is very high, but the number of variables is excessively reduced and/or has little predictive power. Therefore, if needed, depending on the results obtained we could come back to Stage 4 "Data Selection" to reduce the number of variables. As a guideline, to avoid over-parametrization the 1 to 10 ratio between variables (attributes or features) and data (number of instances) should not be exceeded [20,52]. If there was a smaller ratio between the variables and data, a more exhaustive screening of variables would have to be carried or a larger sample would have to be obtained. In terms of classification, having an excessive number of variables will lead to not solving the problem or not achieving the proposed objective because the model will only be able to classify the training data correctly [70].

To select the most suitable algorithm for the project, it is necessary to follow an organization strategy, storing each previous version and modification of the project [52]. In this way, the results are contrasted (training data, validation, errors, etc.). After the selection of the most effective algorithm, we will be able to generate the definitive predictive model that incorporates the already-existing filtered database. If the predictive model were evaluated positively, a continuous learning process could begin by receiving periodic information from the assessment tests performed on future patients, as shown in Figure 3.

Application to Our Case Study

In view of the target of our clinical study to classify the presence of cervical pain, only supervised learning algorithms must be selected, dismissing unsupervised learning algorithms. The algorithms selected in our study were logistic regression [71], decision trees [72], random forests [73], SVM [73], neural networks (MLP neural networks) [74], k-Nearest Neighbors (KNN) [73], and Gradient Boosting Algorithm (GBA) [75]. All these are popular supervised machine learning approaches. The main parameters selected to perform the parameter tuning of those algorithms are shown in Table 3. In our experimental evaluation, we combined the parameters of each algorithm presented in Table 3 using the software tool Weka [76] (v. 3.8); specifically, for the parameter tuning we used the Weka Experimenter user interface.

Table 3. ML approaches considered and their main parameters.

Approach	Main Parameters
Logistic regression	Ridge value in the log-likelihood: from 10^{-4} to 10^{-12} (parameter change every 10^{-2}).
Decision tree (C4 pruned)	Number of instances per leaf: 3/5/10/15/20. Confidence factor for pruning (Conf.): 0.15/0.25/0.35.
Random forest	Maximum depth of the tree: 3/4/5. Number of trees: 25/50/100/200.
Support vector machine (SVM)	Tolerance: 10^{-3}. Kernel function: radial basis function (RBF). Epsilon for round-off error: 10^{-12}. Complexity (C): 0.25/0.5/1/2/4. Gamma (kernel width): 0.01/0.25/0.5/1/2.
Neural Network (MLP neural network)	Type: multilayer perceptron (MLP). Learning Rate (LR, the amount the weights are updated): 0.2/0.3/0.4/0.5. Momentum (Mom., applied to the weights during updating): 0.1/0.2/0.3. Number of epochs for training: 500. Number of hidden layers: 15. Auto-built option in Weka set to true.
K-Nearest Neighbors (KNN)	Number of Neighbors (K): 1/3/5/7/9/11/13/15/20. Distance function: Euclidean distance, Manhattan distance.
Gradient Boosting Algorithm (GBA)	Iterations (Iter.): 10/20/50/100. Weight threshold (W.T.): 50/100/200. AdaBoost implementation provided by Weka.

In our case study, the predictive models generated by applying the previously selected algorithms are shown in Table 3. As mentioned previously, the DM software used in this study was Weka (v. 3.8). Considering the current availability of data for our case study, the performance of each parameter configuration of each algorithm was tested using a validation set which is the same as the test set; using the same set for validation and testing is not the ideal situation, but we decided not to reserve a part of the available dataset for validation because of the moderate size of our sample. We considered the accuracy metric (i.e., the percentage of instances correctly classified) for determining the most suitable algorithm configuration. Figure 5 shows the performance of the algorithms obtained during parameter tuning using a k-fold cross validation (k = 10).

Consequently, the parameter configuration selected for each algorithm is shown in the first row of Table 4. The effectiveness of the models generated by k-fold cross validation (k = 10) was evaluated. The following metrics were computed in order to determine the most suitable algorithms (see Table 4): the accuracy (the percentage of instances correctly classified), the precision (the percentage of patients with pain correctly classified over all the patients labelled by the algorithms as patients with pain), the recall/sensitivity (the percentage of patients with pain correctly classified over all the patients with real pain), the specificity (the percentage of healthy patients correctly classified over all the patients who are really healthy), and the F1-score (the harmonic average of the precision and recall).

We have noticed using the software Weka, which provides the attribute weights of each model in the results display section, that the variables with greater predictive power in all the predictive models evaluated are the following: maximum speed in all the movements, the existence of a traffic accident, and the presence of a contracture. In our case study, there is no indication of over-parametrization; as described in Section 3.4, we have a sample of 302 instances and 28 selected variables, which complies with the 1 to 10 ratio between the variables and data.

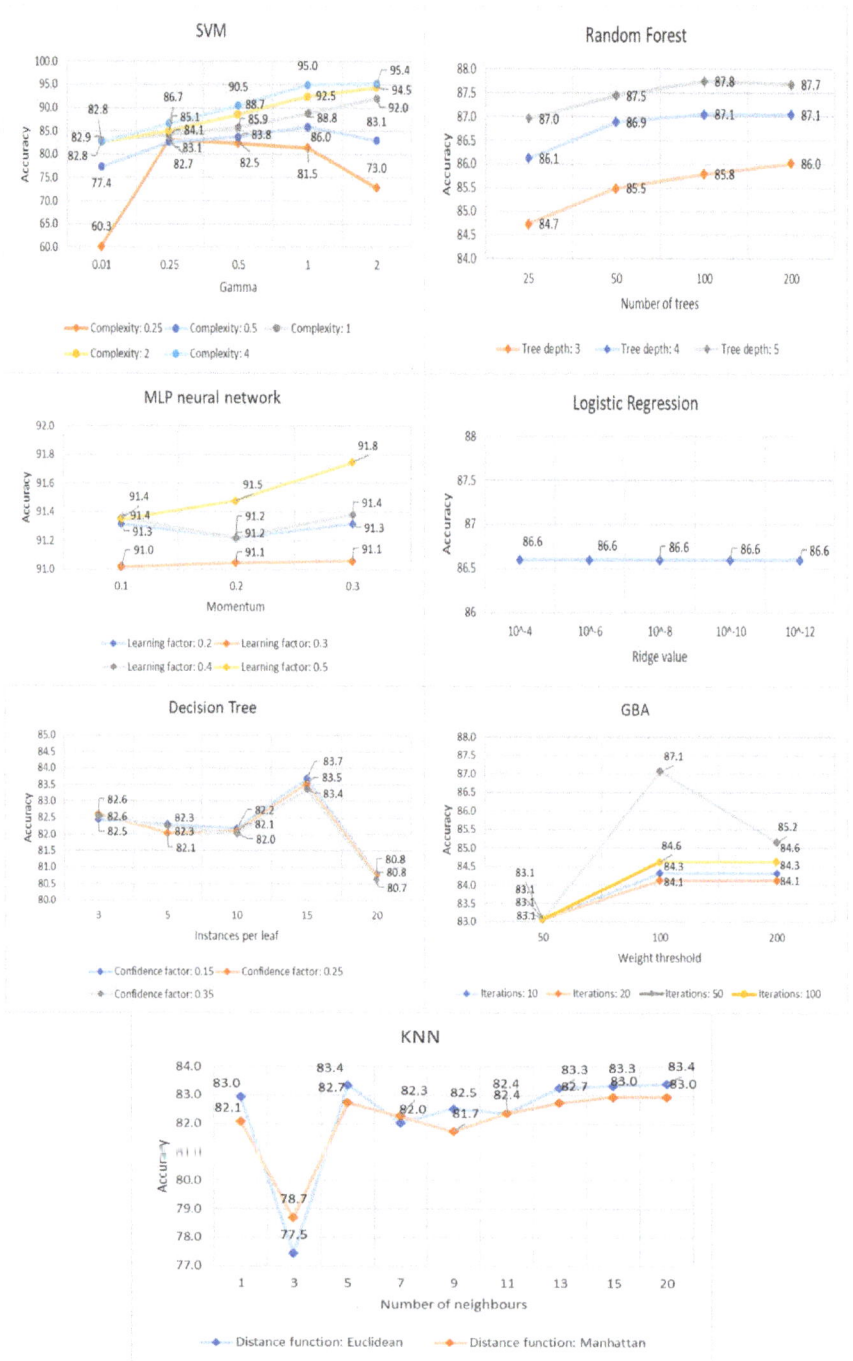

Figure 5. Parameter tuning of the seven algorithms selected.

Table 4. Metrics considered for algorithm selection and the results obtained for each algorithm.

	Logistic Regression	SVM	Decision Tree	Random Forest	MLP Neural Network	KNN	GBA
Parameter Selection	Ridge: 10^{-8}	C: 4; Gamma: 2	Instances per leaf: 15; Conf.: 0.15	Trees: 200 Depth: 5	LR: 0.5; Mom.: 0.3	K: 20; Euclidean	Iterat.: 50 W.T.:100
Accuracy	86.6%	95.4%	83.7%	87.7%	91.8%	83.4%	87.1%
Precision	88.6%	95.4%	86.9%	86.1%	93%	83.5%	87.1%
Recall/Sensitivity	89.6%	97.8%	84.1%	92.3%	92.5%	91.2%	92.9%
Specificity	82.5%	91.7%	80.8%	76.6%	90.5%	71.7%	78.3%
F1 Score	89.1%	95.3%	85.5%	88.9%	92.8%	83.2%	86.9%

3.6. Stage 6: Interpretation of Results and Model Selection

Once a statistically acceptable predictive model has been created, it can be deployed to be used in production, since it can provide predictions with good accuracy to support decision-making (Figure 4, stage 6). However, for the exploitation of the model, it is necessary first to evaluate the degree of correlation between the results obtained and the previously defined clinical target (in our case study, the prediction of cervical pain). Besides, some models (e.g., the tree-based classifiers) could be explored to analyze which particular features are the most decisive factors in the classification model.

If the evaluation of the correlation does not yield satisfactory results—that is, if the consonance of the results with the target is not achieved or the model does not have enough predictive power according to the minimum goals established initially—the previous stages must be repeated with the objective of improving and optimizing the process according to the target initially set, leading to an iterative process (see Figure 4) [20,77]. There can be several causes of low correlation or poor predictive power:

- The target is difficult to achieve or too complex;
- Patients are inadequately characterized;
- The sample is insufficient;
- The data include variables that are not necessary (e.g., irrelevant variables, confounding factors, or redundant variables) or do not include those that are;
- Problems exist in the predictive model generation stage regarding the selected algorithm [78], overfitting, or over-parameterization.

For effective deployment, not only the accuracy of the models but also the resources must be considered. For example, the scalability requirements are key when you have high volumes of data to avoid very long training times, lack of memory, etc. This is important in terms of productivity, portability, cost reduction, the minimization of staff involvement, etc. In cases where large volumes of data have been collected for many years (cancer studies, studies of discharge from the hospital and sick leaves, etc.), scalability acquires a transcendental role [30].

Application to Our Case Study

Based on the results collected in Table 4, a quite good performance of all the algorithms can be observed for most metrics. Considering the large number of variables available initially, the rigor with which all the data were obtained by the multidisciplinary team, and the adequate selection of variables carried out in previous phases (choosing the objective variables and with a greater predictive power), a suitable prediction performance was initially expected.

Considering the minimal target values of the statistical measures established in Stage 1 "Clinical target definition", several algorithms fulfil the requirements in terms of the target metrics:

- Accuracy (>85%): logistic regression, SVM, random forest, MLP neural network, and GBA.
- Precision (>85%): logistic regression, SVM, decision tree random forest, MLP neural network, and GBA.

- Recall (>90%): SVM, random forest, MLP neural network, kNN, and GBA.

According to the results, the four algorithms that fulfil the requirements are SVM, random forest, the MLP neural network, and GBA. From all these algorithms, SVM achieves the best results in all the metrics considered, and therefore it could be the model selected for production.

3.7. Stage 7: Operating Profit and Clinical Use

The last stage (Figure 4, stage 7) concerns the adaptation and organization of the acquired knowledge and the predictive capacity of the system to make it accessible to the physician [47]. At this point, it is important to emphasize the key role played by the expert medical professionals (final decision makers) in interpreting the results, in determining whether certain patterns observed make medical sense and are relevant, or in clearly distinguishing between correlation and causality (as studied for different heath topics [79,80]). The "intelligence" provided is not intended to replace the physician but to advise and guide his/her decisions, which will always prevail [20].

Application to Our Case Study

The results obtained directly by the model may involve difficulties when interpreted by the physicians. That is why the information presented to them must be intuitive, simple, and easily interpretable. In this regard, a concise graphic and clear report, where the results of the test and the prediction of the pathology/target variable to be predicted are presented, can help the clinical to more easily interpret the test performed and the results of the predictive model. This paper is accompanied by a report example as Supplementary Material File S4, showing a possible example of a report for our case study that includes patient data, test results in a tabular and graphic format, and an area showing the prediction of cervical pain obtained by the model.

Once the model enters production, it will be possible to add data regarding new patients both with or without cervical pain and verified diagnosis, which would increase the sample and thus the predictive power.

4. Discussion and Lessons Learnt

In this paper, the particularities of applying ML techniques in the field of healthcare are shown, developing all the stages that comprise it, to generate reliable and stable models. It has been exemplified through a case study of cervical pain evaluation, where we have been able to predict the presence of cervical pain with accuracy, precision, and recall above 85% with the approaches based on SVM, random forest, MLP neural networks, and GBA.

In order to clarify and structure the knowledge acquired during the development of the current study, a summary of some key aspects and lessons learnt regarding DM and ML in the field of healthcare is shown in Table 5. Every key aspect has been categorized in a general classification, followed by a description, the real situation exemplified in our case study, and some important related references.

Table 5. Summary of the key aspects and lessons learnt.

Category	Key Aspect	Description	Case Study	Sample References
Clinical target	Proper selection	Clinical target definition according to the aims and clinical needs. This facilitates the subsequent selection of data.	Presence of cervical pain. Only collaborating subjects and objective variables were selected.	[34,40]
	Definition of statistical measures	Minimum metrics to be fulfilled by the model according to the clinical target. Metrics are checked in stage 6 (interpretation of results) after the predictive model generation.	Performance required: accuracy: greater than 85%; precision: greater than 85%; recall: greater than 90%.	[39]

Table 5. Cont.

Category	Key Aspect	Description	Case Study	Sample References
Data	Identification and understanding	Diversity of the origins of data in healthcare (regarding typology, consistency, and veracity) and need to correctly understand the data. A health expert is required in this stage.	Prior to the field work, relevant clinical information was identified and the tests to perform were determined.	[34]
	Clear and concise structure	Categorization of data using appropriate variables/features, applying classifications motivated by medical needs. This is essential to carry out an adequate analysis of the information.	Data classification motivated by clinical staff and forensic experts: patient characterization data, assessed and reported clinical data, measured clinical data.	[30]
	Data transformations in healthcare	Feature engineering. Reducing the raw data to be handled and adapting them to the required format in order to increase the predictive power.	Variables such as the age, level of studies, weight, height, etc., were transformed into discrete variables. Ranges of variables were associated with a numeric code.	[5,19,47,52]
	Anonymization	Preservation of sensitive patient data by transforming values of data variables into scales or groups, thus avoiding patient identification. This is a key aspect in healthcare data management.	No quantitative variables remained after the anonymization process (through transformation into discrete variables and the removal of identifying attributes) that could be associated with patients.	[58]
	Selection	After data transformation, the selection of variables applying a filter according to the target:ethical and legal issues, manual selection, automated attribute selection.	The volume of data in the case study was reduced from 230 variables to 28 after applying the three successive aforementioned filters.	[19,21]
	Normalization	Normalization of quantitative attributes avoiding situations where variables that can take larger values could end up dominating others.	No quantitative variables remained after anonymization.	[55–57]
	Completeness	Completeness and quality of the data recorded as a key aspect in the health area.	Incomplete data from 5 patients related to specific features were collected through a telephone call.	[81]
	Over-parametrisation	Need not to exceed the 1 to 10 ratio between variables and data to avoid overfitting. The dimensionality is an issue in studies with a high number of variables compared to the total number of samples.	This was a real issue in our case study because of the volume of data provided by sensors. A sample of 302 and 28 variables was finally selected, which complies with the 1 to 10 ratio.	[20]

Table 5. *Cont.*

Category	Key Aspect	Description	Case Study	Sample References
	Scalability	Support for handling large amounts of data (efficient and effective collection, storage, management, and exploitation). Depending on the project duration, and especially if it is intended to have an adaptive character (projects with data collected for many years), scalability is a key issue to consider.	The current project is still in an initial stage, with no large-scale deployment. No scalability problems have been detected.	[30]
Predictive model	High recall and relatively high precision	Minimization of the number of false negatives (increasing recall). This is a key goal in healthcare, since false negatives and false positives have no similar costs in this area. The precision should also be suitable, as a high number of false positives would lead to false alarms, the performance of needless procedures, and increasing costs and discomfort for the patients.	The selected algorithms (SVM, random forest, MLP neural network, and GBA) have recall >90%.	[39]
Project work procedure	Multidisciplinary work as a key point	Composing teams involving technical people and diverse health professionals. This is required, but not always possible. Insufficient collaboration could be diminished by applying the stages assigned to each of the professionals in a concise and structured way.	There was interaction between professionals in almost all the stages. Nevertheless, more interventions could be encouraged because clinical experts were not present in stage 5.	[34,52]
	Continuous data collection	Improvement of the model performance thanks to a continuous learning process.	There is an intention to improve the current system by incorporating data of new collaborating patients.	[30]
MoCap	Sensors/devices in healthcare	Complementary objective tests to help physicians.	We expect the applicability of the proposal in the forensic field as an objective system of application to aid in judicial processes.	[19,82]

Data structuring. A clear and concise structuring of the data is essential to carry out an adequate analysis of the information as well as to make this information really useful for the purposes of the predictive model. In our case study, and prior to the field work, the relevant clinical information was identified and the tests to perform were determined (cervical ROM in three different planes with a MoCap system of inertial sensors), so that its processing and subsequent structuring were easier. It is essential to accurately structure the available information in a suitable way (using appropriate variables/features) when working with large volumes of data, and to classify the different variables in different groups (using appropriate categories) to facilitate access (for all the parties involved) in a more effective and useful way. Data management is so important that the preparation of the data covers three of the seven stages of the methodology (stages 2, 3, and 4).

Selection of variables. Likewise, the selection of the most adequate information to predict a certain characteristic, as well as its transformation in terms of variables, is essential. In relation to this adaptation, sensitive patient data must be anonymized for their use in the generation of a predictive model [19,21]. Although converting continuous predictors to discrete variables (specifically binary variables) is not always recommended [20], the necessary transformation of data for privacy reasons in the field of health conditions the stage of data transformation. The reduction in the volume of data in the case study was from 230 variables to 28 due to the large number of variables provided by the inertial sensors and the clinical data. The variable reduction applied (based on the gain ratio of the variables) after the corresponding selection of the data for ethical and legal issues and the screening made by an expert was necessary to fulfil the 1 to 10 ratio between the variables and data. This key point allowed us to ensure that the predictive models work properly, maximizing the predictive power and avoiding overfitting.

Selection of the predictive model. Regarding the selection of the predictive model, after performing a parameter tuning of the seven selected algorithms and comparing the most suitable configuration of each of them (see Figure 5), it was concluded that the models that meet the established requirements regarding accuracy, precision, and recall for the case study were SVM, random forest, MLP neural networks, and GBA. Our results highlight the low number of false negatives achieved (high recall), a fundamental aspect in healthcare studies [39]. These results are in agreement with other investigations of a similar nature, using the same software (Weka), in terms of the accuracy, precision, recall, and F1 score with the SVM and random forest algorithms [36].

Variability of the measures acquired. It has been detected that it is possible to assess the measurement capacity of our medical equipment in terms of the variability of the measures that it obtains. A *series* variable identifies whether the data are relative to the first measure of each subject or to the second (which was performed consecutively). The results obtained by the predictive models showed that there were no differences between the two series of cervical ROM (this variable had the lowest predictive power among all the variables introduced in the model). This result indicates that the measure has behaved stably in collaborating subjects. This result is interesting in the forensic field due to the following reason. If repeating the cervical ROM test in a patient results in significant differences, they would not be derived from the variability of the test, but by the type of pathology that prevents the patient from repeating the test normally. Alternatively, the patient may try to simulate or magnify the lesion by not showing consistent results between the first and second series. This aspect would be of relevance to judicial experts [29,83].

Data collection in production. Once the system is applied in its context and has been developed, continuous data collection must be planned in production in order to improve the prediction accuracy, resulting in a continuous learning system (Figure 3). In the case study, to increase the sample in the exploitation stage of the model it is possible to include those patients who perform cervical assessment tests in a care or rehabilitation setting; thus, their sincerity can be assumed regarding the degree of cervical pain as well as full collaboration in the performance of the tests. However, for the collection of training data it may be necessary to exclude those patients who are immersed in a judicial and indemnifying process and who report cervical pain because their degree of collaboration or sincerity is unknown. In the future, the system can be used to predict the cervical pain of non-collaborating patients (e.g., patients in a judicial process or patients with a high degree of anxiety or hypochondriacs) from the predictive model previously generated with collaborating patients, serving as objective evidence in judicial proceedings with insurance companies [40].

Multidisciplinarity. For a correct interpretation of the results, multidisciplinary work is a key point, since the contribution of each of the branches of knowledge is necessary in this type of project to optimize the possibilities offered by the model. In this way, it will be possible to assess the statistical quality of the results and their medical utility. For example, in our case study questions were raised regarding the way the data and the results should be represented (solved with the databases defined and the design of a report for physicians, presented as Supplementary Material), the possible interpretation and use of the system by the clinician (problems could have arisen if we had not been worked in close collaboration with the clinicians; however, the target variable and how to present the results were clarified from the beginning of the project), and the overlap with other possible decision-support systems (if other systems could also provide in the future a prediction indicating that a patient suffers cervical pain, both results would be presented to the clinician and he/she would take the final decision). Through collaboration with the medical experts, these issues have been solved. However, multidisciplinary work is not always possible, since professionals participate in different stages of the entire process according to their degree of knowledge, experience, and training, so in some cases there may be no direct or sufficient interaction between them [34]. This lack of interaction among professionals could be diminished by following the stages assigned to each of the professionals in a concise and structured way, thus avoiding problems that may lead to project failure [52]. In the case study, the rigor followed by the different professionals involved in the different stages have resulted in adequate results. Nevertheless, although there has been interaction between them, it could have been done in a more collaborative way, since clinical experts were not present in the generation of the predictive model and the interpretation of the results, which could have improved the quality of the study thanks to its specific medical knowledge.

Exploitation of sensor data. The use of sensors and devices with the use of ML could be implemented as a complementary objective test to help physicians. This type of test could constitute an aid to the decision-making in the diagnosis or treatment, or if there is doubt about the veracity of the information reported by the patient [19,82]. Although we wanted to show the clinical utility of this type of technology, the lack of studies on the application of ML techniques with motion capture sensors in healthcare, and specifically their applicability in the forensic field as an objective system of application in judicial processes, have further motivated the choice of the case study. Therefore, while our case study focuses on the medical legal/forensic field, the procedure proposed to use ML techniques could be applied in any study of the health field (cancer detection, studies of discharge from the hospital and sick leave, etc.).

Use of resources. Regarding the frequency and regularity of data acquisition, it is necessary to previously estimate it to limit the duration of the project [34], as well as to quantify the necessary storage size, which is a factor with high variability between projects. If the project is intended to have an adaptive character that can be applied or expanded for subsequent research, the scalability and magnitude should be considered. If the scalability of the project is not considered, and the intention is to continue acquiring data and adapting the model to the continuous growth of information, there may come a time when the project is no longer viable because it is unable to assimilate the corresponding increase in data size. This situation is common in epidemiological projects of data collection for large periods of time, where the scalability is transcendental for the future of the project [30]. On the other hand, it is important to consider that, in certain projects as in the case study presented in this paper, the ratio between available variables and data can be high. So, not exceeding the 1 to 10 ratio between variables and data is transcendental to avoid overfitting effects [20].

5. Conclusions and Future Work

Through a practical guide, the stages and particularities to consider for the application of ML techniques in the field of healthcare have been described, considering all the stages involved in the process. This procedure is shown through objective cervical functional assessment tests that use MoCap technology with inertial sensors and a predictive model whose goal is to estimate the presence of cervical pain from the data collected with the test. Four models (SVM, random forest, MLP neural network, and GBA) from the seven models initially generated obtained an accuracy and precision of more than 85% and a recall of more than 90% (i.e., the percentage of false negatives is smaller than 10%). The approach and the results obtained could help objectify diagnoses, improve test treatment efficacy, and save resources in healthcare systems. The procedure, which has been applied to data derived from a cervical assessment study for verification and evaluation, is also appropriate for any healthcare field regardless of the origin of the data. It can be useful, for example, in gait studies [82], balance studies [84], cardiac failure studies [85], the prediction of events [86], fertility tests [87], etc.

Despite the great usefulness of ML in the field of healthcare, some limitations have been detected in this field. First, a major limitation is how to achieve a suitable flow of data from health centers and hospitals, as well as the accessibility (in relation to privacy policies and authorizations) [21], gathering, and integration of the data [3]. If a global information collaboration policy were established between hospitals [6,69,88], the problem of access to information could be solved, and it would be possible to share more data and feed the predictive models applied to the field of healthcare more efficiently. The explainability of predictions [89,90] is an important issue in a health care domain, as it could increase the trust in the ML systems (for both clinicians and patients) and even lead to the acquisition of new knowledge; however, more research on how to achieve explainability while considering the potential trade-off with accuracy must be performed, especially in the health domain.

Regarding the limitations of the conclusions obtained with this case study, once the model is in the exploitation stage it would be advisable to carry out an external validation to verify the viability of the model in terms of geography, temporality, etc. [30,77]. Regarding the data sample used in our case study, its size has been large enough to obtain good results, but it would be relevant to see the impact of increasing it, as new data about patients becomes available, to enable a continuous learning process that could lead to better results over time. Besides, a study is currently being conducted to check the accuracy of the proposed models with a sample of non-collaborating patients.

Concerning the target variable (presence of cervical pain), which is a binary variable, it could be defined in a more granular way considering not only the presence of pain but also its intensity (as a continuous variable or as a discrete variable with several pain degrees). The problem with pain intensity is that pain scales are highly dependent on the subjectivity of the patient, and this issue could be further exacerbated with non-collaborating subjects. However, as a future goal of our research, it could be useful to tackle this issue and introduce some statistical techniques, such as the numerical measurement z-score, to normalize the subjective values from pain intensity scales (e.g., the Visual Analogue Scale) provided by the patients. The z-score could help to reduce the bias of patients, allowing us to include pain intensity as a target variable in our proposal.

Finally, as future work, it could also be interesting to extend the range of experiments performed and analyze the potential interest of other ML methods; for example, we could consider applying different classifiers applied over different categories of data proposed in the paper and combine them into an ensemble.

Supplementary Materials: The following materials are available online at http://www.mdpi.com/2076-3417/10/17/5942/s1, File S1: Initial database. File S2: Coded database. File S3: Filtered database. File S4: Report for physician.

Author Contributions: Conceptualization, J.d.l.T., J.M., S.I., and J.J.M.; data curation, J.d.l.T., J.M., and J.J.M.; formal analysis, J.d.l.T., J.M., S.I., and J.J.M.; funding acquisition, S.I. and J.J.M.; investigation, J.d.l.T.; methodology, J.d.l.T., J.M., and J.J.M.; project administration, J.J.M.; resources, S.I. and J.J.M.; software, J.d.l.T. and J.J.M.; supervision, S.I. and J.J.M.; validation, J.d.l.T.; visualization, J.d.l.T.; writing—original draft preparation, J.d.l.T., J.M., and J.J.M.; writing—review and editing, J.d.l.T., J.M., S.I., and J.J.M. All authors have read and agreed to the published version of the manuscript.

Funding: This project was co-funded by the Government of Aragon, the European Regional Development Fund and the University of Zaragoza. We thank the support of the project TIN2016-78011-C4-3-R (AEI/FEDER, UE) and the Government of Aragon (Group Reference T64_20R, COSMOS research group).

Acknowledgments: We thank Mapfre insurance company (Zaragoza, Spain) for allowing us to use their facilities. We also thank the I3A—University Institute of Research of Engineering of Aragon, University of Zaragoza, Zaragoza, Spain—for the materials and support they provided.

Conflicts of Interest: The authors declare no conflict of interest.

Abbreviations

The following abbreviations are used in this manuscript:

BMI	Body Mass Index
CEICA	Bioethics Committee of Aragón
CRISP-DM	CRoss-Industry Standard Process for Data Mining
DLA	Daily life activities
DM	Data Mining
EMG	Surface Electromyography
GBA	Gradient Boosting Algorithm
KDD	Knowledge Discovery in Databases
KNN	K-Nearest Neighbors
MAE	Mean Absolute Error
ML	Machine Learning
MLP	MultiLayer Perceptron
MoCap	Motion Capture
PCA	Principal component analysis
RMSE	Root Mean Squared Error
ROM	Range of Movement
SEMMA	Sample, Explore, Modify, Model, and Assess
SVM	Support Vector Machine
WDQ	Whiplash Scale

References

1. Kayyali, B.; Knott, D.; Van Kuiken, S. *The Big-Data Revolution in US Health Care: Accelerating Value and Innovation*; Mc Kinsey Co.: New York, NY, USA, 2013; Volume 2, pp. 1–13.
2. Tomar, D.; Agarwal, S. A survey on Data Mining approaches for Healthcare. *Int. J. Bio-Sci. Bio-Technol.* **2013**, *5*, 241–266. [CrossRef]
3. Koh, H.C.; Tan, G. Data mining applications in healthcare. *J. Healthc. Inf. Manag.* **2011**, *19*, 65.
4. Maity, N.G.; Das, S. Machine learning for improved diagnosis and prognosis in healthcare. In Proceedings of the 2017 IEEE Aerospace Conference, Big Sky, MT, USA, 4–11 March 2017; pp. 1–9.
5. Yoo, I.; Alafaireet, P.; Marinov, M.; Pena-Hernandez, K.; Gopidi, R.; Chang, J.-F.; Hua, L. Data Mining in Healthcare and Biomedicine: A Survey of the Literature. *J. Med. Syst.* **2012**, *36*, 2431–2448. [CrossRef]
6. Sen, I.; Khandelwal, K. Data Mining in Healthcare. 2018. Available online: https://www.researchgate.net/publication/322754945_DATA_MINING_IN_HEALTHCARE (accessed on 26 August 2020).
7. Clavel, D.; Mahulea, C.; Albareda, J.; Silva, M. A Decision Support System for Elective Surgery Scheduling under Uncertain Durations. *Appl. Sci.* **2020**, *10*, 1937. [CrossRef]
8. Cruz, J.A.; Wishart, D.S. Applications of Machine Learning in Cancer Prediction and Prognosis. *Cancer Inform.* **2006**, *2*, 59–77. [CrossRef]
9. Wang, F.; Stiglic, G.; Obradovic, Z.; Davidson, I. Guest editorial: Special issue on data mining for medicine and healthcare. *Data Min. Knowl. Discov.* **2015**, *29*, 867–870. [CrossRef]
10. Rosales, R.E.; Rao, R.B. Guest Editorial: Special Issue on impacting patient care by mining medical data. *Data Min. Knowl. Discov.* **2010**, *20*, 325–327. [CrossRef]
11. Alotaibi, S.; Mehmood, R.; Katib, I.; Rana, O.; Albeshri, A. Sehaa: A Big Data Analytics Tool for Healthcare Symptoms and Diseases Detection Using Twitter, Apache Spark, and Machine Learning. *Appl. Sci.* **2020**, *10*, 1398. [CrossRef]
12. Huang, Z.; Dong, W.; Bath, P.; Ji, L.; Duan, H. On mining latent treatment patterns from electronic medical records. *Data Min. Knowl. Discov.* **2015**, *29*, 914–949. [CrossRef]
13. Bentham, J.; Hand, D.J. Data mining from a patient safety database: The lessons learned. *Data Min. Knowl. Discov.* **2012**, *24*, 195–217. [CrossRef]
14. Obenshain, M.K. Application of Data Mining Techniques to Healthcare Data. *Infect. Control. Hosp. Epidemiol.* **2004**, *25*, 690–695. [CrossRef] [PubMed]
15. Zhang, P.; Wang, F.; Hu, J.; Sorrentino, R. Towards Personalized Medicine: Leveraging Patient Similarity and Drug Similarity Analytics. *AMIA Summits Transl. Sci. Proc.* **2014**, *2014*, 132. [PubMed]
16. Hamet, P.; Tremblay, J. Artificial intelligence in medicine. *Metab. Clin. Exp.* **2017**, *69*, S36–S40. [CrossRef] [PubMed]

17. Joyner, M.J.; Paneth, N. Seven Questions for Personalized Medicine. *JAMA* **2015**, *314*, 999–1000. [CrossRef]
18. Weiss, J.C.; Natarajan, S.; Peissig, P.L.; McCarty, C.A.; Page, D. Machine Learning for Personalized Medicine: Predicting Primary Myocardial Infarction from Electronic Health Records. *AI Mag.* **2012**, *33*, 33–45. [CrossRef]
19. Mannini, A.; Sabatini, A.M. Machine Learning Methods for Classifying Human Physical Activity from On-Body Accelerometers. *Sensors* **2010**, *10*, 1154–1175. [CrossRef]
20. Moons, K.; Kengne, A.P.; Woodward, M.; Royston, P.; Vergouwe, Y.; Altman, U.G.; Grobbee, D.E. Risk prediction models: I. Development, internal validation, and assessing the incremental value of a new (bio)marker. *Heart* **2012**, *98*, 683–690. [CrossRef]
21. Wilkowska, W.; Ziefle, M. Privacy and data security in E-health: Requirements from the user's perspective. *Heal. Inform. J.* **2012**, *18*, 191–201. [CrossRef]
22. Dolley, S. Big Data Solution to Harnessing Unstructured Data in Healthcare. IBM Report. 2015. Available online: https://assets.sourcemedia.com/31/a6/cb1b019c4d6cb338fab539eea360/ims14428usen.pdf. (accessed on 26 August 2020).
23. Andersen, R.M.; Davidson, P.L.; Baumeister, S.E. Improving access to care. In *Changing the US Health Care System: Key Issues in Health Services Policy and Management*; John Wiley & Sons: Hoboken, NJ, USA, 2013; pp. 33–70.
24. Marin, J.; Blanco, T.; Marin, J.J. Research Lines to Improve Access to Health Instrumentation Design. *Procedia Comput. Sci.* **2017**, *113*, 641–646. [CrossRef]
25. Cassidy, J.D.; Carroll, L.; Côté, P.; Lemstra, M.; Berglund, A.; Nygren, Å. Effect of Eliminating Compensation for Pain and Suffering on the Outcome of Insurance Claims for Whiplash Injury. *N. Engl. J. Med.* **2000**, *342*, 1179–1186. [CrossRef]
26. Moreno, A.J.; Utrilla, G.; Marin, J.; Marin, J.J.; Sanchez-Valverde, M.B.; Royo, A.C. Cervical Spine Assessment with Motion Capture and Passive Mobilization. *J. Chiropr. Med.* **2018**, *17*, 167–181. [CrossRef] [PubMed]
27. Utrilla, G.; Marín, J.J.; Sanchez-Valverde, B.; Gomez, V.; JAuria, J.M.; Marin, J.; Royo, C. *Cervical Mobility Testing in Flexion-Extension and Protraction-Retraction to Evaluate Whiplash Syndrome Through Motion Capture*; Universidad de Zaragoza: Zaragoza, Spain, 2017.
28. Marín, J.J.; Pina, M.J.B.; Gil, C.B. Evaluación de Riesgos de Manipulación Repetitiva a Alta Frecuencia Basada en Análisis de Esfuerzos Dinámicos en las Articulaciones sobre Modelos Humanos Digitales. *Cienc. Trab.* **2013**, *15*, 86–93. [CrossRef]
29. Marín, J.; Boné, M.; Ros, R.; Martínez, M. Move-Human Sensors: Sistema portátil de captura de movimiento humano basado en sensores inerciales, para el análisis de lesiones musculoesqueléticas y utilizable en entornos reales. In Proceedings of the Sixth International Conference on Occupational Risk Prevention, Galicia, Spain, 14–16 May 2008.
30. Steyerberg, E.W. *Clinical Prediction Models: A Practical Approach to Development, Validation, and Updating*; Springer: Berlin, Germany, 2009.
31. Fayyad, U.M.; Piatetsky-Shapiro, G.; Smyth, P.; Uthurusamy, R. *Advances in Knowledge Discovery and Data Mining*; AAAI Press: Menlo Park, CA, USA, 1996.
32. Azevedo, A.I.R.L.; Santos, M.F. KDD, SEMMA and CRISP-DM: A Parallel Overview. ISCAP—Informática—Comunicações em Eventos Científicos. 2008. Available online: https://recipp.ipp.pt/handle/10400.22/136 (accessed on 26 August 2020).
33. Chapman, P.; Clinton, J.; Kerber, R.; Khabaza, T.; Reinartz, T.; Shearer, C.; Wirth, R. *CRISP-DM 1.0 Step-by-Step Data Mining Guide*; SPSS Inc.: Chicago, IL, USA, 2000.
34. McGregor, C.; Catley, C.; James, A. A process mining driven framework for clinical guideline improvement in critical care. In Proceedings of the Learning from Medical Data Streams Workshop, Bled, Slovenia, 6 July 2011.
35. Catley, C.; Smith, K.; McGregor, C.; Tracy, M. Extending CRISP-DM to incorporate temporal data mining of multidimensional medical data streams: A neonatal intensive care unit case study. In Proceedings of the 2009 22nd IEEE International Symposium on Computer-Based Medical Systems, Albuquerque, NM, USA, 3–4 August 2009; pp. 1–5.
36. Araujo, F.H.; Santana, A.M.; Neto, P.S. Using machine learning to support healthcare professionals in making preauthorisation decisions. *Int. J. Med. Inform.* **2016**, *94*, 1–7. [CrossRef]
37. Bose, I.; Mahapatra, R.K. Business data mining—A machine learning perspective. *Inf. Manag.* **2001**, *39*, 211–225. [CrossRef]

38. Bhatla, N.; Jyoti, K. An analysis of heart disease prediction using different data mining techniques. *Int. J. Eng.* **2012**, *1*, 1–4.
39. Raschka, S.; Mirjalili, V. *Python Machine Learning*; Packt Publishing Ltd.: Birmingham, UK, 2017.
40. Schuller, E.; Eisenmenger, W.; Beier, G. Whiplash Injury in Low Speed Car Accidents: Assessment of Biomechanical Cervical Spine Loading and Injury Prevention in a Forensic Sample. *J. Musculoskelet. Pain* **2000**, *8*, 55–67. [CrossRef]
41. Naumann, F. Data profiling revisited. *ACM SIGMOD Rec.* **2014**, *42*, 40–49. [CrossRef]
42. Rahm, E.D.H. Data Cleaning: Problems and Current Approaches. *Bull. Tech. Comm. Data Eng.* **2000**, *23*, 3–13.
43. Jannot, A.-S.; Zapletal, E.; Avillach, P.; Mamzer, M.-F.; Burgun, A.; Degoulet, P. The Georges Pompidou University Hospital Clinical Data Warehouse: A 8-years follow-up experience. *Int. J. Med. Inform.* **2017**, *102*, 21–28. [CrossRef]
44. Evans, R.S.; Lloyd, J.F.; Pierce, L.A. Clinical Use of an Enterprise Data Warehouse. *AMIA Annu. Symp. Proc.* **2012**, *2012*, 189–198.
45. Batista, G.E.A.P.A.; Prati, R.C.; Monard, M.C. A study of the behavior of several methods for balancing machine learning training data. *ACM SIGKDD Explor. Newsl.* **2004**, *6*, 20–29. [CrossRef]
46. Batista, G.E.A.P.A.; Prati, R.C.; Monard, M.C. Balancing Strategies and Class Overlapping. *Lect. Notes Comput. Sci.* **2005**, *3646*, 24–35. [CrossRef]
47. Bhardwaj, R.; Nambiar, A.R.; Dutta, D. A Study of Machine Learning in Healthcare. *2017 IEEE 41st Annu. Comput. Softw. Appl. Conf.* **2017**, *2*, 236–241. [CrossRef]
48. Dörre, J.; Gerstl, P.; Seiffert, R. Text mining: Finding nuggets in mountains of textual data. In Proceedings of the Fifth ACM SIGKDD International Conference on Knowledge Discovery and Data Mining (KDD), San Diego, CA, USA, 23–27 August 1999; pp. 398–401.
49. Aggarwal, C.C.; Zhai, C. *Mining Text Data*; Springer Science & Business Media: Berlin, Germany, 2012.
50. Janasik, N.; Honkela, T.; Bruun, H. Text mining in qualitative research: Application of an unsupervised learning method. *Organ. Res. Methods* **2009**, *12*, 436–460. [CrossRef]
51. Blei, D.M. Probabilistic topic models. *Commun. ACM* **2012**, *55*, 77–84. [CrossRef]
52. Henri, L. *Data Scientist y Lenguaje R Guía de Autoformación Para el uso de Big Data*; Francisco, J., Piqueres, J., Eds.; Colecciones Epsilon: Cornellá de Llobregat, Spain, 2017.
53. Stavrianou, A.; Andritsos, P.; Nicoloyannis, N. Overview and semantic issues of text mining. *ACM SIGMOD Rec.* **2007**, *36*, 23–34. [CrossRef]
54. Carlos, T.; Sergio, I.; Carlos, S. Text Mining of Medical Documents in Spanish: Semantic Annotation and Detection of Recommendations. In Proceedings of the 16th International Conference on Web Information Systems and Technologies (WEBIST 2020), Budapest, Hungary, 3–5 November 2020.
55. Donders, A.R.T.; Van Der Heijden, G.J.; Stijnen, T.; Moons, K.G. Review: A gentle introduction to imputation of missing values. *J. Clin. Epidemiol.* **2006**, *59*, 1087–1091. [CrossRef]
56. Farhangfar, A.; Kurgan, L.; Dy, J. Impact of imputation of missing values on classification error for discrete data. *Pattern Recognit.* **2008**, *41*, 3692–3705. [CrossRef]
57. Bennett, D.A. How can I deal with missing data in my study? *Aust. N. Z. J. Public Health* **2001**, *25*, 464–469. [CrossRef]
58. Arbuckle, L.; El Emam, K. *Anonymizing Health Data*; O'Reilly Media, Inc.: Newton, MA, USA, 2013.
59. Kargupta, H.; Datta, S.; Wang, Q.; Sivakumar, K. On the privacy preserving properties of random data perturbation techniques. In Proceedings of the Third IEEE International Conference on Data Mining, Melbourne, FL, USA, 19–22 November 2003; pp. 99–106.
60. El Emam, K.; Dankar, F.; Issa, R.; Jonker, E.; Amyot, D.; Cogo, E.; Corriveau, J.-P.; Walker, M.; Chowdhury, S.; Vaillancourt, R.; et al. A globally optimal k-anonymity method for the de-identification of health data. *J. Am. Med. Inform. Assoc.* **2009**, *16*, 670–682. [CrossRef]
61. Dankar, F.K.; El Emam, K. The application of differential privacy to health data. *Jt. EDBT/ICDT Workshops EDBT-ICDT* **2012**, *2012*, 158–166. [CrossRef]
62. IBM. SPSS Software. Available online: https://www.routledge.com/IBM-SPSS-Statistics-26-Step-by-Step-A-Simple-Guide-and-Reference/George-Mallery/p/book/9780367174354 (accessed on 16 February 2020).
63. Wu, X.; Kumar, V.; Quinlan, J.R.; Ghosh, J.; Yang, Q.; Motoda, H.; McLachlan, G.J.; Ng, A.; Liu, B.; Yu, P.; et al. Top 10 algorithms in data mining. *Knowl. Inf. Syst.* **2007**, *14*, 1–37. [CrossRef]

64. Gupta, P. Cross Validation in Machine Learning. 2020. Available online: https://towardsdatascience.com/cross-validation-in-machine-learning-72924a69872f (accessed on 26 August 2020).
65. Arlot, S.; Celisse, A. A survey of cross-validation procedures for model selection. *Stat. Surv.* **2010**, *4*, 40–79. [CrossRef]
66. Refaeilzadeh, P.; Tang, L.; Liu, H. Cross-Validation. *Encycl. Database Syst.* **2009**, *5*, 532–538.
67. Xu, Y.; Goodacre, R. On Splitting Training and Validation Set: A Comparative Study of Cross-Validation, Bootstrap and Systematic Sampling for Estimating the Generalization Performance of Supervised Learning. *J. Anal. Test.* **2018**, *2*, 249–262. [CrossRef] [PubMed]
68. McCaffrey, J. Neural Network Train-Validate-Test Stopping. 2020. Available online: https://visualstudiomagazine.com/articles/2015/05/01/train-validate-test-stopping.aspx (accessed on 26 August 2020).
69. Ferber, R.; Osis, S.T.; Hicks, J.L.; Delp, S.L. Gait biomechanics in the era of data science. *J. Biomech.* **2016**, *49*, 3759–3761. [CrossRef] [PubMed]
70. Reed, R.; MarksII, R.J. *Neural Smithing: Supervised Learning in Feedforward Artificial Neural Networks*; Mit Press: Cambridge, MA, USA, 1999.
71. Christodoulou, E.; Ma, J.; Collins, G.S.; Steyerberg, E.W.; Verbakel, J.Y.; Van Calster, B.; Evangelia, C.; Jie, M. A systematic review shows no performance benefit of machine learning over logistic regression for clinical prediction models. *J. Clin. Epidemiol.* **2019**, *110*, 12–22. [CrossRef]
72. Bae, J.M. The clinical decision analysis using decision tree. *Epidemiol. Health* **2014**, *36*. [CrossRef] [PubMed]
73. Noi, P.T.; Kappas, M. Comparison of Random Forest, k-Nearest Neighbor, and Support Vector Machine Classifiers for Land Cover Classification Using Sentinel-2 Imagery. *Sensors* **2018**, *18*, 18. [CrossRef]
74. Penny, W.; Frost, D.; Penny, W. Neural Networks in Clinical Medicine. *Med. Decis. Mak.* **1996**, *16*, 386–398. [CrossRef]
75. Zhang, Z.; Zhao, Y.; Canes, A.; Steinberg, D.; Lyashevska, O.; AME Big-Data Clinical Trial Collaborative Group. Predictive analytics with gradient boosting in clinical medicine. *Ann. Transl. Med.* **2019**, *7*. [CrossRef]
76. Witten, I.; Frank, E.; Hall, M.; Pal, C. Appendix B: The WEKA workbench. In *Data Mining: Practical Machine Learning Tools and Techniques*, 4th ed.; Morgan Kaufmann: Burlington, MA, USA, 2016.
77. Moons, K.; Kengne, A.P.; Grobbee, D.E.; Royston, P.; Vergouwe, Y.; Altman, U.G.; Woodward, M. Risk prediction models: II. External validation, model updating, and impact assessment. *Heart* **2012**, *98*, 691–698. [CrossRef] [PubMed]
78. Murphy, C.K. Identifying Diagnostic Errors with Induced Decision Trees. *Med. Decis. Mak.* **2001**, *21*, 368–375. [CrossRef] [PubMed]
79. Zhao, L. The gut microbiota and obesity: From correlation to causality. *Nat. Rev. Genet.* **2013**, *11*, 639–647. [CrossRef] [PubMed]
80. Dab, W.; Ségala, C.; Dor, F.; Festy, B.; Lameloise, P.; Le Moullec, Y.; Le Tertre, A.; Médina, S.; Quenel, P.; Wallaert, B.; et al. Air pollution and health: Correlation or causality? The case of the relationship between exposure to particles and cardiopulmonary mortality. *J. Air Waste Manag. Assoc.* **2001**, *51*, 220–235. [CrossRef] [PubMed]
81. Liu, C.; Talaei-Khoei, A.; Zowghi, D.; Daniel, J. Data completeness in healthcare: A literature survey. *Pac. Asia J. Assoc. Inf. Syst.* **2017**, *9*, 5. [CrossRef]
82. Mannini, A.; Trojaniello, D.; Cereatti, A.; Sabatini, A.M. A Machine Learning Framework for Gait Classification Using Inertial Sensors: Application to Elderly, Post-Stroke and Huntington's Disease Patients. *Sensors* **2016**, *16*, 134. [CrossRef]
83. Ramírez, P.C.; Ordi, H.G.; Fernández, P.S.; Morales, M.I.C. Detección de exageración de síntomas en esguince cervical: Pacientes clínicos versus sujetos análogos. *Trauma* **2014**, *25*, 4–10.
84. De La Torre, J.; Marin, J.; Marin, J.J.; Auria, J.M.; Sanchez-Valverde, M.B. Balance study in asymptomatic subjects: Determination of significant variables and reference patterns to improve clinical application. *J. Biomech.* **2017**, *65*, 161–168. [CrossRef]
85. Austin, P.C.; Tu, J.V.; Ho, J.E.; Levy, D.; Lee, D.S. Using methods from the data-mining and machine-learning literature for disease classification and prediction: A case study examining classification of heart failure subtypes. *J. Clin. Epidemiol.* **2013**, *66*, 398–407. [CrossRef]
86. Choi, E.; Bahadori, M.T.; Schuetz, A.; Stewart, W.F.; Sun, J. Doctor AI: Predicting Clinical Events via Recurrent Neural Networks. *JMLR Work. Conf. Proc.* **2016**, *56*, 301–318.

87. Uyar, A.; Bener, A.; Ciray, H.N. Predictive modeling of implantation outcome in an in vitro fertilization setting: An application of machine learning methods. *Med. Decis. Mak.* **2015**, *35*, 714–725. [CrossRef] [PubMed]
88. Abdelaziz, A.; Elhoseny, M.; Salama, A.S.; Riad, A. A machine learning model for improving healthcare services on cloud computing environment. *Measurement* **2018**, *119*, 117–128. [CrossRef]
89. Hall, P.; Gill, N. *An Introduction to Machine Learning Interpretability*; O'Reilly Media, Inc.: Sebastopol, CA, USA, 2018.
90. Guidotti, R.; Monreale, A.; Ruggieri, S.; Turini, F.; Giannotti, F.; Pedreschi, D. A Survey of Methods for Explaining Black Box Models. *ACM Comput. Surv.* **2018**, *51*, 1–42. [CrossRef]

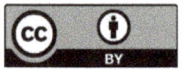

© 2020 by the authors. Licensee MDPI, Basel, Switzerland. This article is an open access article distributed under the terms and conditions of the Creative Commons Attribution (CC BY) license (http://creativecommons.org/licenses/by/4.0/).

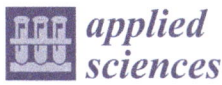

Article

Taylor Bird Swarm Algorithm Based on Deep Belief Network for Heart Disease Diagnosis

Afnan M. Alhassan [1,2,*] and Wan Mohd Nazmee Wan Zainon [1]

1. School of Computer Science, Universiti Sains Malaysia, George Town 11800, Malaysia; nazmee@usm.my
2. College of Computing and Information Technology, Shaqra University, Shaqra 11961, Saudi Arabia
* Correspondence: afnan@student.usm.my

Received: 27 July 2020; Accepted: 18 September 2020; Published: 22 September 2020

Abstract: Contemporary medicine depends on a huge amount of information contained in medical databases. Thus, the extraction of valuable knowledge, and making scientific decisions for the treatment of disease, has progressively become necessary to attain effective diagnosis. The obtainability of a large amount of medical data leads to the requirement of effective data analysis tools for extracting constructive knowledge. This paper proposes a novel method for heart disease diagnosis. Here, the pre-processing of medical data is done using log-transformation that converts the data to its uniform value range. Then, the feature selection process is performed using sparse fuzzy-c-means (FCM) for selecting significant features to classify medical data. Incorporating sparse FCM for the feature selection process provides more benefits for interpreting the models, as this sparse technique provides important features for detection, and can be utilized for handling high dimensional data. Then, the selected features are given to the deep belief network (DBN), which is trained using the proposed Taylor-based bird swarm algorithm (Taylor-BSA) for detection. Here, the proposed Taylor-BSA is designed by combining the Taylor series and bird swarm algorithm (BSA). The proposed Taylor-BSA–DBN outperformed other methods, with maximal accuracy of 93.4%, maximal sensitivity of 95%, and maximal specificity of 90.3%, respectively.

Keywords: deep belief network; heart disease diagnosis; sparse FCM; bird swarm algorithm

1. Introduction

Contemporary medicine depends on a large amount of information accumulated in medical datasets. The extraction of such constructive knowledge can help when making scientific decisions to diagnose disease. Medical data can enhance the management of hospital information and endorse the growth of telemedicine. Medical data primarily focuses on patient care first, and research resources second. The main rationalization to collect medical data is to promote patient health conditions [1]. The accessibility of numerous medical data causes redundancy, which requires effectual and significant techniques for processing data to extract beneficial knowledge. However, the diagnostics of various diseases indicate significant issues in data analysis [2]. Quantifiable diagnosis is performed by adoctor's guidance rather than patterns of the medical dataset; thus, there is the possibility of incorrect diagnosis [3]. Cloud-based services can assist with managing medical data, including compliance management, policy integration, access controls, and identity management [4].

Now a day, heart disease is a foremost source of death. We are moving towards a new industrial revolution; thus, lifestyle changes should take place to prevent risk factors of heart disease, such as obesity, diabetes, hypertension, and smoking [5]. The treatment of disease is a complex mission in medical field. The discovery of heart disease, with different risk factors, is considered a multi-layered issue [6]. Thus, patient medical data are collected to simplify the diagnosis process. Offering a valuable service (at less cost) is a major limitation in the healthcare industry. In [7], valuable quality service refers to the precise diagnosis (and effective treatment) in patients. Poor clinical decisions cause disasters, which may affect the health of patients. Automated approaches, such as the machine-learning approach [8,9] and data mining [10] approach, assist with attaining clinical tests, or diagnoses, at reduced risks [11,12]. The classification and pattern recognition by machine learning algorithms are widely included in prognostic and diagnosis monitoring. The machine learning approach supports decision-making, which increases the safety of the patients and avoids medical errors, so that it can be used in clinical decision support systems (CDSS) [13,14].

Several methods are devised for automatic heart disease detection to evaluate the efficiency of the decision tree and Naive Bayes [15]. Moreover, optimization with the genetic algorithm is employed for minimizing the number of attributes without forfeiting accuracy and efficiency to diagnose heart disease [16]. Data mining methods for heart disease diagnosis include the bagging algorithm, neural network, support vector machine, and automatically defined groups [17]. In [18], the study acquired 493 samples from a cerebrovascular disease prevention program, and utilized three classification techniques (the Bayesian classifier, decision tree, and backpropagation neural network) for constructing classification models. In [19], a method is devised for diagnosing coronary artery disease. The method utilized 303 samples by adapting the feature creation technique. In [20], a methodology is devised for automatically detecting the efficiency of features to reveal heart rate signals. In [21], a hybrid algorithm is devised with K-Nearest Neighbour (KNN), and the genetic algorithm for effectual classification. The method utilized a genetic search as a decency measure for ranking attributes. Then, the classification algorithm was devised on evaluated attributes for heart disease diagnosis. The extraction of valuable information from huge data is a time-consuming task [22]. The size of the medical dataset is increasing in a rapid manner and advanced techniques of data mining help physicians make effective decisions. However, the issues of heart disease data involve feature selection, in which the imbalance of samples and the lack of magnitude of features are just some of the issues [23]. Although there are methods for heart disease detection with real-world medical data, these methods are devised to improve accuracy and time for computation in disease detection [24]. In [25], a hybrid model with the cuckoo search (CS)—and a rough set—is adapted for diagnosing heart disease. The drawback is that a rough set produces an unnecessary number of rules. To solve these challenges in heart disease diagnoses; a novel method, named the Taylor-based bird swarm algorithm–deep belief network (Taylor-BSA–DBN), is proposed for medical data classification.

The purpose of the research is to present a heart disease diagnosis strategy, for which the proposed Taylor-BSA–DBN is employed. The major contribution of the research is the detection of heart disease using selected features. Here, the feature selection is performed using sparse FCM for selecting imperative features. In addition, DBN is employed for detecting heart disease data using the features. Here, the DBN is trained by the proposed Taylor-BSA, in such a way that the model parameters are learned optimally. The proposed Taylor-BSA is developed through the inheritance of the high global convergence property of BSA in the Taylor series. Hence, the proposed Taylor-BSA–DBN renders effective accuracy, sensitivity, and specificity while facilitating heart disease diagnosis.

The major portion of the paper focuses on:

- Proposed Taylor-BSA–DBN for heart disease diagnosis: Taylor-BSA–DBN (a classifier) is proposed by modifying the training algorithm of the DBN with the Taylor-BSA algorithm, which is newly derived by combining the Taylor series and BSA algorithm, for the optimal tuning of weights and biases. The proposed Taylor-BSA–DBN is adapted for heart disease diagnosis.

Other sections of the paper are arranged as follows: Section 2 elaborates the descriptions of conventional heart disease detection strategies utilized in the literature, as well as challenges faced, which are considered as the inspiration for developing the proposed technique. The proposed method for heart disease diagnosis using modified DBN is portrayed in Section 3. The outcomes of the proposed strategy with other methods are depicted in Section 4; Section 5 presents the conclusion.

2. Motivations

This section illustrates eight strategies employed for heart disease diagnosis, along with its challenges.

Literature Survey

Reddy, G.T. et al. [22] devised an adaptive genetic algorithm with fuzzy logic (AGAFL) model for predicting heart disease, which assists clinicians in treating heart disease at earlier phases. The model comprises rough sets with a fuzzy rule-based classification module and heart disease feature selection module. The obtained rules from fuzzy classifiers are optimized by adapting an adaptive genetic algorithm. Initially, the significant features that affect heart disease are chosen using the rough set theory. Then, the second step predicts heart disease with the AGAFL classifier. The method is effective in handling noisy data and works effectively with large attributes. Nourmohammadi-Khiarak et al. [23] devised a method for selecting features and reducing the number of features.

Here, the imperialist competitive algorithm was devised to choose important features from heart disease. This algorithm offers an optimal response in selecting features. Moreover, the k-nearest neighbor algorithm was utilized for classification. The method showed that the accuracy of feature selection was enhanced. However, the method failed to utilize incomplete or missed data. Magesh, G. and Swarnalatha, P. [26] devised a model using Cleveland heart samples for heart disease diagnosis. The method employed cluster-based Decision Tree learning (CDTL) for diagnosing heart disease. Here, the original set was partitioned using target label distribution. From elevated distribution samples, the possible class was derived. For each class set, the features were detected using entropy for diagnosing heart disease. Thiyagaraj, M. and Suseendran, G. [27] developed Particle Swarm Optimization and Rough Sets with Transductive Support Vector Machines (PSO and RS with TSVM) for heart disease diagnosis. This method improved data integrity to minimize data redundancy. The normalization of data was carried out using Zero-Score (Z-Score). Then, the PSO was employed for selecting the optimal subset of attributes, reduce computational overhead, and enhance prediction performance. The Radial Basis Function-Transductive Support Vector Machines (RBF-TSVM) classifier was employed for heart disease prediction. Abdel-Basset, M. et al. [28] devised a model using Internet of Things (IoT) for determining and monitoring heart patients. The goal of the healthcare model was to obtain improved precision for diagnosis. The neutrosophic multi-criteria decision-making (NMCDM) technique was employed for aiding patients (i.e., for observing patients suffering from heart failure). Moreover, the model provided an accurate solution that decreases the rate of death and the cost of treatment. Nilashi, M. et al. [24] devised a predictive technique for heart disease diagnosis with machine learning models. Here, the method adapted unsupervised and supervised learning for diagnosing heart disease. In addition, the method employed Self-Organizing Map, Fuzzy Support Vector Machine (FSVM), and Principal Component Analysis (PCA) for missing value assertion. Moreover, incremental PCA and FSVM are devised for incremental learning of data to minimize the time taken for computation in disease prediction. Shah, S.M.S. et al. [29] devised an automatic diagnostic technique for diagnosing heart disease. The method evaluated the pertinent feature subset by employing the benefits of feature selection and extraction models. For accomplishing the feature selection, two algorithms: accuracy based feature selection algorithm (AFSA) and Mean Fisher based feature selection algorithm (MFFSA) for heart disease diagnosis. However, the method failed to employ PCA for dimension reduction. Acharjya, D.P. [25] devised a hybrid method for diagnosing heart disease. The method combined the cuckoo search (CS) and rough set to infer decision rules. Moreover, the CS was employed for discovering essential features. In addition, three major features were evaluated with rough set rules. The method improved feasibility, but failed to induce an intuitionistic fuzzy rough set and CS for diagnosing heart disease.

3. Proposed Taylor-BSA–DBN for Medical Data Classification

The accessibility of a large amount of medical data led to the requirement of strong data analysis tools for extracting valuable knowledge. Researchers are adapting data mining and statistical tools for improving the analysis of data on huge datasets. The diagnosis of a disease is the foremost application in which data mining tools are offering triumphant results. Medical data tend to be rich in information, but poor in knowledge. Thus, there is a deficiency of effectual analysis tools for discovering hidden relation and trends from medical data generated from clinical records. The processing of medical data brings a manifestation if it has some powerful methods. Thus, the proposed Taylor-BSA–DBN is devised to process medical data for attaining effective heart disease diagnosis. Figure 1 portrays the schematic view of the proposed Taylor-BSA–DBN for heart disease diagnosis. The complete process of the proposed model is pre-processing feature selection, and detection. At first, the medical data is fed as an input to the pre-processing phase, wherein log transformation is applied to pre-process the data. Log transformation is applied for minimizing skew, and to normalize the data. Once the pre-processed data are obtained, then it is further subjected to the feature selection phase. In the feature selection phase, the imperative features are selected with Sparse FCM. After obtaining imperative features, the detection is performed with DBN, wherein the training of DBN is carried out using Taylor-BSA. The proposed Taylor-BSA is devised by combining the Taylor series and BSA. The output produced from the classifier is the classified medical data.

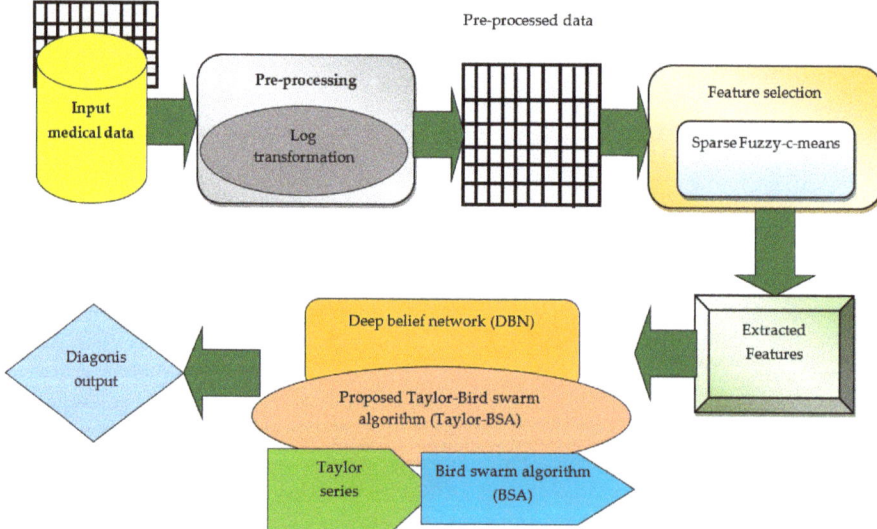

Figure 1. Schematic view of the proposed Taylor-based bird swarm algorithm (Taylor-BSA)–deep belief network (DBN) for heart disease diagnosis.

Consider an input medical data be given as A, with various attributes, and is expressed as

$$A = \{A_{G,H}\}; (1 \leq G \leq B); (1 \leq H \leq C) \tag{1}$$

where $A_{G,H}$ denotes H^{th} attribute in G^{th} data, B specifies a total number of data, and C specifies total attributes in each data. The dimension of the database is represented as $[B \times C]$.

3.1. Pre-Processing

The importance of pre-processing is to facilitate smoother processing of the input data. Additionally, the pre-processing is carried out for eliminating the noise and artefacts contained in the data.

In this method, the pre-processing is carried out by using log transformation, in which data are replaced with a log function, wherein the base of the log is set by the analyst (maybe 2, or 10). The process is used to compress the massive data. In addition, the log transformation has extensively adapted the method to solve skewed data and assist data normalization. The log transformation is formulated as,

$$D = \log_{10}(A) \tag{2}$$

The dimension of pre-processed dataset A becomes $[B \times C]$.

3.2. Selection of Features with Sparse FCM Clustering

The pre-processed data are fed to the feature selection module, considering the Sparse FCM algorithm [30], which is the modification of the standard FCM. The benefit of using Sparse FCM is to provide high dimensional data clustering. The pre-processed data contain different types of attributes, each indicating individual value. In the medical data classification strategy, the sparse FCM is applied for determining the features from the data. The sparse FCM clustering algorithm clusters nodes, to attain communication between nodes through the cluster head, and facilitate effective detection of the attacker node. Generally, in sparse FCM, dimensional reduction is effective, poses the ability to handle disease diagnosis without delay, and is easier with optimization techniques.

3.3. Classification of Medical Data with Proposed Taylor-BSA-Based DBN

In this section, medical data classification using the proposed Taylor-BSA method is presented, and the classification is progressed using the feature vector.

3.3.1. Proposed Taylor-BSA Algorithm

The proposed Taylor-BSA is the combination of the Taylor series and BSA. The Taylor series [31] explains the functions of complex variables, and it is the expansion of a function into an infinite sum of terms. It not only serves as a powerful tool, but also helps in evaluating integrals and infinite sums. Moreover, the Taylor series is aone-step process, and it can deal with higher-order terms. The Taylor series seems to be advantageous for derivations, and can be used to get theoretical error bounds. Above all, the Taylor series ensures the accuracy of classification. Moreover, it is a simple method to solve complex functions. BSA [32] is duly based on the social behaviors of birds that follow some idealistic rules. BSA is more accurate than other standard optimizations with highly efficient, accurate, and robust performances. In addition, there is a perfect balance between exploration and exploitation in BSA. The DBN has recently become a popular approach in machine learning for its promised advantages, such as fast inference and the ability to encode richer and higher order network structures. DBN is used to extract better feature representations, and several related tasks are solved simultaneously by using shared representations. Moreover, it has the advantages of a multi-layer structure, and pre-training with the fine-tuning learning method. The algorithmic steps of the proposed Taylor-BSA are described below:

Step 1. Initialization: the first step is the initialization of population and other algorithmic parameters, including: $F_{i,j}$; $(1 \leq i \leq j)$, where, the population size is denoted as j, h_{max} represent maximal iteration, *prob* indicate the probability of foraging food, and the frequency of flight behavior of birds is expressed as Ft.

Step 2. Determination of objective function: the selection of the best position of the bird is termed as a minimization issue. The minimal value of error defines the optimal solution.

Step 3. Position update of the birds: for updating the positions, birds have three phases, which are decided using probability. Whenever the random number $Rand(0,1) < prob$, then the update is based on foraging behavior, or else the vigilance behavior commences. On the other hand, the swarm splits as scroungers and producers, which is modeled as flight behaviors. Finally, the feasibility of the solutions is verified and the best solution is retrieved.

Step 4. Foraging behavior of birds: the individual bird searches for the food based on its own experience, and the behavior of the swarm, which is given below. The standard equation of the foraging behavior of birds [32] is given by,

$$F_{i,j}^{h+1} = F_{i,j}^h - F_{i,j}^h Rand(0,1)[Z+T] + Rand(0,1)[P_{i,j}Z + Y_j T] \quad (3)$$

where, $F_{i,j}^{h+1}$ and $F_{i,j}^h$ denotes the location of ith bird in j^{th} dimension at $(h+1)$ and h, $P_{i,j}$ refers to the previous best position of the ith bird, $Rand(0,1)$ is independent uniformly distributed numbers, Y_j indicates the best previous location shared by the birds swarm, Z denotes the cognitive accelerated coefficients, and T denotes the social accelerated coefficients. Here, Z and T are positive numbers.

According to the Taylor series [31], the update equation is expressed as,

$$F_{i,j}^{h+1} = 0.5F_{i,j}^h + 1.3591F_{i,j}^{h-1} - 1.359F_{i,j}^{h-2} + 0.6795F_{i,j}^{h-3}$$
$$-0.2259F_{i,j}^{h-4} + 0.0555F_{i,j}^{h-5} - 0.0104F_{i,j}^{h-6} + 1.38e^{-3}F_{i,j}^{h-7} - 9.92e^{-5}F_{i,j}^{h-8} \quad (4)$$

$$F_{i,j}^h = \frac{1}{0.5}\left[\begin{array}{l} F_{i,j}^{h+1} - 1.3591F_{i,j}^{h-1} + 1.359F_{i,j}^{h-2} - 0.6795F_{i,j}^{h-3} + 0.2259F_{i,j}^{h-4} \\ -0.0555F_{I,j}^{h-5} + 0.0104F_{i,j}^{h-6} - 1.38e^{-3}F_{i,j}^{h-7} + 9.92e^{-5}F_{i,j}^{h-8} \end{array}\right] \quad (5)$$

Substituting Equation (5) in Equation (3),

$$F_{i,j}^{h+1} = F_{i,j}^h - \left[\begin{array}{c} 2F_{i,j}^{h+1} - 2.7182F_{i,j}^{h-1} + 2.718F_{i,j}^{h-2} - 1.359F_{i,j}^{h-3} \\ -0.4518F_{i,j}^{h-4} - 0.111F_{i,j}^{h-5} + 0.0208F_{i,j}^{h-6} - 0.00276F_{i,j}^{h-7} + 0.0001984F_{i,j}^{h-8} \\ Rand(0,1)[Z+T] + Rand(0,1)\left[P_{i,j}Z + Y_j T\right] \end{array}\right] \quad (6)$$

$$F_{i,j}^{h+1} + 2F_{i,j}^{h+1} = F_{i,j}^h + \left[\begin{array}{c} 2.7182F_{i,j}^{h-1} - 2.718F_{i,j}^{h-2} + 1.359F_{i,j}^{h-3} \\ +0.4518F_{i,j}^{h-4} + 0.111F_{i,j}^{h-5} - 0.0208F_{i,j}^{h-6} + 0.00276F_{i,j}^{h-7} - 0.0001984F_{i,j}^{h-8} \\ Rand(0,1)[Z+T] + Rand(0,1)\left[P_{i,j}Z + Y_j T\right] \end{array}\right] \quad (7)$$

$$3F_{i,j}^{h+1} = F_{i,j}^h + \left[\begin{array}{c} 2.7182F_{i,j}^{h-1} - 2.718F_{i,j}^{h-2} + 1.359F_{i,j}^{h-3} \\ +0.4518F_{i,j}^{h-4} + 0.111F_{i,j}^{h-5} - 0.0208F_{i,j}^{h-6} + 0.00276F_{i,j}^{h-7} - 0.0001984F_{i,j}^{h-8} \\ Rand(0,1)[Z+T] + Rand(0,1)\left[P_{i,j}Z + Y_j T\right] \end{array}\right] \quad (8)$$

$$F_{i,j}^{h+1} = \frac{1}{3}\left[F_{i,j}^h + \left[\begin{array}{c} 2.7182F_{i,j}^{h-1} - 2.718F_{i,j}^{h-2} + 1.359F_{i,j}^{h-3} \\ +0.4518F_{i,j}^{h-4} + 0.111F_{i,j}^{h-5} - 0.0208F_{i,j}^{h-6} + 0.00276F_{i,j}^{h-7} - 0.0001984F_{i,j}^{h-8} \\ Rand(0,1)[Z+T] + Rand(0,1)[P_{i,j}Z + Y_j T] \end{array}\right]\right] \quad (9)$$

Step 5. Vigilance Behavior of Birds: the birds move towards the center, during which, the birds compete with each other; the vigilance behavior of birds is modeled as,

$$F_{i,j}^{h+1} = F_{i,j}^h + V_1\left(\mu_j - F_{i,j}^h\right) \times Rand(0,1) + V_2\left[U_{oj} - F_{i,j}^h\right] \times Rand(-1,1) \quad (10)$$

$$V_1 = w_1 \times \exp\left(\frac{-RQ(U)_i}{\Sigma RQ + \psi} \times v\right) \quad (11)$$

$$V_2 = w_2 \times \exp\left[\left(\frac{RQ(U)_i - RQ(U)_T}{|RQ(U)_T - RQ(U)_i| + \psi}\right) \frac{v \times RQ(U)_T}{\Sigma RQ + \psi}\right] \quad (12)$$

where, V represents the number of birds, w_1 and w_2 are the positive constants lying in the range of $[0,2]$, $RQ(U)_i$ denotes the optimal fitness value of ith bird, and ΣRQ corresponds to the addition of the best fitness values of the swarm. ψ be the constant that keeps optimization away from zero-division error. T signifies the positive integer.

Step 6. Flight Behavior: this behavior is of the birds' progress, when the birds fly to another site in case of any threatening events and foraging mechanisms. When the birds reach a new site, they search for food. Some birds in the group act as producers and others as scroungers. The behavior is modeled as,

$$F_{i,j}^{h+1} = F_{i,j}^h + Rand\ r(0,1) \times F_{i,j}^h \tag{13}$$

$$F_{i,j}^{h+1} = F_{i,j}^h + \left(F_{\gamma,j}^h - F_{i,j}^h\right) \times Fl \times Rand(0,1) \tag{14}$$

where, $Random\ (0,1)$ refer to the Gaussian distributed random number with zero-mean and standard deviation.

Step 7. Determination of best solution: the best solution is evaluated based on error function. If the newly computed solution is better than the previous one, then it is updated by the new solution.

Step 8. Terminate: the optimal solutions are derived in an iterative manner until the maximum number of iterations is reached. The pseudo-code of the proposed Taylor-BSA algorithm is illustrated in Algorithm 1.

Algorithm 1. Pseudocode for the proposed Taylor-BSA algorithm

Input: Bird swarm population $W_{k,l}$; $(1 \leq k \leq b)$
Output: Best solution

Procedure:
Begin
  Population initiation: $F_{i,j}$; $(1 \leq i \leq p)$
  Read the parameters: b – population size; h_{max}
maximal iteration, $prob$–probability of foraging food, Fl-frequency of flight behavior of birds
  Determine the fitness of the solutions
  While $h < h_{max}$
  For $k = 1 : b$
    If $Rand(0,1) < prob$
      Foraging behavior using Equation (3)
    Else
      Vigilance behavior using Equation (12)
    End if
  End for
  Else
  Split the swarm as scroungers and producers
    For $k = 1 : b$
      If k is a producer
        Update using Equation (13)
      Else
        Update using Equation (14)
      End if
    End for
  Check the feasibility of the solutions
  Return the best solution
  $h = h + 1$
  End while
  Optimal solution is obtained
End

3.3.2. Architecture of Deep Belief Network

The DBN [33] is a subset of Deep Neural Network (DNN) and comprises different layers of Multilayer Perceptrons (MLPs) and Restricted Boltzmann Machines (RBMs). RBMs comprise of visible and hidden units that are associated with weights. The basic structural design of the DBN is illustrated in Figure 2.

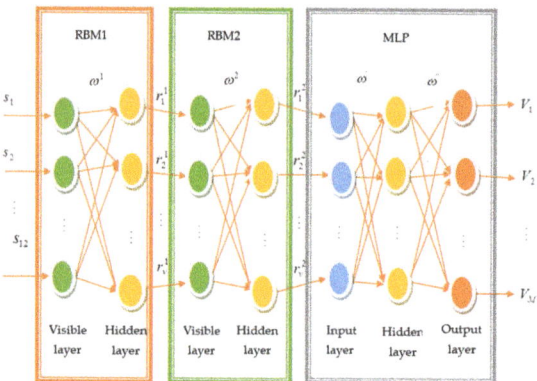

Figure 2. Architectural view diagram of DBN classifier.

Training of Deep Belief Network

This section elaborates on the training process of the proposed Taylor-BSA–DBN classifier. A RBM has unsupervised learning based on the gradient descent method, whereas MLP performs a supervised learning method using the standard backpropagation algorithm. Therefore, the training of DBN is based on a gradient descent–backpropagation algorithm. Here, the most appropriate weights are chosen optimally for the update. The training procedure of the proposed DBN classifier is described below,

I. Training of RBM Layers A training sample N is given as the input to the first layer of RBM. It computes the probability distribution of the data and encodes it into the weight parameters. The steps involved in the training process of RBM are illustrated below.

1. The input training sample is read and the weight vector is produced randomly.
2. The probability function of each hidden neuron in the first RBM is calculated.
3. The positive gradient is computed using a visible vector and the probability of the hidden layer.
4. The probability of each visible neuron is obtained by reconstructing the visible layer from the hidden layer.
5. The probability of reconstruction of hidden neurons is obtained by resampling the hidden states.
6. The negative gradient is computed.
7. Weights are updated by subtracting the negative gradient from the positive gradient.
8. Weights are updated for the next iteration, using the steepest or gradient descent algorithm.
9. Energy is calculated for a joint configuration of the neurons in the visible and the hidden layers.

II. Training of MLP The training procedure in MLP is based on a backpropagation approach by feeding the training data, which are the hidden output of the second RBM layer through the network. Analyzing the data, the network is adjusted iteratively until the optimal weights are chosen. Moreover, Taylor-BSA is employed to compute the optimal weights, which are determined using the error function. The training procedure is summarized below.

1. Randomly initialize the weights.

2. Read the input sample from the result of the preceding layer.
3. Obtain the average error, based on the difference between the obtained output and the desired output.
4. Calculate the weight updates in the hidden and the visible layers.
5. Obtain the new weights from the hidden and the visible layers by applying gradient descent.
6. Identify the new weights using the updated equation of Taylor-BSA.
7. Estimate the error function using gradient descent and Taylor-BSA.
8. Choose the minimum error and repeat the steps.

4. Results and Discussion

This section elaborates on the assessment of the proposed strategy with classical strategies for medical data classification using accuracy, sensitivity, and specificity. The analysis is done by varying training data. In addition, the effectiveness of the proposed Taylor-BSA–DBN is analyzed.

4.1. Experimental Setup

The implementation of the proposed strategy is carried out using Java libraries via Java Archive (JAR) files, utilizing a PC, Windows 10 OS, 2GB RAM, and an Intel i3 core processor. The simulation setup of the proposed system is depicted in Table 1.

Table 1. Simulation setup.

Parameter	Value
Number of input layers	2
Number of hidden layers	2
Number of output layers	1
Cluster size	5 to 9
Number of selected features in Cleveland dataset	123
Number of selected features in Hungarian dataset	139
Number of selected features in Switzerland dataset	139
Learning rate	0.1

4.2. Dataset Description

The experimentation is done using Cleveland, Hungarian, and Switzerland datasets taken from healthcare data based on University of California Irvine (UCI) machine learning repository [34], which is commonly used for both detection and classification. The Cleveland database is taken from the Cleveland Clinical Foundation contributed by David W. Aha. The Hungarian dataset is obtained from the Hungarian Institute of Cardiology. The Switzerland dataset is obtained from the University Hospital, Basel, Switzerland. The dataset comprises of 303 number of instances and 75 attributes, ofwhich, 13 attributes are employed for experimentation. Furthermore, the dataset is characterized as multivariate with integer and real attributes. The attributes (features), such asresting blood pressure (trestbps), maximum heart rate achieved (thalach), the slope of the peak exercise ST segment (slope), age (age), sex (sex), fasting blood sugar (fbs), ST depression induced by exercise relative to rest (oldpeak), chest pain (cp), serum cholesterol (chol), exercise-induced angina (exang), resting electrocardiographic results (restecg), number of major vessels (0–3) colored by fluoroscopy (ca), and 3 = normal; 6 = fixed defect; 7 = reversible defect (thal).

4.3. Evaluation Metrics

The performance of the proposed Taylor-BSA–DBN is employed for analyzing the methods, including accuracy, sensitivity, and specificity.

4.3.1. Accuracy

The accuracy is described as the degree of closeness of an estimated value with respect to its original value in optimal medical data classification, and it is represented as,

$$Accuracy = \frac{T^p + T^n}{T^p + T^n + F^p + F^n} \tag{15}$$

where, T^p represent true positive, F^p indicate false positive, T^n indicate true negative, and F^n represents false negative, respectively.

4.3.2. Sensitivity

This measure is described as the ratio of positives that are correctly identified by the classifier, and it is represented as,

$$Sensitivity = \frac{T^p}{T^p + F^n} \tag{16}$$

4.3.3. Specificity

This measure is defined as the ratio of negatives that are correctly identified by the classifier, and is formulated as,

$$Specificity = \frac{T^n}{T^n + F^p} \tag{17}$$

4.4. Comparative Methods

The methods employed for the analysis include the Support Vector Machine (SVM) [35], Naive Bayes (NB) [36], DBN [33], and the proposed Taylor-BSA–DBN.

4.5. Comparative Analysis

The analysis of the proposed Taylor-BSA–DBN, with the conventional methods, with accuracy, sensitivity, and specificity parameters, is evaluated. The analysis is performed by varying the training data using Cleveland, Hungarian, and Switzerland databases.

4.5.1. Analysis with Cluster Size = 5

The analysis of methods, considering cluster size = 5, using Cleveland, Hungarian, and Switzerland databases are specified below:

Analysis Considering Cleveland Database

Table 2 elaborates the analysis of methods using the Cleveland database, considering training data with accuracy, sensitivity, and specificity parameters. The maximum accuracy, sensitivity, and specificity is considered as the best performance. Here, the proposed system offers better performances than the existing methods, such as SVM, NB, and DBN, respectively.

Table 2. Analysis of methods with cluster size = 5 using the Cleveland database. Abbreviations: SVM, Support Vector Machine; NB, Naive Bayes; DBN, deep belief network.

Methods Training Percentage	SVM	NB	DBN	Proposed Taylor-BSA–DBN
		Accuracy		
50	0.7590	0.7603	0.7874	0.8625
60	0.7143	0.7682	0.7851	0.8632
70	0.7460	0.7627	0.8122	0.8531
80	0.7236	0.7619	0.7869	0.8644
90	0.7538	0.7647	0.7742	0.8710
		Sensitivity		
50	0.7535	0.7613	0.7908	0.8693
60	0.7120	0.7611	0.7886	0.8699
70	0.7473	0.7558	0.8172	0.8602
80	0.7167	0.7656	0.7903	0.8710
90	0.7576	0.7667	0.7714	0.8788
		Specificity		
50	0.7566	0.7667	0.7838	0.8551
60	0.7165	0.7750	0.7815	0.8559
70	0.7447	0.7692	0.8068	0.8452
80	0.7302	0.7581	0.7833	0.8571
90	0.7500	0.7576	0.7813	0.8621

Analysis Considering Hungarian Database

Table 3 elaborates the analysis of methods using the Hungarian database, considering training data with accuracy, sensitivity, and specificity parameters. The proposed system offers the best performance when considering 90% of training data.

Table 3. Analysis of methods with cluster size = 5 using the Hungarian database.

Methods Training Percentage	SVM	NB	DBN	Proposed Taylor-BSA–DBN
		Accuracy		
50	0.7810	0.8043	0.8428	0.9200
60	0.7906	0.7976	0.8595	0.8907
70	0.7674	0.8143	0.8182	0.8551
80	0.7576	0.8095	0.8710	0.8710
90	0.6957	0.7500	0.7647	0.9130
		Sensitivity		
50	0.8160	0.8456	0.8776	0.9388
60	0.8300	0.8347	0.8908	0.9160
70	0.8052	0.8539	0.8571	0.8876
80	0.8065	0.8400	0.8795	0.9000
90	0.7500	0.8000	0.8125	0.9333
		Specificity		
50	0.7294	0.7326	0.7805	0.8846
60	0.7143	0.7500	0.8030	0.8438
70	0.7115	0.7451	0.7500	0.7959
80	0.6757	0.7647	0.8182	0.8182
90	0.6111	0.6667	0.6842	0.8750

Analysis Considering Switzerland Database

Table 4 elaborates the analysis of methods using the Switzerland database considering training data with accuracy, sensitivity, and specificity parameters. The better performances of the proposed system, with values, are 0.8462, 0.8571, and 0.8333 for performance metrics, such as accuracy, sensitivity, and specificity.

Table 4. Analysis of methods with cluster size = 5 using the Switzerland database.

Methods Training Percentage	SVM	NB	DBN	Proposed Taylor-BSA–DBN
Accuracy				
50	0.7619	0.7710	0.7895	0.8644
60	0.7009	0.7374	0.7800	0.8557
70	0.7073	0.7568	0.7895	0.8904
80	0.7551	0.7647	0.7778	0.8400
90	0.6774	0.7037	0.7143	0.8462
Sensitivity				
50	0.7656	0.7742	0.7818	0.8710
60	0.6981	0.7292	0.7843	0.8627
70	0.7073	0.7500	0.7948	0.8974
80	0.7500	0.7692	0.7857	0.8462
90	0.6875	0.6923	0.7143	0.8571
Specificity				
50	0.7581	0.7667	0.7966	0.8571
60	0.7037	0.7451	0.7755	0.8478
70	0.7073	0.7632	0.7838	0.8823
80	0.7600	0.7600	0.7692	0.8333
90	0.6667	0.7143	0.7143	0.8333

4.5.2. Analysis with Cluster Size = 9

The analysis of methods considering cluster size = 9, using Cleveland, Hungarian, and Switzerland databases are specified below:

Analysis Considering Cleveland Database

Table 5 depicts the analysis of methods using the Cleveland database, considering training data with accuracy, sensitivity, and specificity parameters. The maximum accuracy, sensitivity, and specificity are considered as the best performances. Here, the proposed system offers better performance than the existing methods, such as SVM, NB, and DBN, respectively.

Analysis Considering Hungarian Database

Table 6 shows the analysis of methods using the Hungarian database, considering training data with accuracy, sensitivity, and specificity parameters. The proposed system offers the best performance when considering 90% of training data.

Table 5. Analysis of methods with cluster size = 9 using the Cleveland database.

Methods Training Percentage	SVM	NB	DBN	Proposed Taylor-BSA–DBN
Accuracy				
50	0.7590	0.7603	0.7993	0.8690
60	0.7166	0.7430	0.7851	0.8632
70	0.7354	0.7363	0.8123	0.8857
80	0.7419	0.7607	0.7619	0.8475
90	0.7460	0.7910	0.8710	0.9016
Sensitivity				
50	0.7535	0.7613	0.8039	0.8758
60	0.7107	0.7440	0.7886	0.8699
70	0.7303	0.7368	0.8172	0.8925
80	0.7419	0.7544	0.7656	0.8548
90	0.7419	0.8000	0.8788	0.9091
Specificity				
50	0.7566	0.7667	0.7945	0.8613
60	0.7222	0.7419	0.7815	0.8559
70	0.7340	0.7419	0.8068	0.8780
80	0.7419	0.7581	0.7667	0.8393
90	0.7500	0.7813	0.8621	0.8929

Table 6. Analysis of methods with cluster size = 9 using the Hungarian database.

Methods Training Percentage	SVM	NB	DBN	Proposed Taylor-BSA–DBN
Accuracy				
50	0.7500	0.7957	0.8515	0.9200
60	0.7513	0.7870	0.8075	0.8907
70	0.7777	0.8273	0.8500	0.9118
80	0.7755	0.8298	0.8974	0.9341
90	0.7674	0.8000	0.8298	0.8696
Sensitivity				
50	0.7907	0.8389	0.8844	0.9388
60	0.8017	0.8218	0.8487	0.9160
70	0.8242	0.8652	0.8732	0.9326
80	0.8226	0.8667	0.9130	0.9500
90	0.8077	0.8438	0.8667	0.9000
Specificity				
50	0.6897	0.7209	0.7927	0.8846
60	0.6667	0.7353	0.7353	0.8438
70	0.6981	0.7600	0.8163	0.8723
80	0.6944	0.7647	0.8750	0.9032
90	0.7059	0.7222	0.7647	0.8125

Analysis Considering Switzerland Database

Table 7 depicts the analysis of methods using the Switzerland database considering training data with accuracy, sensitivity, and specificity parameters. The better performance of the proposed system with values is 0.7778, 0.7857, and 0.7692, for the performance metrics, such as accuracy, sensitivity, and specificity.

Table 7. Analysis of methods with cluster size = 9 using the Switzerland database.

Methods	SVM	NB	DBN	Proposed Taylor-BSA–DBN
Training Percentage				
Accuracy				
50	0.7460	0.7479	0.8017	0.8644
60	0.7170	0.7624	0.7684	0.8947
70	0.7368	0.7500	0.7662	0.8904
80	0.6786	0.7551	0.8200	0.8400
90	0.7333	0.7600	0.7679	0.7778
Sensitivity				
50	0.7414	0.7500	0.8065	0.8710
60	0.7170	0.7609	0.7647	0.9020
70	0.7297	0.7561	0.7692	0.8974
80	0.6786	0.7500	0.8300	0.8462
90	0.7300	0.7500	0.7667	0.7857
Specificity				
50	0.7419	0.7541	0.7966	0.8571
60	0.7170	0.7600	0.7755	0.8864
70	0.7436	0.7436	0.7632	0.8824
80	0.6786	0.7600	0.8200	0.8333
90	0.7143	0.7300	0.7556	0.7692

4.5.3. Analysis Based on Receiver Operating Characteristic (ROC) Curve

Table 8 depicts the comparative analysis based on ROC curve, using Cleveland, Hungarian, and Switzerland databases. In the Cleveland dataset, when the false positive rate (FPR) is 5, the corresponding true positive rate (TPR) of the methods, such as SVM, NB, DBN, and the proposed Taylor-BSA–DBN is 0.8857, 0.9119, 0.9535, and 0.9684, respectively. By considering the Hungarian dataset, when the FPR is 4, the corresponding TPR of the proposed method is a maximum of 0.9348. For the same FPR, the TPR of the methods, such as SVM, NB, and DBN is 0.9030, 0.9130, and 0.9233, respectively. By considering the Switzerland dataset, when the FPR is 6, the TPR of the methods, such as SVM, NB, DBN, and the proposed Taylor-BSA–DBN is 0.9105, 0.9443, 0.9569, and 0.9794, respectively.

4.5.4. Analysis Based on k-Fold

Table 9 depicts the comparative analysis based on k-fold using the Cleveland, Hungarian, and Switzerland databases, for cluster size = 5. The Hungarian datasets offer the maximum accuracy of 0.9021, when k-fold = 8. By considering k-fold = 7, the specificity offered by the Cleveland datasets for the methods, such as SVM, NB, DBN, and the proposed Taylor-BSA–DBN, is 0.8032, 0.8189, 0.8256, and 0.8321, respectively. The proposed Taylor-BSA–DBN offers maximum accuracy, sensitivity, and specificity, when considering k-fold = 8.

4.6. Comparative Discussion

Table 10 portrays the analysis of methods using accuracy, sensitivity, and specificity parameter with varying training data. The analysis is done with Cleveland, Switzerland, and Hungarian databases. Using cluster size = 5, and considering the Cleveland database, the proposed Taylor-BSA–DBN showed maximal accuracy of 0.871, which is 13.43%, 12.17%, and 11.14%, better than the existing methods, such as SVM, NB, and DBN, respectively. In the existing methods, the DBN offers maximum sensitivity of 0.771, but the proposed method is 12.29% better than the existing DBN. The proposed method has a maximum specificity of 0.862. The percentage of improvement of the proposed method with the existing methods, such as SVM, NB, and DBN, is 12.99%, 12.06%, and 9.40%, respectively. Considering the Hungarian database, the proposed Taylor-BSA–DBN showed maximal accuracy of 0.913, maximal sensitivity of 0.933, and maximal specificity of 0.875. Considering the Switzerland database, the proposed Taylor-BSA–DBN showed maximal accuracy of 0.846, which is 19.98%, 16.78%, and 15.60% better than the existing methods, such as SVM, NB, and DBN, respectively. Similarly, the proposed system has a maximum sensitivity of 0.857. The percentage of improvement of the proposed system sensitivity, with the existing methods, such as SVM, NB, and DBN is 19.72%, 19.25%, and 16.69%, respectively. Likewise, the proposed Taylor-BSA–DBN showed maximal specificity of 0.833.

Table 8. Analysis based on ROC.

Methods	SVM	NB	DBN	Proposed Taylor-BSA–DBN
FPR			TPR	
Cleveland				
1	0	0	0	0
2	0.7913	0.7949	0.8429	0.8761
3	0.7961	0.8330	0.8523	0.8798
4	0.8462	0.8753	0.9149	0.9284
5	0.8857	0.9119	0.9535	0.9684
6	0.9153	0.9569	0.9788	0.9847
7	0.9710	0.9783	0.9895	0.9975
8	0.9952	0.9989	1	1
9	1	1	1	1
10	1	1	1	1
Hungarian				
1	0	0	0	0
2	0.8233	0.8410	0.8553	0.8941
3	0.8286	0.8647	0.8734	0.8953
4	0.9030	0.9130	0.9233	0.9348
5	0.9246	0.9417	0.9596	0.9789
6	0.9521	0.9697	0.9803	0.9999
7	0.9793	0.9800	0.9946	1
8	0.9981	0.9985	1	1
9	1	1	1	1
10	1	1	1	1
Switzerland				
1	0	0	0	0
2	0.7593	0.7682	0.8024	0.8258
3	0.7620	0.7923	0.8399	0.8682
4	0.8452	0.8735	0.8781	0.9101
5	0.8725	0.9184	0.9194	0.9564
6	0.9105	0.9443	0.9569	0.9794
7	0.9701	0.9722	0.9865	0.9924
8	0.9946	0.9953	0.9994	1
9	1	1	1	1
10	1	1	1	1

Table 9. Analysis based on k-fold.

Metrics	Methods k-Fold	SVM	NB	DBN	Proposed Taylor-BSA–DBN
			Cleveland		
Accuracy	5	0.7021	0.7088	0.7126	0.7239
	6	0.7122	0.7189	0.7245	0.7365
	7	0.7345	0.7543	0.7634	0.7843
	8	0.7528	0.7843	0.7965	0.8132
Sensitivity	5	0.7567	0.7678	0.7898	0.7956
	6	0.7834	0.8045	0.8156	0.8232
	7	0.8032	0.8189	0.8256	0.8321
	8	0.8145	0.8229	0.8365	0.8448
Specificity	5	0.7586	0.7656	0.7699	0.7865
	6	0.7854	0.7745	0.7965	0.8043
	7	0.7940	0.8088	0.8124	0.8227
	8	0.8021	0.8178	0.8249	0.8339
			Hungarian		
Accuracy	5	0.7960	0.8758	0.8791	0.8822
	6	0.8071	0.8413	0.8838	0.8854
	7	0.7985	0.8030	0.8324	0.8917
	8	0.7982	0.8626	0.8948	0.9021
Sensitivity	5	0.7959	0.8027	0.8197	0.8231
	6	0.7857	0.7891	0.7925	0.8367
	7	0.7891	0.7925	0.7959	0.8393
	8	0.7857	0.7925	0.8061	0.8458
Specificity	5	0.7494	0.7513	0.7645	0.7656
	6	0.7146	0.7343	0.7645	0.7760
	7	0.7433	0.7535	0.7645	0.7719
	8	0.7530	0.7645	0.7697	0.7873
			Switzerland		
Accuracy	5	0.7528	0.7789	0.7799	0.7896
	6	0.7658	0.7828	0.7925	0.8012
	7	0.7712	0.7958	0.8028	0.8156
	8	0.7828	0.8128	0.8159	0.8259
Sensitivity	5	0.7428	0.7689	0.7847	0.7956
	6	0.7625	0.7758	0.7858	0.8028
	7	0.7748	0.7896	0.7952	0.8125
	8	0.7828	0.7986	0.8078	0.8225
Specificity	5	0.7658	0.7589	0.7750	0.7896
	6	0.7758	0.7832	0.7962	0.8020
	7	0.7841	0.7911	0.8025	0.8196
	8	0.7950	0.8002	0.8178	0.8319

Table 10. Comparative analysis.

Cluster Size	Database	Metrics	SVM	NB	DBN	Proposed Taylor-BSA–DBN
Cluster size = 5	Cleveland	Accuracy	0.754	0.765	0.774	0.871
		Sensitivity	0.758	0.767	0.771	0.879
		Specificity	0.750	0.758	0.781	0.862
	Hungarian	Accuracy	0.696	0.750	0.765	0.913
		Sensitivity	0.750	0.800	0.813	0.933
		Specificity	0.611	0.667	0.684	0.875
	Switzerland	Accuracy	0.677	0.704	0.714	0.846
		Sensitivity	0.688	0.692	0.714	0.857
		Specificity	0.667	0.714	0.714	0.833
Cluster size = 9	Cleveland	Accuracy	0.776	0.830	0.897	0.934
		Sensitivity	0.823	0.867	0.913	0.950
		Specificity	0.694	0.765	0.875	0.903
	Hungarian	Accuracy	0.746	0.791	0.871	0.902
		Sensitivity	0.742	0.800	0.879	0.909
		Specificity	0.750	0.781	0.862	0.893
	Switzerland	Accuracy	0.679	0.755	0.820	0.840
		Sensitivity	0.679	0.750	0.830	0.846
		Specificity	0.679	0.760	0.820	0.833

Using cluster size = 9, and considering the Cleveland database, the proposed Taylor-BSA–DBN showed maximal accuracy of 0.934, which is 16.92%, 11.13%, and 3.96%, better than the existing methods, such as SVM, NB, and DBN, respectively. In the existing methods, the DBN offers maximum sensitivity of 0.913, but the proposed method is 3.89% better than the existing DBN. The proposed method has a maximum specificity of 0.903. The percentage of improvement of the proposed method with the existing methods, such as SVM, NB, and DBN, is 23.15%, 15.28%, and 3.10%, respectively. Considering the Hungarian database, the proposed Taylor-BSA–DBN showed maximal accuracy of 0.902, maximal sensitivity of 0.909, and maximal specificity of 0.893. Considering the Switzerland database, the proposed Taylor-BSA–DBN showed maximal accuracy of 0.840, which is 19.17%, 10.12%, and 2.38%, better than the existing methods, such as SVM, NB, and DBN, respectively. Similarly, the proposed system has a maximum sensitivity of 0.846. The percentage of improvement of the proposed system sensitivity with the existing methods, such as SVM, NB, and DBN is 19.74%, 11.35%, and 1.89%, respectively. Likewise, the proposed Taylor-BSA–DBN showed maximal specificity of 0.833.

Table 11 shows the computational time of the proposed system and the existing methods, such as SVM, NB, and DBN, in which the proposed Taylor-BSA–DBN has a minimum computation time of 6.31 sec.

Table 11. Computational Time.

Methods	SVM	NB	DBN	Proposed Taylor-BSA–DBN
Time (Sec)	10.08	8.79	7.56	6.31

Table 12 shows the statistical analysis of the proposed work and the existing methods based on mean and variance.

Table 12. Statistical Analysis.

Dataset	Methods	Accuracy	Mean	Variance	Sensitivity	Mean	Variance	Specificity	Mean	Variance
				Cluster size = 5						
Cleveland	SVM	0.754	0.752	0.002	0.758	0.754	0.004	0.750	0.748	0.002
	NB	0.765	0.761	0.004	0.767	0.765	0.002	0.758	0.754	0.004
	DBN	0.774	0.771	0.003	0.771	0.768	0.003	0.781	0.779	0.002
	Proposed Method	0.871	0.869	0.002	0.879	0.878	0.001	0.862	0.860	0.002
Hungarian	SVM	0.696	0.693	0.003	0.750	0.748	0.002	0.611	0.608	0.003
	NB	0.750	0.746	0.004	0.800	0.799	0.001	0.667	0.665	0.002
	DBN	0.765	0.763	0.002	0.813	0.810	0.003	0.684	0.682	0.002
	Proposed Method	0.913	0.911	0.002	0.933	0.932	0.001	0.875	0.873	0.002
Switzerland	SVM	0.677	0.675	0.002	0.688	0.684	0.004	0.667	0.665	0.002
	NB	0.704	0.702	0.003	0.692	0.690	0.002	0.714	0.711	0.003
	DBN	0.714	0.711	0.003	0.714	0.713	0.001	0.714	0.712	0.002
	Proposed Method	0.846	0.844	0.002	0.857	0.855	0.002	0.833	0.831	0.002
				Cluster size = 9						
Cleveland	SVM	0.776	0.773	0.003	0.823	0.822	0.001	0.694	0.691	0.003
	NB	0.830	0.826	0.004	0.867	0.865	0.002	0.765	0.761	0.004
	DBN	0.897	0.895	0.002	0.913	0.911	0.002	0.875	0.873	0.002
	Proposed Method	0.934	0.932	0.002	0.950	0.948	0.002	0.903	0.901	0.002
Hungarian	SVM	0.746	0.743	0.003	0.742	0.740	0.002	0.750	0.748	0.002
	NB	0.791	0.790	0.001	0.800	0.797	0.003	0.781	0.780	0.001
	DBN	0.871	0.868	0.003	0.879	0.878	0.001	0.862	0.860	0.002
	Proposed Method	0.902	0.900	0.002	0.909	0.907	0.002	0.893	0.891	0.002
Switzerland	SVM	0.679	0.677	0.002	0.679	0.675	0.004	0.679	0.677	0.002
	NB	0.755	0.752	0.003	0.750	0.748	0.002	0.760	0.758	0.002
	DBN	0.820	0.818	0.002	0.830	0.827	0.003	0.820	0.819	0.001
	Proposed Method	0.840	0.838	0.002	0.846	0.844	0.002	0.833	0.832	0.001

5. Conclusions

Contemporary medicine depends on a huge amount of information contained in medical databases. The obtainability of large medical data leads to the requirement of effective data analysis tools for extracting constructive knowledge. This paper proposes a novel, fully automated DBN for heart disease diagnosis using medical data. The proposed Taylor-BSA is employed to train DBN. The proposed Taylor-BSA is designed by combining the Taylor series and BSA algorithm, which can be utilized for finding the optimal weights for establishing effective medical data classification. Here, the sparse-FCM is employed for selecting significant features. The incorporation of sparse FCM for the feature selection process provides more benefits for interpreting the models, as this sparse technique provides important features for detection, and can be utilized for handling high dimensional data. The obtained selected features are fed to DBN, which is trained by the proposed Taylor BSA. The proposed Taylor BSA is designed by integrating the Taylor series and BSA in order to generate optimal weights for classification. The proposed Taylor-BSA–DBN outperformed other methods with maximal accuracy of 93.4%, maximal sensitivity of 95%, and maximal specificity of 90.3%, respectively. The proposed method does not classify the type of heart disease. In the future, other medical data classification datasets will be employed for computing efficiency of the proposed method. In addition, the proposed system will be further improved to classify heart diseases, such as congenital heart disease, coronary artery disease, and arrhythmia.

Author Contributions: Conceptualization, A.M.A. methodology, A.M.A.; software, A.M.A.; validation, A.M.A.; resources, A.M.A.; data curation, A.M.A.; writing—original draft preparation, A.M.A. and W.M.N.W.Z.;

writing—review and editing, A.M.A. and W.M.N.W.Z.; visualization, A.M.A. and W.M.N.W.Z.; supervision, W.M.N.W.Z. All authors have read and agreed to the published version of the manuscript.

Funding: This research received no external funding.

Conflicts of Interest: The authors declare no conflict of interest.

References

1. Abdel-Basset, M.; Gamal, A.; Manogaran, G.; Long, H.V. A novel group decision making model based on neutrosophic sets for heart disease diagnosis. *Multimed. Tools Appl.* **2019**, *79*, 9977–10002. [CrossRef]
2. Acharjya, D.P. A Hybrid Scheme for Heart Disease Diagnosis Using Rough Set and Cuckoo Search Technique. *J. Med. Syst.* **2020**, *44*, 27.
3. Ahn, G.J.; Hu, H.; Lee, J.; Meng, Y. Representing and Reasoning about Web Access Control Policies. In Proceedings of the IEEE 34th Annual Computer Software and Applications Conference, Seoul, Korea, 19–23 July 2010; pp. 137–146.
4. Alizadehsani, R.; Habibi, J.; Hosseini, M.J.; Mashayekhi, H.; Boghrati, R.; Ghandeharioun, A.; Bahadorian, B.; Sani, Z.A. A data mining approach for diagnosis of coronary artery disease. *Comput. Methods Programs Biomed.* **2013**, *11*, 52–61. [CrossRef] [PubMed]
5. Alzahani, S.M.; Althopity, A.; Alghamdi, A.; Alshehri, B.; Aljuaid, S. An overview of data mining techniques applied for heart disease diagnosis and prediction. *Lect. Notes Inf. Theory* **2014**, *2*, 310–315. [CrossRef]
6. Babič, F.; Olejár, J.; Vantová, Z.; Paralič, J. Predictive and descriptive analysis for heart disease diagnosis. In Proceedings of the Federated Conference on Computer Science and Information Systems (FedCSIS), Prague, Czech Republic, 3–6 September 2017; pp. 155–163.
7. Chang, X.; Wang, Q.; Liu, Y.; Wang, Y. Sparse Regularization in Fuzzy c-Means for High-Dimensional Data Clustering. *IEEE Trans. Cybern.* **2017**, *47*, 2616–2627. [CrossRef]
8. Fatima, M.; Pasha, M. Survey of Machine Learning Algorithms for Disease Diagnostic. *J. Intell. Learn. Syst. Appl.* **2017**, *9*, 1–16. [CrossRef]
9. Ghumbre, S.; Patil, C.; Ghatol, A. Heart disease diagnosis using support vector machine. In Proceedings of the International Conference on Computer Science and Information Technology (ICCSIT), Mumbai, India, 10–12 June 2011.
10. Ghumbre, S.U.; Ghatol, A.A. Heart Disease Diagnosis Using Machine Learning Algorithm. In Proceedings of the International Conference on Information Systems Design and Intelligent Applications, Visakhapatnam, India, 5–7 January 2012; Volume 132, pp. 217–225.
11. Giri, D.; Acharya, U.R. Automated diagnosis of Coronary Artery Disease affected patients usingLDA, PCA, ICA and Discrete WaveletTransform. *Knowl. Based Syst.* **2013**, *37*, 274–282. [CrossRef]
12. Heart Disease Data Set. Available online: http://archive.ics.uci.edu/ml/datasets/Heart+Disease (accessed on 22 April 2020).
13. Jabbar, M.A.; Deekshatulu, B.; LandChandra, P. Classification of Heart Disease Using K- Nearest Neighbor and Genetic Algorithm. *Procedia Technol.* **2013**, *10*, 85–94. [CrossRef]
14. Jabbar, M.A.; Deekshatulu, B.L.; Chandra, P. Heart disease classification using nearest neighbor classifier with feature subset selection. *An. Ser. Inform.* **2013**, *11*, 47–54.
15. Kukar, M.; Kononenko, I.; Groselj, C.; Kralj, K.; Fettich, J. Analysing and Improving the Diagnosis of Ischaemic Heart Disease with Machine Learning. *Artif. Intell. Med.* **1999**, *16*, 25–50. [CrossRef]
16. Magesh, G.; Swarnalatha, P. Optimal feature selection through a cluster-based DT learning (CDTL) in heart disease prediction. *Evol. Intell.* **2020**, 1–11. [CrossRef]
17. Mangai, S.A.; Sankar, B.R.; Alagarsamy, K. Taylor Series Prediction of Time Series Data with Error Propagated by Artificial Neural Network. *Int. J. Comput. Appl.* **2014**, *89*, 41–47.
18. Mannepalli, K.; Sastry, P.N.; Suman, M. A novel Adaptive Fractional Deep Belief Networks for speaker emotion recognition. *Alex. Eng. J.* **2017**, *56*, 485–497. [CrossRef]
19. Medhekar, D.S.; Bote, M.P.; Deshmukh, S.D. Heart disease prediction system using naive Bayes. *Int. J. Enhanc. Res. Sci. Technol. Eng.* **2013**, *2*, 1–5.
20. Meng, X.; Gao, X.Z.; Lu, L.; Liu, Y.; Zhang, H. A new bio-inspired optimisation algorithm: Bird Swarm Algorithm. *J. Exp. Theor. Artif. Intell.* **2016**, *28*, 673–687. [CrossRef]

21. Mohan, S.; Thirumalai, C.; Srivastava, G. Effective Heart Disease Prediction Using Hybrid Machine Learning Techniques. *IEEE Access* **2019**, *7*, 81542–81554. [CrossRef]
22. Nilashi, M.; Ahmadi, H.; Manaf, A.A.; Rashid, T.A.; Samad, S.; Shahmoradi, L.; Aljojo, N.; Akbari, E. Coronary Heart Disease Diagnosis Through Self-Organizing Map and Fuzzy Support Vector Machine with Incremental Updates. *Int. J. Fuzzy Syst.* **2020**, *23*, 1376–1388. [CrossRef]
23. Nourmohammadi-Khiarak, J.; Feizi-Derakhshi, M.R.; Behrouzi, K.; Mazaheri, S.; Zamani-Harghalani, Y.; Tayebi, R.M. New hybrid method for heart disease diagnosis utilizing optimization algorithm in feature selection. *Health Technol.* **2019**, *10*, 667–678. [CrossRef]
24. Oyyathevan, S.; Askarunisa, A. An expert system for heart disease prediction using data mining technique: Neural network. *Int. J. Eng. Res. Sports Sci.* **2014**, *1*, 1–6.
25. Palaniappan, S.; Awang, R. Intelligent heart disease prediction system using data mining techniques. In Proceedings of the International Conference on Computer Systems and Applications, Doha, Qatar, 31 March–4 April 2008.
26. Palaniappan, S.; Awang, R. Intelligent Heart Disease Prediction System Using Data Mining Techniques. *Int. J. Comput. Sci. Netw. Secur.* **2008**, *8*, 343–350.
27. Patil, S.B.; Kumaraswamy, Y.S. Extraction of significant patterns from heart disease warehouses for heart attack prediction. *Int. J. Comput. Sci. Netw. Secur.* **2009**, *9*, 228–235.
28. Pattekari, S.A.; Parveen, A. Prediction system for Heart Disease using Naive Bayes. *Int. J. Adv. Comput. Math. Sci.* **2012**, *3*, 290–294.
29. Ranganatha, S.; Raj, H.P.; Anusha, C.; Vinay, S.K. Medical data mining and analysis for heart disease dataset using classification techniques. In Proceedings of the National Conference on Challenges in Research & Technology in the Coming Decades (CRT), Ujire, India, 27–28 September 2013.
30. Reddy, G.T.; Reddy, M.P.K.; Lakshmanna, K.; Rajput, D.S.; Kaluri, R.; Srivastava, G. Hybrid genetic algorithm and a fuzzy logic classifier for heart disease diagnosis. *Evol. Intell.* **2019**, *13*, 185–196. [CrossRef]
31. Safdar, S.; Zafar, S.; Zafar, N.; Khan, N. Machine learning based decision support systems (DSS) for heart disease diagnosis: A review. *Artif. Intell. Rev.* **2018**, *50*, 597–623. [CrossRef]
32. Shah, S.M.S.; Shah, F.A.; Hussain, S.A.; Batool, S. Support Vector Machines-based Heart Disease Diagnosis using Feature Subset, Wrapping Selection and Extraction Methods. *Comput. Electr. Eng.* **2020**, *84*, 106628. [CrossRef]
33. Shouman, M.; Turner, T.; Stocker, R. Using data mining techniques in heart disease diagnosis and treatment. In Proceedings of the IEEE Japan-Egypt Conference on Electronics, Communications and Computers, Alexandria, Egypt, 6–9 March 2012; pp. 173–177.
34. Subbalakshmi, G. Decision support in heart disease prediction system using naive bayes. *Indian J. Comput. Sci. Eng.* **2011**, *2*, 170–174.
35. Thiyagaraj, M.; Suseendran, G. Enhanced Prediction of Heart Disease Using Particle Swarm Optimization and Rough Sets with Transductive Support Vector Machines Classifier. In *Data Management, Analytics and Innovation*; Springer: Singapore, 2020; Volume 2, pp. 141–152.
36. Yeh, D.Y.; Cheng, C.H.; Chen, Y.W. A predictive model for cerebrovascular disease using data mining. *Expert Syst. Appl.* **2011**, *38*, 8970–8977. [CrossRef]

© 2020 by the authors. Licensee MDPI, Basel, Switzerland. This article is an open access article distributed under the terms and conditions of the Creative Commons Attribution (CC BY) license (http://creativecommons.org/licenses/by/4.0/).

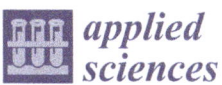

Article

A Decision Support System for Elective Surgery Scheduling under Uncertain Durations

Daniel Clavel [1], Cristian Mahulea [1,*], Jorge Albareda [2] and Manuel Silva [1]

[1] Department of Computer Science and Systems Engineering, University of Zaragoza, 50018 Zaragoza, Spain; clavel@unizar.es (D.C.); silva@unizar.es (M.S.)
[2] "Lozano Blesa" Hospital of Zaragoza, 50009 Zaragoza, Spain; jcalbareda@salud.aragon.es
* Correspondence: cmahulea@unizar.es; Tel.: +34-976-762517

Received: 22 January 2020; Accepted: 9 March 2020; Published: 12 March 2020

Featured Application: A software tool for helping doctors in the automatic scheduling of elective patients is proposed. The tool has been developed considering the organizational structure of Spanish hospitals. However, it may be easily extended to any hospital (public or private) working under operation room block booking criterion.

Abstract: The *operation room* (OR) is one of the most expensive material resources in hospitals. Additionally, the demand for surgical service is increasing due to the aging population, while the number of surgical interventions performed is stagnated because of budget reasons. In this context, the importance of improving the efficiency of the surgical service is accentuated. The main objective of this work is to propose and to evaluate a *Decision Support System* (DSS) for helping medical staff in the automatic scheduling of elective patients, improving the efficiency of medical teams' work. First, the scheduling criteria are fixed and then the scheduling problem of elective patients is approached by a mathematical programming model. A heuristic algorithm is proposed and included in the DSS. Moreover, other different features are implemented in a software tool with a friendly user interface, called CIPLAN. Considering realistic data, a simulation comparison of the scheduling obtained using the approach presented in this paper and other similar approaches in the bibliography is shown and analyzed. On the other hand, a case study considering real data provided by the Orthopedic Surgical Department (OSD) of the "Lozano Blesa" hospital in Zaragoza (HCU) is proposed. The simulation results show that the approach presented here obtains similar occupation rates and similar confidence levels of not exceeding the available time than approaches in the bibliography. However, from the point of view of respecting the order of the patients in the waiting list, the approach in this paper obtains scheduling much more ordered. In the case of the Orthopedic Surgical Department of the "Lozano Blesa" hospital in Zaragoza, the occupation rate may be increased by 2.83%, which represents a saving of 110,000 euros per year. Moreover, medical doctors (who use this tool) consider CIPLAN as an intuitive, rapid and efficient software solution that can make easier the corresponding task.

Keywords: decision support system; heuristic approach; surgery scheduling; software tool; case study

1. Introduction

The *Operation Room* (OR) is one of the most expensive material resources of the hospitals (in Spain being about 40% of the total hospitalization cost [1]) and approximately 60% of patients need it at some point during their hospital stay [2]. On the other hand, the demand for surgical services is increasing due to the aging population. In Spain, the average life expectancy is about 81.8 years being one of the highest in Europe [3].

Moreover, as a result of the economic crisis in 2008, the number of surgical interventions performed annually in Spanish public hospitals has stagnated at 3.5 million. This situation has also contributed to a continuous increment in the number of patients in the surgical waiting lists, reaching 600,000 in 2017 [4]. In some cases, these huge lists lead into waiting times greater than six months, which is becoming a serious problem for the healthcare system. Being difficult to increase the surgical resources, the importance of improving the efficiency is accentuated. New management techniques, scheduling methods, and specific information systems could help to improve the efficiency of the surgical services and, consequently, could reduce the surgical waiting lists.

The main objective of this work is to provide a DSS for managing surgical services in hospitals. In particular, a software tool (called CIPLAN from the Spanish words *PLANificación de CIrugías*) is presented that may be used by medical doctors to automatically perform a scheduling of the patients. It is assumed that the uncertain parameters (surgery duration and cleaning time) follow a normal distribution and, consequently, the expected total duration of a surgical block also follows a normal distribution. In this way, the probability of exceeding the working time can be introduced as a capacity chance constraint. Even if the lognormal distribution may give better approximations of the surgery times [5], the optimization problem has nonlinear constraints, being difficult to solve. Since, in general, acceptable error is obtained for normal distribution, this work assumes this type of distribution.

The following three criteria have been considered for the scheduling problem.

C1. Maximize the occupation of the ORs. Since the ORs with their associated cost constitute the bottleneck of the system (they can be open only during a given period of time every working day and their cost is high), the first scheduling criterion is to maximize the occupation of the ORs. In this way, the underutilization of the ORs is prevented and the use of resources is maximized.

C2. Ensure with a minimum confidence level that the total available time in a time block is not going to be exceeded. On contrary to C1, an over-scheduling of the ORs is not desired since the last scheduled surgeries can be canceled if the medical personnel believes that the time of the time block will be exceeded. Among other problems, such cancellations reduce the *real* occupation rate in the ORs.

C3. Respect as much as possible the order of the patients in the waiting list. Due to ethical and common sense reasons, patients with the same urgency level should spend a similar time in the waiting list. For that, once the patients in a waiting list are ordered depending on the urgency level and the admission date, the third scheduling criterion is to respect as much as possible the order of the patients in the waiting list. For example, in the Orthopedic Department of the HCU, each team has assigned two time blocks per week for the elective patients, so the difference of scheduling a patient in the first time block with the sixth one is 21 days.

Mathematical programming is an optimization technique [6] commonly used in managing hospitals [7], not only for surgery scheduling problems [8], but also for other problems such as bed management [9], nurse scheduling [10], or management policy decisions [11]. This paper proposes first an *Mixed Integer Quadratic Constrained Programming* problem for performing the scheduling of patients based on the three criteria presented before. It is well known that the computational complexity to obtain the optimal solution is high and a heuristic method is proposed called *Specific Heuristic Algorithm* (SHA) [12]. The software tool, in addition to helping doctors in the scheduling task, has also been developed for managing medical doctors, medical teams, OR timetable, and patients.

A preliminary version of this work has been reported in [12] where a first version of the SHA has been proposed. In this paper, the heuristic SHA is improved by adding a post arranging of the time scheduled blocks. This improvement provides solutions respecting the order of the patients in the waiting list more. Additionally, the DSS is explained (not only the part related to surgery scheduling but also related to management tasks), and the solution is compared using real data from the HCU with two other methods in literature.

2. Related Work

In literature, many researchers studied the problem of planning and scheduling of elective patients (see [8,13] and the references herein for an overview while for an overview of the problems see [14]). Almost all the works consider criterion C1 presented before. Criterion C2 (of using chance constraints for the scheduling) is considered also in some contributions presented in the last years. For example, in [15], integer stochastic formulations are proposed for two sub-problems in which the original problem is decomposed. The approach to solve them is based on neighborhood search techniques and Monte Carlo simulation. In [16], a two-stage robust optimization model is proposed that is solved based on a column-and-constraint generation method. A similar method is used by the authors in [17] to deal with uncertain surgery duration and emergency demand, while, in [18], the authors use particle swarm optimization for the scheduling of surgeries.

The approaches presented in [19,20] are the most related to the one presented in this paper. The authors in [19] present an optimization framework for batch scheduling within a block booking system that maximizes the expected utilization of ORs subject to a set of probabilistic capacity constraints. They propose an algorithm that iteratively solves a series of mixed-integer programs that are based on a normal approximation of cumulative surgery duration. In [20], constructive and local search heuristics for maximization of ORs utilization and minimization of the overcoming risk are proposed. In their model, to address the randomness of surgery processing times, a planned time slack is reserved in each scheduling block, which is a function of total mean and variance of surgeries assigned to the corresponding block. When determining an appropriate size of the planned slacks, the authors assume that the sum of surgery duration follows a normal distribution.

Both approaches in [19,20] require setting in advance the patients that are going to be scheduled in the next blocks. Therefore, in these approaches, all considered patients must be scheduled in one of the available blocks. For this, both approaches start with an initial scheduling obtained through the scheduling rule: *first-fit probabilistic*. Following this rule, sequentially each surgery is assigned to the first available block for which the probabilistic capacity constraint is satisfied after the assignment. Once the initial scheduling is obtained, the expected occupation rate of the first blocks is improved by rescheduling the surgeries. In this way, the last blocks are totally or partially released.

Unlike [19,20], the approach presented in this paper does not require to know in advance the set of patients that should be scheduled in the next surgical blocks, since any patient on the waiting list may or may not be scheduled. Another big difference with [19,20] consists of the usage of two balanced terms in the cost function that favor patients to be scheduled in an orderly manner at the same time that the expected occupation rate of the OR is maximized. An exhaustive numerical comparison using realistic data is performed and analyzed showing that the approach presented in this manuscript provides better solutions to the considered problem than the one in [19,20]. In particular, even if the results show similar occupation rates and similar confidence levels, the approach presented in this paper respect the preference order of the patients in the waiting list more. Therefore, criterion C3 is better considered. In the case of the hospital in which the approach is implemented, the number of available time blocks per week for each medical team is equal to two, while, on average, three patients are scheduled in a time block, making it very important to keep, if possible, the order of patients in the waiting lists. This is one of the main differences of the approach presented in this paper with the other approaches.

DSS are used for managing tasks in different fields of applications, as for example in stormwater management [21], dental manufacturing production line [22], offshore wind farms [23] and healthcare systems [24,25]. Moreover, a DSS for OR scheduling was proposed in [26] based on a Mixed Integer Linear Programming (MILP) problem [27,28] that takes into account the preference order of the patients. However, this approach does not consider the variability on the uncertain parameters (surgery duration, cleaning time, etc.) and consequently can not manage the risk of exceeding the total time. The DSS proposed in this work uses an heuristic algorithm allowing to impose a minimum confidence level of not exceeding the total time in a surgical block. In this way, doctors not only can manage the risk but also can know in advance the probability that each block exceeds the available time. The DSS proposed in this paper can also perform the management of medical teams and OR time table. Moreover, it is possible to perform iterative scheduling which is useful if, for example, after obtaining a first scheduling, some patients can not attend the day of their surgeries. Furthermore, after a surgery is performed, the DSS automatically updates and customizes the average and standard deviation of the surgery duration. Finally, in order to provide a safe environment to work and better security of the medical data, different access levels are provided to every user.

The second main contribution of this paper is the presentation of a DSS that can help medical doctors not only for scheduling of surgeries, but also it can be used for management tasks of patients, medical teams, hospital resources, etc. Finally, the scheduling approach presented is compared with real historical data from the studied hospital, this being a third contribution of this manuscript.

3. Preliminaries and Problem Definition

Let us assume that each surgical team of a hospital department has some surgical blocks booked for performing the surgeries of their elective patients list. Thus, the problem of scheduling can be divided into different independent sub-problems: one for each medical team. In this process, some patients are assigned from the waiting list to the next time blocks previously booked. Currently, in many Spanish hospitals, the scheduling is performed manually, so the schedulers (normally medical doctors) are guided by their own intuition and experience to assign the patients.

3.1. Scheduling Problem Statement

In this subsection, the **Scheduling problem** is introduced formally. First, the notation, terminology, and assumptions are fixed and then the scheduling criteria are transformed to cost function and constraints.

Let $S = \{s_1, s_2, \ldots, s_{|S|}\}$ be the set of surgery types that can be performed in the medical department and let us assume that the duration $d(s_k)$ of each type of surgery $s_k \in S$ is a random variable with normal probability density function (pdf) $d(s_k) = N(\mu_{d(s_k)}, \sigma_{d(s_k)})$, where $\mu_{d(s_k)}$ is the average and $\sigma_{d(s_k)}$ is the standard deviation.

On the other hand, let Dt be the delay with respect to the starting time of a block and let Ct be the cleaning time duration of the OR after a surgery is performed. It is assumed that Dt and Ct are also random variables with normal pdf, i.e., $Dt = N(\mu_{Dt}, \sigma_{Dt})$ and $Ct = N(\mu_{Ct}, \sigma_{Ct})$.

Furthermore, let us consider $\mathcal{W} = \{w_1, w_2, \ldots, w_{|\mathcal{W}|}\}$ an ordered list of patients such that, if $w_j \in \mathcal{W}$, j is the preference order of the patient w_j in the waiting list.

In addition, let us assume an ordered set of time blocks $\mathcal{B} = \{b_1, \ldots, b_{|\mathcal{B}|}\}$ to schedule, where $b_{|\mathcal{B}|}$ is the block corresponding to the latest date. Each block $b_i \in \mathcal{B}$ has a fixed duration denoted by $l(b_i)$.

For each time block $b_i \in \mathcal{B}$ to schedule, there exists a binary decision vector $S_i \in \{0,1\}^{1 \times |\mathcal{W}|}$ with a dimension equal to the number of the patients in the waiting list. If $S_i[j] = 1$, then surgery of patient w_j should be performed in working day $i \leq |\mathcal{B}|$.

Let S_{b_i} be the set of surgeries scheduled in the time block b_i; then, the total duration T_{b_i} of the time block b_i can be computed by Equation (1). That is the sum of: (i) the delay with respect to the starting time (i.e., Dt), (ii) the duration of the surgeries scheduled in the time block b_i, and (iii) the cleaning time duration Ct between two consecutive surgeries. Notice that the cleaning time after the last surgery is not considered:

$$T_{b_i} = Dt + (|S_{b_i}| - 1) \cdot Ct \sum_{s_k \in S_{b_i}} [d(s_k)]. \tag{1}$$

Because all these variables are assumed to follow a normal distribution, the total duration T_{b_i} of the time block b_i also follows a normal distribution $T_{b_i} = N(\mu_{T_{b_i}}, \sigma_{T_{b_i}})$.

The goal of the scheduling problem is the assignment of the patients from the waiting list $\mathcal{W}$ to the set of time blocks $\mathcal{B}$ considering the scheduling criteria C1, C2 and C3. Let us define the following further notations:

- μ_w be a row vector containing the average duration of surgeries of the patients in the waiting list $\mathcal{W}$. For example, $\mu_w(j)$ represents the average duration of the surgery corresponding to the patient w_j.
- Po be a row vector containing the preference order of the patients. Assuming that patients are ordered according to their priority, then $Po(j) = j$.
- Cl is the minimum confidence level of not exceeding the total time.

then:

Criterion C1 is formalized by objective **O1** given by Equation (2). This equation maximizes the expected surgery time in each block ($\mu_w \cdot S_i$) giving more importance to the first ones ($|\mathcal{B}| + 1 - i$):

$$max \sum_{i=1}^{|\mathcal{B}|} [\mu_w \cdot S_i \cdot (|\mathcal{B}| + 1 - i)]. \quad (2)$$

Criterion C2 is imposed by the chance probability constraint given by Equation (3). It ensures with a minimum confidence level Cl that the total duration T_{b_i} in each time block $b_i \in \mathcal{B}$ does not exceed the available time $l(b_i)$:

$$P[T_{b_i} \leq l(b_i)] \geq Cl, \forall i = 1, 2, \ldots, |\mathcal{B}|. \quad (3)$$

Finally, criterion C3 is formalized by the objective **O2** given by Equation (4). Here, by minimizing the sum of the preference order of the patients scheduled in each time block ($Po \cdot S_i$), preference to the first patients in the waiting list is given. Moreover, multiplying by the term ($|\mathcal{B}| + 1 - i$), first patients should be scheduled in the first time blocks:

$$min \sum_{i=1}^{|\mathcal{B}|} [Po \cdot S_i \cdot (|\mathcal{B}| + 1 - i)], \quad (4)$$

3.2. Optimal Mathematical Programming Model

A Mixed-Integer Quadratic Constrained Programming (MIQCP) model is proposed (5) for solving the patients **Scheduling problem**. In this model, the objectives given in Equations (2) and (4) are mixed in a linear cost function with two terms balanced by the value of the parameter β:

$$min \sum_{i=1}^{|\mathcal{B}|} [-\mu_w \cdot S_i \cdot (|\mathcal{B}| - i + 1) + \beta \cdot Po \cdot S_i \cdot (|\mathcal{B}| - i + 1)]$$

Subject to: (5)

$$\begin{cases} P[T_{b_i} \leq l(b_i)] \geq Cl, & \forall i = 1, 2, \ldots, |\mathcal{B}|. \\ \sum_{i=1}^{|\mathcal{B}|} S_i[j] \leq 1, & \forall j = 1, 2, \ldots, |\mathcal{W}| \\ S_i \in \{0,1\}^{1 \times |\mathcal{W}|}, & \forall i = 1, 2, \ldots, |\mathcal{B}|. \end{cases}$$

The MIQCP model has two sets of constraints. The first one is related to the chance probability constraint given in Equation (3), while the second one imposes that each patient in the waiting list is scheduled at most once. Development of the chance constraint (3) quadratic constraints is obtained [29].

Moreover, the decision variables S_i are binary, so the computational complexity of the MIQCP model is really high. In order to obtain scheduling in a reasonable time, heuristic approaches are needed.

4. Proposed Solution

4.1. Specific Heuristic Algorithm

Two heuristic approaches have been discussed for implementation in the DSS. The first one is a *Receding Horizon Strategy* (RHS) which obtains a sub-optimal solution sequentially (similar to [30]), while the second one is a *Specific Heuristic Algorithm* (SHA) based on list scheduling techniques [31–33].

The SHA for the scheduling of patients problem is composed of three parts: (i) a previous data analysis; (ii) the scheduling of the time blocks; and (iii) a re-assignment of time blocks.

Part (i): A previous data analysis. This part is composed of two steps executed sequentially once at the beginning of the scheduling.

Step 1. Classify the set of surgeries S in a given number t of disjoint subsets such that $S = \overline{S_1} \cup \ldots \cup \overline{S_t}$, t being an input parameter. This classification is done based on two conditions: (1) the average duration of all surgeries in a subset $\overline{S_i} \in S, i = 1, 2, \ldots, t-1$ must be less than or equal to the average duration of all surgeries in subset $\overline{S_{i+1}} \in S$, and (2) the expected number of patients in each subset $S_i \in S$ should be similar. In order to compute the expected number of patients for each $\overline{S_i} \in S$, the probability of occurrence of all surgeries in S should be known, and it is obtained using historical data of the studied department.

For example, if there exist three types of surgeries $S = \{s_1, s_2, s_3\}$ with $\mu_d(s_1) < \mu_d(s_2) < \mu_d(s_3)$ and the occurrence probabilities are 0.25 for s_1 and s_2 and 0.5 for s_3, a valid classification for $t = 2$ is $S = \{\overline{S_1}, \overline{S_2}\}$ where $\overline{S_1} = \{s_1, s_2\}$ and $\overline{S_2} = \{s_3\}$. However, if $\mu_d(s_1) < \mu_d(s_3) < \mu_d(s_2)$, a valid classification could be $\overline{S_1} = \{s_1, s_3\}$ and $\overline{S_2} = \{s_2\}$ but also $\overline{S_1} = \{s_1\}$ and $\overline{S_2} = \{s_2, s_3\}$ is a valid solution.

Step 2: Obtain the set of possible scheduling types for each time block $b_i \in \mathcal{B}$. In this step, all multisets from set $S = \{\overline{S_1}, \overline{S_2}, \ldots, \overline{S_t}\}$ are obtained from the possible scheduling type for the time block b_i. Formally, a possible scheduling type is a tuple (S, m), where S is the underlying set of the multiset and $m : S \to \mathbb{N}_{\geq 1}$ is a function giving the multiplicity of the elements in the multiset. A multiset belonging to the possible scheduling type of block b_i should satisfy the chance constraint (3). In order to check that the chance constraint (3) is satisfied, the surgeries with lower average duration are considered.

For example, a possible scheduling type for time block b_i could be $\{\overline{S_k}, \overline{S_k}, \overline{S_j}\}$ meaning that, in block b_i, two surgeries from set $\overline{S_k}$ may be scheduled and another one from set $\overline{S_j}$. If s_k^1 is the surgery type with the lowest average duration from $\overline{S_k}$ and s_j^1 is the surgery type with the lowest average duration from $\overline{S_j}$, according to the total duration in (1), the minimum total duration of the time block b_i is

$$T_{b_i} = \left(Dt + s_k^1 + s_k^1 + s_j^1 + 2 \cdot Ct\right),$$

where Dt is the delay with respect to the starting time and Ct is the cleaning time duration after each surgery.

As observed before, T_{b_i} is following a normal distribution with mean

$$\mu_{T_{b_i}} = \mu_{Dt} + 2 \cdot \mu_d(s_k^1) + \mu_d(s_j^1) + 2 \cdot \mu_{Ct}$$

and standard deviation

$$\sigma_{T_{b_i}} = \sqrt{(\sigma_{Dt})^2 + 2 \cdot (\sigma_d(s_k^1))^2 + (\sigma_d(s_j^1))^2 + 2 \cdot (\sigma_{Ct})^2}.$$

Since $\{\overline{S_k}, \overline{S_k}, \overline{S_j}\}$ is a possible scheduling type, the chance constraint (3) is satisfied. In order to check this equation, based on normal distribution property [34], the following inequality is equivalent to

$$\frac{l(b_i) - \mu_{T_{b_i}}}{\sigma_{T_{b_i}}} \geq V_{Cl},$$

$$P[T_{b_i} \leq l(b_i)] \geq Cl$$

where V_{Cl} is the value corresponding to the normal variable ($x \sim N(0,1)$) with a cumulative distribution function Cl, i.e., $P[x \leq V_{Cl}] = Cl$ and this value is tabulated.

Part (ii): Scheduling of the time blocks, consisting of the following four steps executed sequentially for each time block b_i to schedule.

Step 3: For each possible scheduling type of time block b_i, obtain the sets of real scheduling. Given a possible scheduling type, a real scheduling is composed by a set of patients with the types of surgeries equal to the possible scheduling types.

For example, considering the scheduling type $\{\overline{S_k}, \overline{S_k}, \overline{S_j}\}$, a real scheduling is composed from two patients w' and w'' on which a surgery $s_k \in \overline{S_k}$ should be performed and one patient w''' on which a surgery $s_j \in \overline{S_j}$ should be performed. The first real scheduling corresponding to $\{\overline{S_k}, \overline{S_k}, \overline{S_j}\}$ is chosen by taking the patients with a lower number of preference order (corresponding to the higher preference). However, all other combinations of patients satisfying the chosen scheduling type having no patients with preference order greater than the maximum preference order of the patient in the first real scheduling will be considered.

Let us assume, for example, the list of patients given in Table 1 with $W = \{w_1, w_2, w_3, w_4, w_5, w_6\}$ such that patients w_1, w_3, and w_5 have assigned the surgery s_1, the patient w_2 has assigned the surgery s_2, the patient w_4 the surgery s_3, and the patient w_6 the surgery s_4. Assuming the set of surgeries $S = \{\overline{S_1}, \overline{S_2}, \overline{S_3}\}$ with $\overline{S_1} = \{s_1, s_2\}$, $\overline{S_2} = \{s_3\}$ and $\overline{S_3} = \{s_4\}$ and two possible scheduling types $\{\overline{S_1}, \overline{S_1}, \overline{S_2}\}$ and $\{\overline{S_1}, \overline{S_2}, \overline{S_3}\}$, the first real scheduling considered for $\{\overline{S_1}, \overline{S_1}, \overline{S_2}\}$ is $\{w_1, w_2, w_4\}$. The maximum order of patients in this real scheduling is 4 (corresponding to w_4), hence the following real scheduling will be considered as well: $\{w_1, w_3, w_4\}$ and $\{w_2, w_3, w_4\}$. For the scheduling type $\{\overline{S_1}, \overline{S_2}, \overline{S_3}\}$, the first real scheduling is $\{w_1, w_4, w_6\}$. Since the maximum preference order of patients is 6, the following real scheduling will be considered as well: $\{w_2, w_4, w_6\}$, $\{w_3, w_4, w_6\}$ and $\{w_4, w_5, w_6\}$. All of this real scheduling is shown in Table 2.

Table 1. Surgery data and waiting list of patients used for explaining part 2 of the SHA.

	Surgeries Data		Waiting List						
S	Types	Average Duration							
$\overline{S_1}$	s_1	90	Patient	w_1	w_2	w_3	w_4	w_5	w_6
	s_2	110	Surgery type	s_1	s_2	s_1	s_3	s_1	s_4
$\overline{S_2}$	s_3	125							
$\overline{S_3}$	s_4	135							

Table 2. Motivation example for explaining part 2 of the SHA.

Possible Scheduling Types	Real Scheduling	r (%)	Ap	H (Step 4)	H (Step 5)
	$w_1 w_2 w_4$	77.38	2.33	0	10.71
$\overline{S_1}\,\overline{S_1}\,\overline{S_2}$	$w_1 w_3 w_4$	72.61	2.66	5.62	-
	$w_2 w_3 w_4$	77.38	3	1.74	-
	$w_1 w_4 w_6$	83.33	3.66	4.76	-
$\overline{S_1}\,\overline{S_2}\,\overline{S_3}$	$w_2 w_4 w_6$	88.09	4	0.88	4.34
	$w_3 w_4 w_6$	83.33	4.33	6.50	-
	$w_4 w_5 w_6$	83.33	5	8.24	-

Step 4: Evaluate the real scheduling and select the best one for each scheduling type. First, the real scheduling not fulfilling the chance constraint (3) is removed and the check is similar to the one in Step 2. For the remaining real scheduling, the expected occupation rate r is computed by summing the average duration of all surgeries in the real scheduling divided by the time block duration $l(b_i)$ (multiplied by 100 if percentage). Furthermore, the average preference order Ap is computed by summing the preference order of all patients in the real scheduling divided by the number of patients in the real scheduling. The real scheduling with the minimum value of the following fitness function is chosen:

$$H = (Ap - Min_{Ap}) \cdot \beta + (Max_r - r), \qquad (6)$$

where Min_{Ap} is the minimum average preference order of all real scheduling; Max_r is the maximum occupation rate r of all real scheduling; and β is a balancing parameter between the two terms (one for preference order and one for occupation rate).

For example, in Table 2, the computations of the occupation rates are given, preference order, and fitness function (fifth column) for the set of real scheduling considered before. In this example, a value of $\beta = 2.6$ is used and the time block duration are assumed to be $l(b_i) = 420$ (min), corresponding to 7 h. In this step, the real scheduling $w_1 w_2 w_4$ is chosen for the possible scheduling type $\overline{S_1 S_1 S_2}$ and $w_2 w_4 w_6$ is chosen for $\overline{S_1 S_2 S_3}$.

Step 5: Evaluate the best real scheduling chosen in Step 4 (one for each scheduling type) and select the best one for the current time block b_i. From the set of selected real scheduling in the previous step, the one with minimum value of the fitness function (6) is chosen. Notice that the value of the fitness function of a real scheduling in this step is, in general, different by the one computed in step 4. In particular, Min_{Ap} and Max_r have different values since are computed based only on the best real scheduling computed in step 4.

The sixth column of Table 2 is showing the computation of the fitness function on the two selected real scheduling instances on the previous step. Hence, in this step, $Min_{Ap} = 2.33$ corresponding to $w_1 w_2 w_4$ while $Max_r = 88.09$ corresponding to $w_2 w_4 w_6$. According to them, patients $w_2 w_4 w_6$ are selected for the time block $l(b_i)$.

Step 6: Remove the scheduled patients. The patients scheduled in Step 5 are removed from the waiting list, and the procedure is iterated for time block b_{i+1} from Step 3.

By using the case study in the HCU hospital, it has been observed that values of $t = 3$ and of $\beta = 2.6$ are appropriate. However, for different medical departments, a previous study is necessary in order to better choose these design parameters.

Part (iii): Sorting the time blocks with the same available time. First, the time blocks are grouped depending on their available time $l(b_i)$. Then, the time blocks of each group are sorted in ascending order according to the average preference order of the scheduled patients (indicator Ap). At the end, for each date, a time block is assigned sequentially starting with the closest one.

4.2. Decision Support System

In this section, the main features of the proposed DSS are discussed. Each doctor in the hospital department has his own list of patients and the waiting list of a team is composed by the union of list of doctors belonging to the team. Each team must schedule the patients from its waiting list during the time blocks previously booked by the head of the department. Thus, the main objective of the DSS is to help medical doctors perform a fast efficient and dynamic scheduling of the elective patients. The DSS uses as a core for the scheduling of patients the SHA approach presented in the previous subsection. However, other features are also included which enable (a) managing the medical teams and the OR time-table; (b) updating the waiting lists; (c) dynamic planning; and (d) improving the problem parameter by updating the surgeries duration.

Manage medical team and OR time-table. Normally, the medical teams are composed of the same medical doctors. However, sometimes medical doctors could move from one team to another. The head of the department is responsible for updating the medical teams and including this information in the DSS. Moreover, the head of the department should define the ORs time-table in the DSS. The OR, the date, the starting time, and the ending time of each time block assigned to each team is the information that must be included in the DSS.

Updating the waiting list. Generally, the new arrived patients are included at the end of the waiting list. However, depending on medical criteria, the surgeon could decide to advance the patient into a higher position in the waiting list. The DSS automatically orders the waiting list of patients. There are two parameters influencing directly the position of the patient in the waiting list.

1. The first parameter is related to the waiting time for surgery. A score S_1 of 10 is given to the patient with the highest number of waiting days, while the newest patient has a score of 0. A proportional score between 10 and 0 is given to other patients. In the calculation of total score (denoted S_T), the score S_1 has a weight of p.
2. The second parameter has to do with the surgery priority. Although non-urgent surgeries are scheduled with the DSS, three levels of priorities 1, 2, and 3 are considered by doctors depending on the urgency. A corresponding score (S_2) of 0, 5, and 10 is associated respectively.

The final score is obtained as follows:

$$S_T = p \cdot S_1 + S_2 \qquad (7)$$

Finally, the patients are ordered according to their total score. The patient with the highest total score will be the first, while the patient with the lowest punctuation will be the last one.

Iterative planning. The scheduler of each medical team performs the scheduling for the next $|\mathcal{B}|$ time blocks (this is done by using the SHA). The secretary calls the patients scheduled and asks them for their availability on the scheduled date. The secretary gives back this information to the team scheduler who should schedule the empty gaps again. This process is repeated until the $|\mathcal{B}|$ time blocks are completely scheduled with all patients confirmed.

During the iterative scheduling, if a patient confirms the attendance, she/he is fixed in the corresponding time block. However, in the case that a patient cannot be contacted or she/he cannot be hospitalized, then the patient is not considered for the scheduling of the next $|\mathcal{B}|$ time blocks.

Thus, in the next iteration, the patients previously confirmed and the patients who cannot be hospitalized are not considered in the waiting list. The SHA schedules new patients in the gaps of the uncompleted time blocks.

Updating and customizing the average duration. The average duration and standard deviation of each type of surgery should be computed using historical data from the hospital department. Considering two years, a sufficiently high number of surgeries of each type is obtained, and the average duration is representative. However, depending on the skills and experience of the surgeons, significant differences could exist between their average duration. Moreover, for the same medical doctor, a continuous decrease of the average duration, due to the experience occurring, so these input values should be dynamically updated.

When a surgery is finished, the name of the surgeon and the time spent are introduced in the DSS. The DSS registers this information in a database and updates the average duration.

Overview of the DSS. All the previously explained features are integrated into the DSS whose flowchart is given in Figure 1.

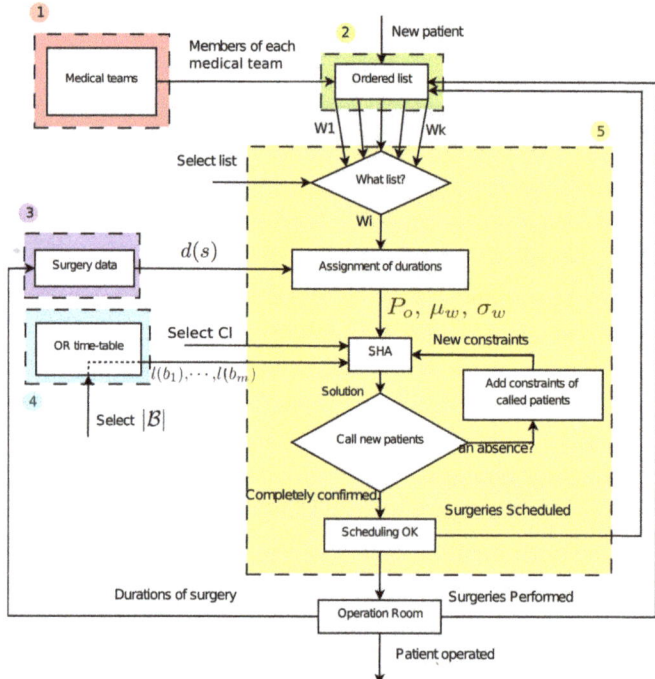

Figure 1. Flowchart of the DSS. The steps form the moment when a patient arrives until she/he is surgically operated are shown. The discontinuous colored boxes reference the five main panels included in the developed software tool: (1) Medical teams; (2) Patients; (3) Surgeries; (4) OR timetable; and (5) Scheduling.

When a new patient arrives at the service, she/he is introduced into the waiting list of a medical doctor. Each surgeon is responsible for including their patients in the system. The DSS recognizes the surgeon (using a personal password) and she/he must enter some personal information of the patient, the pathology and the priority of the surgery. Additionally, the DSS saves the actual date (to compute the waiting time in the list) and the surgeon to whom the patient belongs. When a team scheduler wants to perform a scheduling, she/he is recognized by the DSS and automatically composes the ordered waiting list of his patients.

The DSS has a database, which is updated every time that a surgery is performed. The pathology and its surgery durations are saved in the database. Thus, considering this information, the tool assigns average theoretical duration and standard deviation to each surgery in the waiting list. In this way, the vectors μ_w and σ_w are generated. On the other hand, the DSS saves the OR time-table introduced previously by the head of the department—that is, the time blocks booked for each team as well as their duration defined as $l(b_i)$. The DSS performs an operation scheduling in an iterative way. The input data that the team's manager has to introduce in the DSS to schedule the next time blocks are: (i) the minimum confidence level Cl and (ii) the number of time blocks to schedule $|B|$.

When a patient has been scheduled, his/her state changes from "pending" to "scheduled". Once a specific surgery is performed, the surgeon indicates this situation in the DSS and the corresponding patient is removed from the waiting list. Additionally, the surgeon introduces the operating time in the tool and these new input data are used to update the average duration. If finally a scheduled surgery is not performed, the DSS changes the state of this surgery from "scheduled" to "pending".

Based on the previously described DSS, a Software tool for scheduling elective patients in Spanish Hospitals called CIPLAN has been developed. A first version of this software was described in [12].

CIPLAN has been developed in JAVA language and has a SQL database. Moreover, in order to provide a safe work environment and a better security of the medical data, different access levels are provided to the users. The preferences and concerns of medical doctors in the OSD have been considered not only at the surgery scheduling level but also at the user interface level. Thus, a friendly interface divided into six main panels was proposed. These panels are based on the DSS and the first five are shown with color boxes in the flowchart of Figure 1: (1) *Medical teams*, (2) *Patients*, (3) *Surgeries*, (4) *OR timetable*, (5) *Scheduling*, and (6) *User*. Figure 2 shows the interface of the scheduling panel.

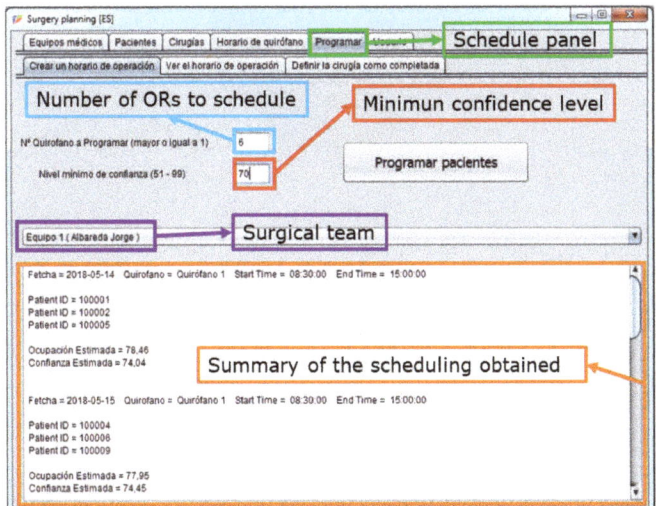

Figure 2. Scheduling panel. The main interface of the software tool is shown. Particularly, the scheduling panel where once the number of blocks to schedule, the minimum confidence level, and the surgical team are introduced, a summary of the scheduling performed is shown at the bottom part.

5. Simulations

In this section, some scheduling results derived of simulation are described and analyzed. The approach presented here is compared with two approaches in literature.

5.1. Simulation Methodology

In order to test the SHA and to compare it with the approaches proposed in [19,20], a discrete event simulation model of the scheduling has been implemented. It is used to simulate scheduling decision for a medical team in the Orthopedic Surgery Department (OSD) at the HCU. One year and the half length (78 weeks) is set for each simulation run. The new patients are assumed to arrive according to a Poisson distribution with an average of six per week. We assume initially a waiting list of 100 patients and every week the new arrived patients are added to the list.

During the last two years, considering historical data in the OSD, the occurrence probability of each surgery type and their duration have been computed. These values are considered in the simulation for generating the surgery of the arrival patients. Figure 3 shows the occurrence of the most common surgeries performed in the OSD while Table 3 indicates their average and standard deviation. Notice that seven types of surgeries represent around 73% of the total surgeries performed; however, all of them are used in the simulations.

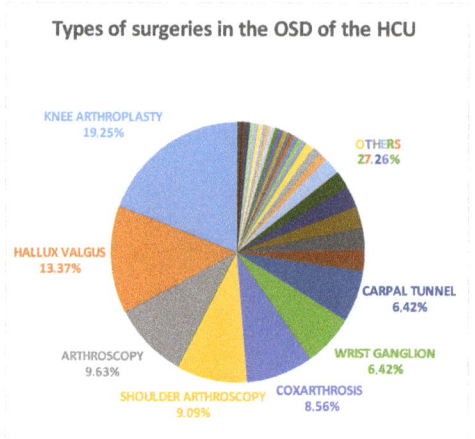

Figure 3. Occurrence of surgeries. The occurrence of some types of surgery that can be performed in the OSD of the LBH are shown.

Table 3. Duration of the surgeries performed in the OSD of the LBH.

Surgery Type	Avg. Duration [min]	Std. Deviation [min]
Knee arthroplasty	123.3	20.95
Hallux Valgus	99.4	17.67
Arthroscopy	79.8	17.97
Shoulder Arthroscopy	115.2	24.76
Coxarthrosis	125.9	32.10
Wrist Ganglion	47.5	21.16
Carpal Tunnel	32.9	7.53

For each set of simulations, 50 replications are performed. Each replication is a schedule of 156 time blocks (78 weeks × 2 time blocks per week) all of them having the same time duration of $l(b_i) = 390$ min (6.5 h). The average values of the probability of not exceeding the total time (confidence level) and the occupation rate are computed. Moreover, the total overtime and the total number of treated patients per year are considered.

In order to be able to compare two different schedules from the point of view of the order of the patients, indicator Ω is defined. This indicator measures the disorder of the patients in the obtained scheduling, so, the smaller it is, the more ordered are the patients. To compute this value, for each time block, an interval $[f_i, l_i]$ is defined. If the preference order of the surgeries scheduled in the time block b_i belongs to the interval $[f_i, l_i]$, Ω is not increased. On the contrary, each patient w_j with a preference order j outside the interval increases the value of Ω. The formal calculation of Ω is given in Algorithm 1, where Np is the total number of patients scheduled and $Pd = \frac{Np}{|B|}$ is the average number of patients scheduled per time block.

Algorithm 1 computes first the lower (f_i) and upper (l_i) preference orders of the patients that should be ideally scheduled in the time block b_i. However, we allow one block before and one block after without any penalization and, for this reason, $f_i = Pd \cdot (i - 2)$ and $l_i = Pd \cdot (i + 1)$. Then, for all patients scheduled in b_i, if their preference order in the waiting list does not belong to $[f_i, l_i]$, Ω parameter is increased with a value depending on the deviation (step 4).

Algorithm 1 Calculation of Ω parameter in a scheduling of $|\mathcal{B}|$ time blocks
---
Input: $\mathcal{B}, Pd$
Output: Ω
1 $\Omega := 0$
   forall $b_i \in \mathcal{B}$ **do**
2      $f_i := (1, \lfloor Pd \cdot (i-2) \rfloor);$
     $l_i := \lceil Pd \cdot (i+1) \rceil;$
     forall *patient* (w_j) *scheduled in block* b_i **do**
3   **if** *the preference order* $(j) \notin [f_i, l_i]$ **then**
4          $\Omega := \Omega + \min(|j - f_i|, |j - l_i|)$

5.2. Simulation Results

Table 4 shows a comparison between the scheduling obtained by using: (1) the first-fit probabilistic rule (commonly used in hospitals), (2) the batch scheduling approach in [19], (3) the constructive algorithm proposed in [20], and (4) the SHA approach presented in this paper. The scheduling is obtained following the simulation methodology explained in the previous subsection for a minimum confidence level $Cl = 70\%$. The average value of probability of not exceeding the total time, occupation rate, and the order of the patients (Ω) are analyzed. Moreover, the total overtime and the total number of treated patients per year are shown.

Table 4. Comparison of the one and the half years scheduling using different chain-constrained approaches with a minimum confidence level of 70%.

Approach	Avg. Confidence Level	OVERTIME (Total) [min]	Avg. Occupation Rate (%)	Total # of Surgeries	Average Ω
first-fit rule	81.98	806.41	76.12	429.9	1935.9
Constructive Alg. [20]	80.43	922	76.69	432.02	2840
Batch Scheduling [19]	75	1183	79.06	447.78	3993.1
SHA (this paper)	77.31	1059	78.28	438.3	395.4

The three approaches analyzed in Table 4 improve the occupation rates obtained by using the first-fit probabilistic rule. However, the improvement in the occupation rate of the time block implies a decrement in the confidence level. For example, the Batch Scheduling approach [19] achieves the highest occupation rate (79.06%) and the highest number of treated patients (447.78), and, consequently, the lower confidence level (75%) and the highest total overtime (1183 [min]) are obtained. Taking into account the pairs of values occupation rate and confidence level, the Batch Scheduling approach obtains the better solution with: (1) the highest occupation rate and (2) a confidence level within the allowed.

The SHA approach presented in this paper obtains a little worse occupation rate (78.28%) than the Batch Scheduling (79.06%). However, considering the order of the patients given by the indicator Ω, it can be checked that the SHA approach by far obtains the best scheduling ($\Omega = 395$). Medical doctors of the OSD consider that the scheduling obtained using the SHA approach is the best one since it maintains the order of the waiting list better. Due to patients having more orders with SHA scheduling, it is possible to provide an estimation period for the patients in the list and this is a possible extension.

6. Case Study Results

This section presents a comparison between a scheduling obtained manually in the OSD and the scheduling obtained by using CIPLAN.

6.1. Case Study Description

Hospital Description. The HCU is a public hospital located in Zaragoza, Spain providing health services to around 325,000 people, and it is a reference center of specialized attention of a population over 1 million inhabitants. The hospital has 800 beds and 15 ORs for major surgery, which is performed by eight different surgical departments. The case study considers the Orthopedic Surgical Department (OSD).

The OSD is composed of five medical teams and has assigned 3 ORs (OR_1, OR_2 and OR_3) from 8:30 a.m. to 3:00 p.m. every day. Although there are other time blocks available for the department, the case study considers only these three ORs because the other ones have a variable time-table depending on the urgent surgeries. OR_1 and OR_2 are used to perform surgeries of elective patients, while OR3 is assigned to perform urgent surgeries. Table 5 shows an example of the weekly OR time-table of this OSD.

Table 5. OR time-table in the Orthopedic Surgical Department of the HCU.

	OR 1	OR 2	OR 3
Mon	team 1	team 2	team 3
Tue	team 4	team 5	team 1
Wed	team 2	team 3	team 4
Thu	team 5	team 1	team 2
Fri	team 3	team 4	team 5

According to Table 5, each medical team has two time blocks per week for performing surgeries on the elective patients.

Methodology of the case study. The main objective of the developed software tool is to improve the efficiency and quality of the surgical service. Thus, in the case study, the scheduling obtained manually is compared with the scheduling obtained by using CIPLAN. The methodology is as follows:

1. Analysis of manual scheduling. Considering historical data of one medical team of the OSD, 36 consecutive OR time blocks of elective patients are analyzed. For each time block, the following information is obtained:

- the type of surgeries performed,
- the starting and ending time of each surgery (real duration),
- the expected and real occupation rate,
- the confidence level of not exceeding the available time,
- the real ending time of each block.

The effective time in a surgery block is the time of using the OR for surgeries; therefore, the occupation rate in a time block is computed as the effective time divided by the total time.

2. Create the waiting list. The manual scheduling and consequently the surgery types in the waiting list are known. However, the preference order of each surgery in the waiting list is unknown. In order to be able to obtain an ordered waiting list from which the scheduling using CIPLAN is performed, it is assumed that the position of the patients (surgeries) in the list corresponds to the order in which they were operated by using the manual scheduling. That is, the first patient in the waiting list is the first patient operated in the first time block. Thus, considering the surgeries performed in the 36 time blocks, an ordered waiting list containing 111 patients is created.

3. Scheduling using CIPLAN. The data necessary to perform the scheduling using CIPLAN are included in the tool and then the scheduling is performed:

- All elective surgery types are added to CIPLAN including their average duration and standard deviation (computed considering historical data of the team during last two years).
- A new medical team (team 1) is added to the tool. Moreover, a new doctor is added to the team.

- All patients in the waiting list constructed using the 36 time blocks are assigned to the doctor.
- For the next three months, two time blocks are booked weekly from 8:30 a.m. to 3:00 p.m., in total being 24 time blocks.
- Using CIPLAN, the 24 time blocks previously booked are scheduled considering a minimum confidence level of not exceeding the total time equal to 69%. This value is fixed by doctors.

4. Analysis of the scheduling performed using CIPLAN. For each time block scheduled, the following parameters are obtained:

- the expected occupation rate,
- the confidence level of not exceeding the total time,
- the real occupation rate,
- the real ending time.

The scheduling obtained by using CIPLAN has not been applied in practice. Thus, to compute the real occupation rate, the time spent when the surgeries were performed (manual scheduling) has been considered. Moreover, in order to obtain the real ending time, 20 min of cleaning time between two consecutive surgeries and 10 min of delay with respect the starting time have been considered.

6.2. Real Case Study

Figure 4a shows the *expected occupation rate* in each time block. The average value obtained using CIPLAN (77.44%) is greater than using the manual method (75%). Moreover, in the scheduling obtained using CIPLAN, the values of the expected occupation rate in each time block are more concentrated around the average value ($\sigma = 3.61$) than using the manual scheduling ($\sigma = 7.42$).

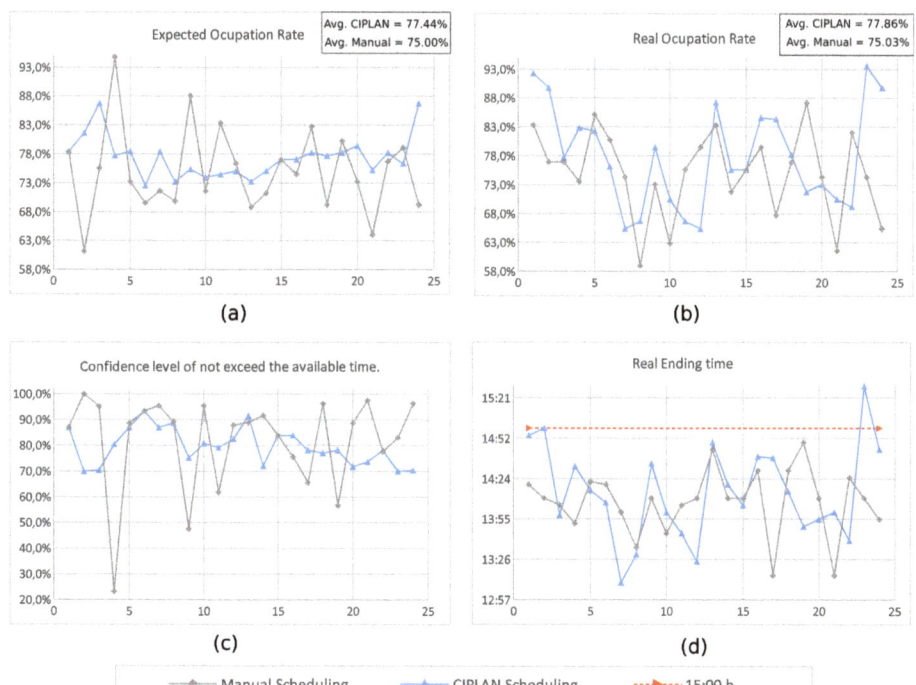

Figure 4. Comparison of manual and CIPLAN scheduling. A set of 24 time blocks has been scheduled manually and using CIPLAN. The following values are shown: (**a**) expected occupation rate; (**b**) real occupation rate; (**c**) confidence level of not exceeded the available time; (**d**) ending time.

In Figure 4b, the *real occupation rate* obtained in each time block is shown. Again, the average value obtained using CIPLAN (77.86%) is greater than the average value using the manual method (75.03%). Using CIPLAN, the improvement in the occupation rate with respect to use the manual method is 2.83%.

In Figure 4b, it is also possible to see that using CIPLAN there are some time blocks (1, 2, 23, and 24) with occupation rates too high (about 90%) and could lead to exceeding the available time. This does not happen in manual scheduling. Analyzing the results, it has been observed that it happens because the scheduler (in the manual method) knows the surgery skill of the surgeon and can estimate better the expected duration of the surgery depending on the surgeon. However, the CIPLAN scheduling algorithm initially uses the average duration of the surgeries. These average durations are computed considering historical data, independently from the surgeon. As the tool is used, the time spent in each surgery as well as the surgeon who performs it will be registered in CIPLAN. Thus, the surgery duration will be more and more customized depending on the surgeon and better results will be obtained.

In Figure 4c, the confidence level of not exceeding the available time is shown. The corresponding values are computed by considering the average duration and the standard deviation of each surgery. It can be seen that using CIPLAN does not exist time blocks with a confidence level lower than 69%. However, using the manual method, there are several time blocks with a really low confidence level. For example, in time block 4, the confidence level of not exceeding the available time is only 23.3%. Again, these low values are obtained since the scheduler knows the surgery skills of the surgeon. Particularly, in time block 4, three knee arthroplasties have been scheduled. Considering the average duration and the standard deviation based on historical data, the expected occupation rate is 94.8% and the confidence level that will not exceed the available time is 23.3%. However, the scheduler knows that the surgeon who has to perform the knee arthroplasties needs 25 min less than the average duration of the team. Consequently, the real occupation rate obtained is 73.3% and the time block ends at 13:52.

Figure 4d shows the ending time of each block. It can be observed that, using CIPLAN, there are four time blocks (1, 2, 13, and 24) ending around 3:00 p.m. and the time block 23 exceeding the available time 30 min (ending 15:30). This situation does not happen in manual scheduling.

According to the results obtained in the case study, the quality of the service decreases, because some blocks exceed the available time. However, this situation will be solved when the average duration and standard deviation of the surgeries will be customized depending on the surgeon. This customization will allow that the real occupation rate will be more similar to the expected one and, consequently, not only the number of blocks exceeding the available time will decrease, but also the total exceeding time.

In Figure 5, the time execution of the manual (a) and automatic (b) scheduling are shown by two bar-graphs.

Each row is composed by boxes that represent different actions in one surgical time block. Colored boxes represent surgeries while white boxes are idle times. The idle time could be: (i) delay regarding the starting time if the box is at the beginning or (ii) cleaning time if the box is between two surgeries. On the other hand, to check how much the order of patients in the waiting list is respected, the preference order of the patients inside the colored boxes has been included. Since the waiting list of patients has been constructed considering real surgeries, in Figure 5a, the patients are perfectly ordered. However, considering the automatic method (Figure 5b), although the SHA tries to make the scheduling respecting as much as possible, the order of the patients in the waiting list results in being a little disorderly. In order to see it visually, three colors have been used with a different meaning:

- The patients delayed or advanced at most a time block respect to the manual scheduling (perfectly ordered) are given in green boxes.
- The patients delayed or advanced two or three time blocks with respect to the manual scheduling are shown in orange or red boxes, respectively.

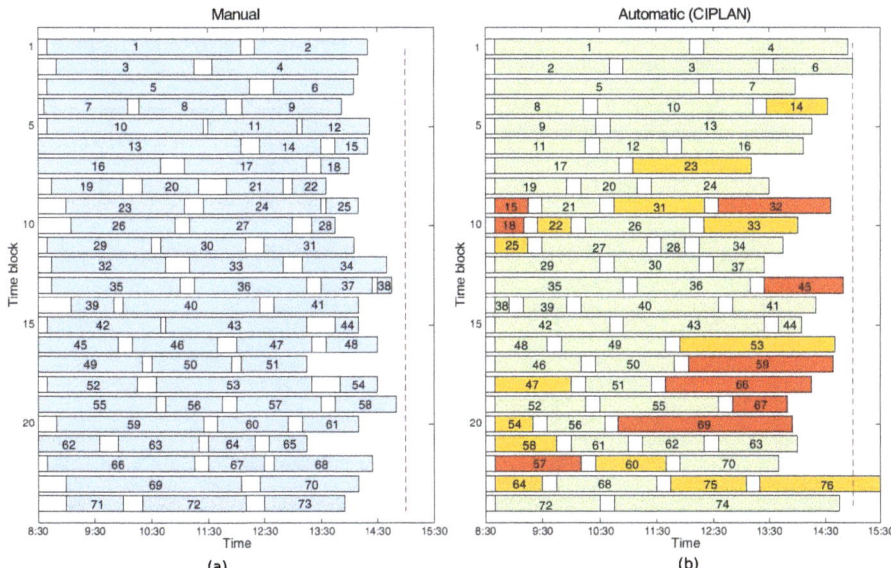

Figure 5. Comparison of the time execution of the surgical blocks. The time execution of the 24 time blocks scheduled (**a**) manually and (**b**) using CIPLAN are compared. Numbers inside the boxes represent the preference order of the patients. In case (**b**) color green/orange/red means that the patient has been advanced or delayed at most 1/2/3 time blocks with respect to the manual scheduling.

Remember that the waiting list has been constructed considering the real surgeries performed in 36 surgical blocks, obtaining a waiting list composed of 111 patients. Considering the manual scheduling, patients with preference order from 1 to 73 have been scheduled in the first 24 time blocks. Using CIPLAN, patients with preference order from 1 to 76 (except 65 and 71) have been scheduled in 24 time blocks. The number of patients advanced or delayed two time blocks (orange) is 14 while the number of patients advanced or delayed three time blocks (red) is 9. However only three patients (15, 18, and 57) have been delayed three time blocks and seven patients (22, 25, 47, 54, 58, 60, and 64) have been delayed two time blocks. This means:

- 4.05% of the patients are delayed three time blocks with respect to the preference order;
- 9.45% of the patients are delayed two time blocks with respect to the preference order.

7. Discussion

7.1. The Use and Experiences with the Scheduling Software Tool

Medical doctors who have used CIPLAN consider it an intuitive, rapid, and efficient software solution that can make easier the scheduling task. With the manual method, the confidence level of not exceeding the available time is unknown before building the schedule. However, with CIPLAN, they find an important advantage that the input parameter is the confidence level and the tool maximizes the occupation rate respecting this confidence level. Moreover, they said that the time spent for scheduling is drastically reduced, a check of the obtained solution being necessary.

Using CIPLAN, from an economic point of view, the improvement in the occupation rate using the manual method is 2.83%. Only considering the OSD, this 2.83% implies an increment Δ_{Oc} of 95.65 effective hours per year in the use of the ORs:

$$\Delta_{Oc} = 0.0283 \cdot 6.5 \left[\frac{hours}{block}\right] \cdot 2 \left[\frac{block}{team \cdot week}\right]$$
$$\cdot 52 \left[\frac{week}{year}\right] \cdot 5[team] = 95.65 \left[\frac{effe.\ hours}{year}\right] \quad (8)$$

Assuming an occupation rate of 77.86% and time blocks of 6.5 h, these 95.65 effective hours are equivalent to an increment Δ_{Tb} of 18.89 blocks per year:

$$\Delta_{Tb} = \frac{95.65 \left[\frac{effe.\ h}{year}\right]}{0.7786 \left[\frac{effe.\ h}{h}\right] \cdot 6.5 \left[\frac{h}{block}\right]} = 18.89 \left[\frac{blocks}{year}\right] \quad (9)$$

Considering that the cost to open an OR during 6.5 h is 5850 euros, the use of CIPLAN in the surgical scheduling could suppose a saving of about 110,000 euros per year. The savings could be really greater extending the use of CIPLAN to other Departments.

7.2. Future Work

Doctors propose two new features that could improve significantly the tool. The first one is a new panel to give the possibility of performing virtual scheduling in which all patients included in a waiting list are scheduled. These provisional scheduling will allow doctors to give patients an estimated date of surgery from the moment when he/she is included in the waiting list. On the other hand, the virtual scheduling allows the head of the department to know the number of time blocks necessary to schedule all patients in the waiting list. Thus, he/she will be able to demand from the health administration the exact blocks needed to operate all patients in a certain period of time.

The second feature proposed is to include a new panel in the tool that, once a time block has finished and the starting and ending time of each surgery performed has been introduced in the tool; a comparison between the expected scheduling and the real execution of the time block is shown. In this way, it will be possible to detect the causes of time deviation between the expected and the real durations.

8. Conclusions

In Spanish hospitals, doctors are responsible for scheduling of elective patients. Currently, this task is performed manually and has three main problems: (i) doctors need to spend their time in the administrative task (scheduling); (ii) usually under or overutilization of the ORs is obtained; and (iii) objectivity can be questioned due to fact that the scheduling is done by a human. This paper presents a *Decision Support System* (DSS) that uses a *specific heuristic algorithm* SHA, in order to help the hospital managers in the scheduling of the elective patients.

Considering the duration of the surgeries and of the cleaning time as random variables with normal probability density function, the SHA with some statistics concepts can be used to schedule the elective patients from the waiting list to the next time blocks in such a way that: (i) the occupation rate of the time block is maximized; (ii) ensures a minimum confidence level of not exceeding the available time; and (iii) respect as much as possible the order of the patients in the waiting list. In addition, the DSS also includes features enabling the management of the medical teams and the OR time-table, updating the waiting list of patients, iterative planning, and automatic improvement of the input data.

In collaboration with the Orthopedic Surgery Department of the "*Lozano Blesa*" Hospital in Zaragoza, a software tool (CIPLAN) based on the proposed DSS has been developed. The preferences and concerns of doctors have been considered not only at the surgery scheduling level, but also at the user interface level. Thus, a friendly interface divided into six main panels is proposed in CIPLAN. It has been developed in Java language and uses a SQL database. Moreover, in order to provide a safe environment to work and better security of the medical data, different access levels are provided to every user.

Finally, in order to check the impact of the software tool in the efficiency and the quality of the surgical service, a case study considering real data from the Orthopedic Department of the HCU has been discussed. The results show that, using CIPLAN, an improvement in the occupation rate of the ORs can be reached.

However, it has been observed that there are significant differences in the surgery duration depending on the experience and on the surgery skill of the surgeon. Thus, if the SHA works with general average duration, over and under occupation rates are obtained more frequently than if it works with customized data. It would be convenient to customize the data of the surgical durations depending on each specific surgeon. In this way, the expected occupation rate and the expected ending time will be more similar to the real ones improving the quality of the service.

As future work, a new panel in CIPLAN can be developed that, once a time block has been finished, allows doctors to compare in a visual way the expected scheduling and the real execution. On the other hand, a new feature in CIPLAN can be included that enables them to perform virtual scheduling in which all patients in the waiting list are scheduled. In this way, an approximated date could be given to patients from the moment when they are included in the system. Moreover, other extensions can be developed—among others, an app connected to CIPLAN allowing patients to know the approximated date of their surgeries.

9. Patents

The developed software tool has been registered by the Office of Transfer of Research Result (OTRI) at the University of Zaragoza.

Author Contributions: All authors contributed to the design of the mathematical model and the conceptual design of the decision support system. J.A. was responsible for collecting the necessary surgical data to analyze the mathematical models and perform the case study. D.C., C.M. and M.S. were involved in the development of the proposed heuristic method as well as the implementation of the DSS. All authors have read and agreed to the published version of the manuscript.

Funding: This work has been partially supported by CICYT-FEDER (Spain-EU) under Grant DPI2014-57252-R and by the Aragonese Government (Spain).

Acknowledgments: We would like to acknowledge with much appreciation Lidia Castan's help in the collection of the necessary surgical data.

Conflicts of Interest: The authors declare no conflict of interest.

Abbreviations

The following abbreviations are used in this manuscript:

OR	Operation Room
DSS	Decision Support System
SHA	Specific Heuristic Algorithm
RHS	Receding Horizon Strategy
HCU	"Lozano Blesa" Hospital in Zaragoza
MIQCP	Mixed Integer Quadratic Constrained Programming
Ap	Average Preference Order
OSD	Orthopedic Surgery Department
CIPLAN	Developed Software Tool
MILP	Mixed Integer Linear Programming.

References

1. Antares Consulting. *Libro Blanco de la Actividad y Gestion del Bloque Quirurgico en España.* Available online: https://www.antares-consulting.com/uploads/TPublicaciones/356f8ea46ff1e222fbcdcdafb4415c0363c9c9aa.pdf (accessed on 11 March 2020).
2. OECD. *Health Data 2005—Statistics and Indicators for 30 Countries*; OECD: Paris, France, 2005.
3. C.I.A. The World Factbook. 2017. Available online: https://www.cia.gov/~library/publications/the-world-factbook/ (accessed on 11 March 2020).
4. Ministerio de Sanidad, Consumo y Bienestar Social. *Crisis Económica y Salud en España*; Informes, Estudios e Investigación; Ministerio de Sanidad, Consumo y Bienestar Social: Madrid, Spain, 2018.
5. Spangler, W.E.; Strum, D.P.; Vargas, L.G.; May, J.H. Estimating Procedure Times for Surgeries by Determining Location Parameters for the Lognormal Model. *Health Care Manag. Sci.* **2004**, *7*, 97–104. [CrossRef] [PubMed]
6. Boyd, S.; Vandenberghe, L. *Convex Optimization*; Cambridge University Press: Cambridge, MA, USA, 2004.
7. Capan, M.; Khojandi, A.; Denton, B.T.; Williams, K.D.; Ayer, T.; Chhatwal, J.; Kurt, M.; Lobo, J.M.; Roberts, M.S.; Zaric, G.; et al. From Data to Improved Decisions: Operations Research in Healthcare Delivery. *Med. Decis. Mak.* **2017**, *37*, 849–859. doi:10.1177/0272989X17705636. [CrossRef] [PubMed]
8. Cardoen, B.; Demeulemeester, E.; Belien, J. Operating room planning and scheduling: A literature review. *Eur. J. Oper. Res.* **2010**, *201*, 921–932. [CrossRef]
9. Schmidt, R.; Geisler, S.; Spreckelsen, C. Decision support for hospital bed management using adaptable individual length of stay estimations and shared resources. *BMC Med. Inform. Decis. Mak.* **2013**, *13*, 3. [CrossRef] [PubMed]
10. Miller, H.E.; Pierskalla, W.P.; Rath, G.J. Nurse scheduling using mathematical programming. *Oper. Res.* **1976**, *24*, 857–870. [CrossRef]
11. Epstein, D.M.; Chalabi, Z.; Claxton, K.; Sculpher, M. Efficiency, Equity, and Budgetary Policies: Informing Decisions Using Mathematical Programming. *Med. Decis. Mak.* **2007**, *27*, 128–137. [CrossRef] [PubMed]
12. Clavel, D.; Botez, D.; Mahulea, C.; Albareda, J. Software Tool for Operating Room Scheduling in a Spanish Hospital Department. In Proceedings of the 22nd International Conference on System Theory, Control and Computing, Sinaia, Romania, 10–12 October 2018.
13. Zhu, S.; Wenjuan, F.; Shanlin, Y.; Jun, P.; Panos, M.P. Operating room planning and surgical case scheduling: A review of literature. *J. Comb. Optim.* **2019**, *37*, 757–805. [CrossRef]
14. Samudra, M.; Van-Riet, C.; Demeulemeester, E.; Cardoen, B.; Vansteenkiste, N.; Rademakers, F.E. Scheduling operating rooms: Achievements, challenges and pitfalls. *J. Sched.* **2016**, *19*, 493–525. [CrossRef]
15. Landa, P.; Aringhieri, R.; Soriano, P.; Tanfani, E.; Testi, A. A hybrid optimization algorithm for surgeries scheduling. *Oper. Res. Health Care* **2016**, *8*, 103–114. [CrossRef]
16. Neyshabouri, S.; Berg, B.P. Two-stage robust optimization approach to elective surgery and downstream capacity planning. *Eur. J. Oper. Res.* **2017**, *260*, 21–40. [CrossRef]
17. Wang, Y.; Tang, J.; Fung, R.Y.K. A column-generation-based heuristic algorithm for solving operating theater planning problem under stochastic demand and surgery cancellation risk. *Int. J. Prod. Econ.* **2014**, *158*, 28–36. [CrossRef]
18. Wang, Y.; Tang, J.; Pan, Z.; Yan, C. Particle swarm optimization-based planning and scheduling for a laminar-flow operating room with downstream resources. *Soft Comput.* **2015**, *19*, 2913–2926. [CrossRef]
19. Shylo, O.V.; Prokopyev, O.A.; Schaefer, A.J. Stochastic operating room scheduling for high-volume specialties under block booking. *INFORMS J. Comput.* **2012**, *25*, 682–692. [CrossRef]
20. Hans, E.; Wullink, G.; Van Houdenhoven, M.; Kazemier, G. Robust surgery loading. *Eur. J. Oper. Res.* **2008**, *185*, 1038–1050. [CrossRef]
21. Kazak, J.; Chruściński, J.; Szewrański, S. The Development of a Novel Decision Support System for the Location of Green Infrastructure for Stormwater Management. *Sustainability* **2018**, *12*, 4388. [CrossRef]
22. Cheng, Y.J.; Chen, M.H.; Cheng, F.C.; Cheng, Y.C.; Lin, Y.S.; Yang, C.J. Developing a Decision Support System (DSS) for a Dental Manufacturing Production Line Based on Data Mining. In Proceedings of the 2018 IEEE International Conference on Applied System Invention (ICASI), Chiba, Japan, 13–17 April 2018; Volume 7.
23. Seyr, H.; Muskulus, M. Decision Support Models for Operations and Maintenance for Offshore Wind Farms: A Review. *Appl. Sci.* **2019**, *9*, 278. [CrossRef]

24. Bernardi, S.; Mahulea, C.; Albareda, J. Toward a decision support system for the clinical pathways assessment. *Discret. Event Dyn. Syst. Theory Appl.* **2019**, *29*, 91–125. [CrossRef]
25. Mahulea, C.; Mahulea, L.; Garcia-Soriano, J.M.; Colom, J.M. Modular Petri Net Modeling of Healthcare Systems. *Flex. Serv. Manuf. J.* **2018**, *30*, 329–357. [CrossRef]
26. Dios, M.; Molina-Pariente, J.M.; Fernandez-Viagas, V.; Andrade-Pineda, J.L.; Framinan, J.M. A Decision Support System for Operating Room scheduling. *Comput. Ind. Eng.* **2015**, *88*, 430–443. [CrossRef]
27. Karlof, J. *Integer Programming: Theory and Practice*; Operations Research Series; CRC Press: Boca Raton, FL, USA, 2005.
28. Apt, K. *Principles of Constraint Programming*; Cambridge University Press: Cambridge, MA, USA, 2003.
29. Clavel, D.; Mahulea, C.; Albareda, J.; Silva, M. *Robust Scheduling of Elective Patients under Block Booking by Chance Constrained Approaches*; Technical Report RR-18-01; Universidad de Zaragoza: Zaragoza, Spain, 2018. Available online: http://webdiis.unizar.es/~cmahulea/papers/rr_2018.pdf (accessed on 11 March 2020).
30. Camacho, E.; Bordons, C. *Model Predictive Control*; Advanced Textbooks in Control and Signal Processing; Springer: London, UK, 2004.
31. Johnson, D.S. Near-Optimal Bin Packing Algorithms. Ph.D. Thesis, Massachusetts Institute of Technology, Cambridge, MA, USA, 1973.
32. Klement, N.; Grangeon, N.; Gourgand, M. Medical Imaging: Exams Planning and Resource Assignment: Hybridization of a Metaheuristic and a List Algorithm. In Proceedings of the 10th International Joint Conference on Biomedical Engineering Systems and Technologies (BIOSTEC 2017), Porto, Portugal, 21–23 February 2017; pp. 260–267.
33. Arabnejad, H.; Barbosa, J.G. List Scheduling Algorithm for Heterogeneous Systems by an Optimistic Cost Table. *IEEE Trans. Parallel Distrib. Syst.* **2014**, *25*, 682–694. doi:10.1109/TPDS.2013.57. [CrossRef]
34. Siegel, A.F. (Ed.) *Practical Business Statistics*, 7th ed.; Academic Press: Cambridge, MA, USA, 2016; pp. 549–552.

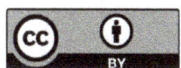

© 2020 by the authors. Licensee MDPI, Basel, Switzerland. This article is an open access article distributed under the terms and conditions of the Creative Commons Attribution (CC BY) license (http://creativecommons.org/licenses/by/4.0/).

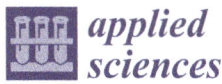

Article

A Prostate MRI Segmentation Tool Based on Active Contour Models Using a Gradient Vector Flow

Joaquín Rodríguez [1], Gilberto Ochoa-Ruiz [2] and Christian Mata [3,*]

1. Vibot ERL Laboratory, Université de Bourgogne Franche-Comté, IUT Le Creusot, 12 rue de la Fonderie, 71200 Le Creusot, France; Joaquin_Rodriguez@etu.u-bourgogne.fr
2. Tecnologico de Monterrey, School of Engineering and Sciences, Ave. Eugenio Garza Sada 2501, Monterrey, N.L., México 64849, Mexico; gilberto.ochoa@tec.mx
3. Centre for Technological Risk Studies, Universitat Politècnica de Catalunya, 08034 Barcelona, Spain
* Correspondence: christian.mata@upc.edu

Received: 28 July 2020; Accepted: 2 September 2020; Published: 4 September 2020

Abstract: Medical support systems used to assist in the diagnosis of prostate lesions generally related to prostate segmentation is one of the majors focus of interest in recent literature. The main problem encountered in the diagnosis of a prostate study is the localization of a Regions of Interest (ROI) containing a tumor tissue. In this paper, a new GUI tool based on a semi-automatic prostate segmentation is presented. The main rationale behind this tool and the focus of this article is facilitate the time consuming segmentation process used for annotating images in the clinical practice, enabling the radiologists to use novel and easy to use semi-automatic segmentation techniques instead of manual segmentation. In this work, a detailed specification of the proposed segmentation algorithm using an Active Contour Models (ACM) aided with a Gradient Vector Flow (GVF) component is defined. The purpose is to help the manual segmentation process of the main ROIs of prostate gland zones. Finally, an experimental case of use and a discussion part of the results are presented.

Keywords: Active Contour Models; snake segmentation; GVF; prostate imaging

1. Introduction

Prostate cancer (PCa) remains one of the most commonly diagnosed solid organ tumor types among men. Early diagnosis and an active follow-up can allow improved prognosis and prevent life-threatening conditions. Once the decision of treatment has been taken, having the most complete information for treatment and follow up is crucial. In 2020, there will be approximately 1,806,590 cancer cases diagnosed and 606,520 cancer deaths are projected to occur in the United States. This classification has been reported by the ICD-O, excepting childhood and adolescent cancers, which were classified according to the ICCC [1]. On the other hand, PCa is the third predicted cause of death in EU with 78,800 death in 2020 [2]. This entails a rate estimation of 10.0/100,000 men.

Medical support systems used to assist in the diagnosis of prostate lesions generally focus on prostate segmentation [3–6]. They rely on computerized techniques for prostate cancer detection applied to ultrasound, magnetic resonance and computed tomodensitometric images [7]. For example, Vos et al. [8] used 3D-T2 imaging to define a specific Region of Interest (ROI), which was subsequently used on diffusion- and perfusion-weighted images to extract relevant features. MRI has been established as the best imaging modality for the detection, localization and staging of PCa on account of its high resolution and excellent spontaneous contrast of soft tissues and the possibilities of multi-planar and multi-parametric scanning [9]. Among the techniques used to detect PCa, MRI also allows non-invasive analysis of the anatomy and the metabolism in the entire prostate gland.

Furthermore, many recent works confirm that the combination of several MRI techniques facilitates the evaluation of prostate diagnoses according to the PI-RADS classification, both for radiologists and medical experts [10]. For instance, a thorough evaluation of various prostate cancer studies was presented in [11]; this study highlights that the correct localization of ROI-containing tumor tissue as the most prevalent problem encountered in the diagnosis of a prostate cancer and other related tasks. Traditionally, clinical experts use different software tools to validate the diagnoses and make annotations in several files. This approach is far from being efficient when managing and dealing with abundant medical data. For the reasons stated above, we propose a new software tool to provide support for the time consuming segmentation process used for annotating images in the clinical practice. Additionally, it enables radiologists to make use of novel semi-automatic segmentation techniques instead of the traditional manual segmentation approaches.

The contributions of this paper are two-fold: we introduce a novel prostate cancer segmentation graphical user interface on which several segmentation algorithms can be easily implemented. In order to demonstrate the strengths and the potential applications of the proposed tool, we included several segmentation algorithms with the software:

- We implemented a modified version of the snake-based active contours segmentation (ACS) algorithm presented in [12] to work with prostate images, which we will refer as *Basic ACS*.
- A simplified version of the *Basic ACS* algorithm, referred as *Simplified ACS*, is included with the program, that runs faster, but with less accuracy.
- Finally, we extended the *Basic ACS* model in order to integrate a Gradient Vector Flow (GVF) component to improve the segmentation process, which we will refer as *GVF ACS* in this paper.

The extensions of original algorithm, in tandem with the novel graphical user interface greatly simplify the segmentation process as it enables a boosted semi-automatic interaction with the clinicians who, eventually, can validate the correctness of the ROI generated by the different methods. Finally, a quantitative study to validate the correctness of the generated segmentation compared to the ground truth and the algorithms is provided. It is worth to mention that the developed program serves as an initial version of a tool that we hope, will create a lot of opportunities to contribute with newer algorithms or improvements to the existing ones in the field of prostate segmentation.

The rest of this paper is organized as follows: in Section 2 we introduce the used dataset and we explain the implementation and features of the proposed Graphical User Interface. Then we describe the Basic ACS and the modifications we introduced to make it work in prostate images. Finally, we present details about the Gradient Vector Flow (GVF) model and its implementation into our tool. In Section 3, we include a single experimental case study to demonstrate the advantages of the proposed approach. In Section 4 we discuss the results in the light of the clinical perspective, and in Section 5 we present the conclusions as well as future works.

2. Materials and Methods

In this section we present the source database and the main contributions of the article, namely the proposed GUI for prostate segmentation process and later on, the integration of the Basic ACS model and its extensions using GVF, the GVF ACS model.

2.1. Database and ROIs References

A database with prostate MRI, based on clinical data with tumor and healthy cases was used. The examinations used in our study contained three-dimensional T2-weighted fast spin-echo (TR/TE/ETL: 3600 ms/143 ms/109, slice thickness: 1.25 mm) images acquired with sub-millimetric pixel resolution in an oblique axial plane. Each study comprises a set of 64 slice images. This database was used in previous works [11] and it has been facilitated for testing the software.

The ground truth annotations were performed using the ProstateAnalyzer tool [11], that allows the drawing of an annotation in a given MRI. For this task, experts with more than 10 years of experience on prostate imaging were asked to provide the annotations using the tool. All the dataset and ground truth data are provided from the medical imaging department of the University Hospital of Dijon

(France). The institutional committee on human research approved the study, with a waiver for the requirement for written consent, because MRI and MRSI were included in the workup procedure for all patients referred for brachytherapy or radiotherapy.

The prostate is composed of a peripheral zone (PZ), central zone (CZ), transitional zone (TZ) and an anterior fibromuscular tissue (AFT) depicted in Figure 1. Most cancer lesions occur in the peripheral zone of the gland, fewer occur in the TZ and almost none arise in the CZ. A detailed description of the influence of the prevalence factor risk according the prostate zone is described in [13]. The T2WI modality was chosen because it provides the best depiction of the prostate's zonal anatomy.

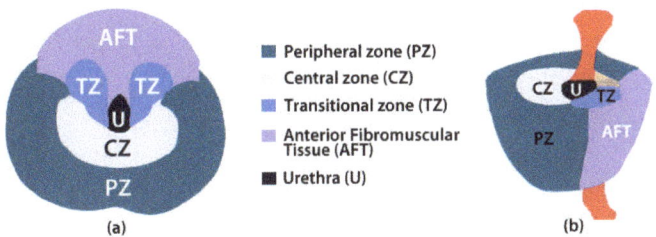

Figure 1. Anatomy of the prostate in (**a**) transversal and (**b**) sagittal planes [11].

The PZ represents up to 70% of a normal prostate gland and around 75% of prostate cancers originate in this zone. The CZ represents about 25% of a normal healthy prostate gland in young adults. Even though the frequency of cancers originating here is much lower, they tend to be of the more aggressive type [14]. An example of a real study case provided by the panel visualization of the prostate tool [11] is depicted in Figure 2. All the overlays are annotated with manual drawings made by radiologists. Each region is represented by different colors (CZ in white and PZ in blue) focusing on a tumor area represented in red (Tum). This example shows the importance of making annotations in regions of interest. In this case, a manual segmentation is validated by experts.

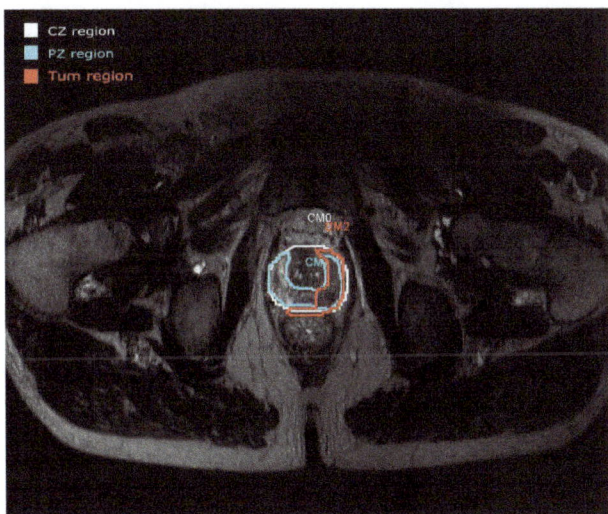

Figure 2. An example of the anatomy (T2WI) panel visualization of the tool developed in [11] with the ROIs annotated by radiologists.

Therefore, one of the main motivations of this work is to develop a new tool focused on improving the results of this initial manual segmentation using Active Contour Models (ACM), facilitating the task of the experts.

In order to attain the above-mentioned goals, we have implemented a novel Graphical User Interface that permits to import, analyze and annotate prostate MR images. The program requires an initial annotation from the user, that does not require to be perfect, and the outcome is an annotation more accurate than the initial one. The modular design of the software allows for integrating segmentation methods as plug-ins or extensions that can be used for testing and clinical purposes. Additionally, this design enables easy performance comparisons between already integrated methods and new methods. In what follows, we will discuss the design of this GUI and subsequently, we will present a study case using three implementations of an ACS model for segmenting the different prostate sections in MR images. It is important to note that this tool and the developed algorithms have not yet been clinically tested and the results presented here represent a proof of concept. However, for the design of the GUI, the expertise and suggestions of clinical experts have been taken into account.

2.2. Implementation of the Graphical User Interface for Prostate Segmentation

In this section, the code organization and the user interface of the program will be explained. The main window of the program is shown in Figure 3. All the code has been developed in Python, using the modules PyQt for the user interface and PyDicom to open the files included in the testing dataset. The code has been organized in modules that do not interact with each other. The integration of all of them has been made in the Main Window class.

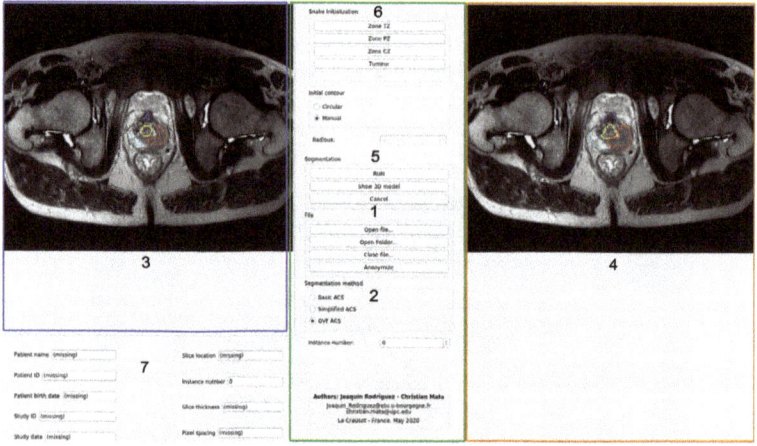

Figure 3. GUI interface of the developed active contour segmentation tool using a prostate MR image.

Each module is placed in folders as follows:

- **DICOM.** This module contains the code that is in charge of handling the Digital Imaging and Communication On Medicine (DICOM) formatted files. It can open either a folder or a single DICOM image. Each file is assumed to contain only one image. The read information will be stored locally on RAM, and after the file or files has/have been opened, a signal will be emitted, and the information can be requested as many times as the user wants.

  The data available to the user includes the images and the patient data fields. This module is also in charge of anonymizing the files and writing them into disc. The functionalities of this module can be accessed through the buttons in the Section 1 of the Figure 3.
- **Image segmentation.** This module stores all the Python code related to the segmentation procedure. The main class in this module is Segmentation-Hub, which is in charge of selecting

the right class for the object that will produce the segmentation, according to the method chosen by the user. The selection of the segmentation method can be done in Section 2 of Figure 3. By implementing the methods in this manner, the actual implementation of the segmentation task is completely transparent for other classes that make use of this module. To select certain segmentation method, only a label that defines the method must be provided.

This module also contains two other files with useful functions:

1. A specific MatLab module which implements some functions that are found in MatLab but not in Python, and their names are the same as in this program.
2. The other file corresponds to a class that finds the ellipse parameters that better fits to a set of points. This code is used for the shape prior of the snake algorithm (Basic ACS) which will be explained in Section 2.3.

- **Image widget.** This module is in charge of showing the image, as well as the initial and the resulting contours from the segmentation. The same module is used for both, left and right images. It also captures the clicks from the user to generate either the circular or the manual initial contour. Both types of initialization will be explained later. The image widget is represented in Sections 3 and 4 of Figure 3.
- **Model 3D widget.** It shows a 3D representation of the output segmentation, based on the Python module Matplotlib. This process is relatively simple as it only replicates the given contour vertically. If the spatial resolution is given in the input DICOM file, the scale of the axis will be given in millimeters. It can be accessed through the button *Show 3D Model* located in Section 5 of Figure 3.
- **Snake init widget.** This widget is in charge of handling all the functionalities of the Snake initialization group, placed at the top of the central control panel of the application.

  Each button will request the main window to ask the user to enter the initial contour in the left image. Once the user has finished, the gathered contours are returned back to this module.

  Afterwards, the corresponding masks for those contours can be generated for the snake algorithm (the mask consists of an image with values of 1 in the interior of the contour, and zeros outside of it). The interface for this module is represented in Section 6 of Figure 3.
- **User data widget.** It is implemented as an efficient and easy to use manner to handle all the user information as an object, and to show it. This class stores all the information related to the patient or the study, retrieved from the DICOM file. It also contains the corresponding widgets that are shown below the left image area, where the gathered information is displayed (see Section 7 of Figure 3).

A block diagram of the proposed tool components is depicted on Figure 4.

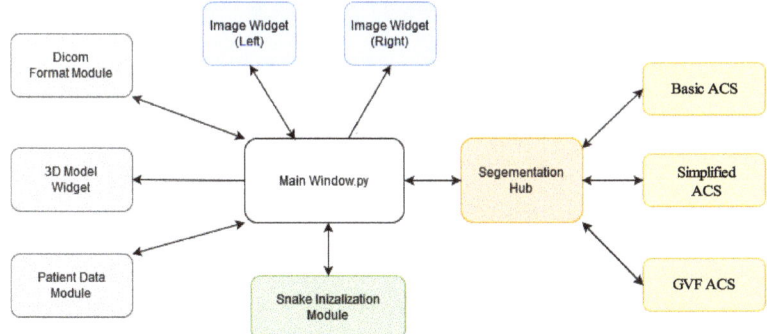

Figure 4. Main software components of the proposed tool. The Segmentation-Hub module can be extended with new modules seamlessly.

Finally, regarding the user interface showed in Figure 3, this program has four well-defined sections:

- **Left panel.** In this area (highlighted in blue), the loaded images are shown, and the user can draw the initial contours of the snake of the different areas of the prostate. Each prostate zone is surrounded with a different color to make it easily distinguishable (see Figure 3)
- **Right panel.** This area (highlighted in orange) shows the loaded images, and the results of the evolution of the selected snake algorithm. Each prostate zone has a pre-defined color, and they match with the colors used for the initial contours (see Section 4 of Figure 3).
- **Bottom area.** The patient information retrieved from the DICOM file is shown (highlighted in blue). Moreover, information related to the spatial resolution and thickness of the gathered slice are included (Section 7 of Figure 3)
- **Central area.** This is the control panel area (highlighted in green). All the functionalities and possible configurations of the program are located in this area. It is represented in the Sections 1, 2, 5 and 6 of Figure 3.

To the best of our knowledge, tools as the proposed in this work, which integrate a Graphical User Interface and semi-automated segmentation algorithms for image annotation do not exist (at least not for prostate MR images). Therefore, a preliminary effort to develop a GUI that includes several active contour model implementations is very important and has driven the development of this work. On the other hand, from the implementation point of view, this program represents an excellent tool to deploy new snake-based algorithms: given that the initial contour and the original image are available in the Segmentation-Hub module, new algorithms can be created using Python, and added as an standalone file to the Image Segmentation folder. This procedure will add another option to the GUI, and the new algorithm's performance and accuracy can be compared with the already existing techniques. This code-base is now available as a GitHub repository to the community [15].

In order to demonstrate how different segmentation methods can be integrated into the proposed tool, we have implemented various versions of an Active Counter Model within the Image Segmentation module of our tool. These methods have been included not only for demonstration purposes, but also to serve as a baseline for future developments in prostate MRI segmentation research (people can improve them, or develop new methods based on them). The proposed Active Contour Model, to be discussed in the following section, also represents a novel contribution, as it has not been previously reported to be used for prostate segmentation purposes.

2.3. Implementation of the Proposed Active Contour Model

The base method implemented is inspired on [12,16]. Both of them are active contours—level-set algorithms. Particularly, the model by Pluempitiwiriyawej et al. [12] was conceived and customized to work with MR images. The general idea of snake algorithms is to modify a curve based on certain forces that push the boundaries of such curve until it reaches the border of the object of interest. A particular feature of this type of segmentation algorithm is that they are unsupervised methods, given that there is not feedback on whether the boundary is following the correct borders or not. Due to this assumption of snake-based methods, an initial contour must be provided, and the closer this initial contour is to the real object, the better the result of the segmentation.

Typically, most snake-based algorithms follow the information about the gradient of the image, which means the curve will try to evolve towards the edges of the object. Nonetheless, if the object does not contain well defined edges, or it has been previously smoothed in order to reduce the noise, this algorithm might fail in following the shape of the object. As a consequence, the outcome will be either a contour that is smaller or larger than the object's boundaries, or in the worst case, the contour will be reduced until it disappears. This is the reason why several researchers developed specific algorithms depending on the type of object to detect, and the type of image to deal with. This is done adding different terms called *priors*. Each constraint added to the algorithm defines a prior, and its corresponding weight will define its contribution to the force.

In this previous work [12], the goal is to segment the shape of the left ventricle of the heart, but since it is aimed to work with MR images, and the priors are similar to the assumptions that can be done for the prostate zones, we considered it as a good starting point for carrying out our experiments and implement the GVF extension to demonstrate its viability in this image modality. The basic assumption of the developed algorithm is that the contour will split the image into two areas, the target object and the background. The evolution of the curve will be driven trying to minimize an energy functional that in this case, it is composed of four components. Each of them will define the priors the final contour must comply with [12]:

1. **Model matching.** it is assumed that the pixel values inside and outside the object follow different statistical models, specified as M1 and M2, respectively.
2. **Edge information.** the contour must be attracted to certain clues that describe the limits of the object, i.e., the strongest edge values of the image should attract the curve.
3. **Shape prior.** Besides certain possible variations between patients, each prostatic zone has a general shape. This shape information can be thought as a function $C_H(\theta)$, with $\theta = [\theta_1, \theta_2, ..., \theta_n]^T$. The parameters θ_i define a model of the actual shape and size of the requested zone, and depending of how distant is the contour from this estimated shape, this prior will contribute more or less to the snake evolution.
4. **Contour smoothness**: The contour is supposed to not be jagged or too noisy, so this parameter controls that.

Then the functional that defines the energy described above, depending on the contour C, can be expressed as:

$$J(C) = \lambda_1 J_1(C) + \lambda_2 J_2(C) + \lambda_3 J_3(C) + \lambda_4 J_4(C) \quad (1)$$

where λ_i are the weights of each prior included in the energy function. This function will be used to make evolve the contour. It follows that it is possible to transform the information of the contour in a level set function, i.e., the information about the contours can be expressed as a function, where the pixels that belong to the object have certain value (or level), the background ones have another level, and the frontier, which is the contour C, is represented by another level. In the case of this paper, the contour is expressed through the level set function as in Equation (2). As it can be seen, the contour is in the level where the function ϕ is equal to zero. Ω represents the space of the image.

$$C = \{(x,y) \in \Omega : \phi(x,y) = 0\} \quad (2)$$

Then, the energy functional can be expressed as depending on ϕ.

$$J(\phi) = \lambda_1 J_1(\phi) + \lambda_2 J_2(\phi) + \lambda_3 J_3(\phi) + \lambda_4 J_4(\phi) \quad (3)$$

This function ϕ evolves with each iteration (i.e., time), depending on the direction in which the forces push the contour. In the following sections the particularities of each term will be described.

2.3.1. Region-Based Model Matching—Term $J_1(\phi)$

The aim of this term is to split the image space Ω into two regions that contain homogeneous pixels: the object and the background. Let's call them Ω_1 and Ω_2, respectively. These two regions are separated by the contour C. An homogeneous region implies a region where all the pixels that are contained in it are described by the same stochastic model. The points that belong to the object have intensities $u_1 = \{u_{i,j} : (i,j) \in \Omega_1\}$, and they are described by the model M_1, and the ones that belong to the background have values $u_2 = \{u_{i,j} : (i,j) \in \Omega_2\}$, and they are represented by the model M_2.

The idea of the model is as follows: let's consider the image u_0 to be formed by two regions, of piecewise-constant intensities c_1 and c_2, and that the intensities of the object are represented by

c_1. The boundary of this region is C_0. Then, the pixel values of the image u_0 are c_1 inside C_0, and c_2 outside of it. Given this, it is possible to build the following fitting term:

$$F(C) = F_1(C) + F_2(C) = \int_{inside(C)} |u_0(x,y) - c_1|^2 dxdy + \int_{outside(C)} |u_0(x,y) - c_2|^2 dxdy \quad (4)$$

where C is any variable curve, and c_1 and c_2 are two constants that depend on the contour C. Based on the previous explanation, if $C = C_0$, then $F(C)$ is approximately zero, because each distance between the image value and the constant c_i are approximately zero for each region. If the curve C is outside C_0, then its interior contains parts of the object and parts of the background, while the exterior of C contains only elements of the background. Because of this, $F_1(C) > 0$ and $F_2(C) \approx 0$. In the backwards case, i.e., the contour C is smaller than C_0, the outside contains parts of the object and the background, whilst the inside only contains parts of the object. It follows that $F_1(C) \approx 0$ and $F_2(C) > 0$. Finally, this fitting function can be used to find the boundaries of the object, by minimizing its value such as

$$\inf_C \{F_1(C) + F_2(C)\} \approx 0 \approx F_1(C_0) + F_2(C_0) \quad (5)$$

In order to achieve this boundary, the evolution of the curve C is done by moving pixels from the exterior to the interior of the contour, and vice-versa. The first estimation of the energy function for this prior is in Equation (6):

$$J_0(C) = p(u|C, M_1, M_2) \quad (6)$$

where p is the probability density function of the image intensities u, given the contour C, and the models M_1 and M_2. Over these probabilities, it is assumed that each element, object and background, are statistically independent, and they have pdfs p_1 and p_2, respectively. Moreover, the pixel intensities are considered to be independent from each other. With these assumptions, and taking the negative of the logarithm of the pdfs, the Equation (6) becomes Equation (7).

$$J_1(C) = \sum_{(i,j) \in \Omega_1} -\ln(p_1(u_{ij})) + \sum_{(i,j) \in \Omega_2} -\ln(p_2(u_{ij})) \quad (7)$$

Assuming a continuous function, the contour embedded in the zero level-set function ϕ, and considering the Heaviside function in order to create a single integral over all the domain of the image, the Equation (7) can be generalized as shown in Equation (8).

$$J_1(\phi) = \int_\Omega -\ln[p_1(u(x,y))]H(\phi(x,y)) - \ln[p_2(u(x,y))](1 - H(\phi(x,y))) dxdy \quad (8)$$

It is assumed that both elements in the image follow a Gaussian distribution, with means m_1 and m_2, and variances σ_1^2 and σ_2^2, which are unknowns, and for each contour C, they will be estimated.

2.3.2. Edge Based Function Term $J_2(\phi)$

This term will push the contour towards the edges of the object. The computation of this type of force is done through the edge-map $Y(x,y)$ generated from the image $u(x,y)$. The most common implementation is the gradient of the smoothed image.

$$Y(x,y) = -|\nabla G_\sigma * u(x,y)| \quad (9)$$

where G_σ is a Gaussian kernel of parameter σ, ∇ is the gradient operator and $(.) * (.)$ is the convolution operator. Finally, the energy functional, depending on the level set function ϕ, which corresponds to this prior is given by the Equation (10).

$$J_2(\phi) = \int_\Omega Y(x,y)\delta(\phi(x,y))|\nabla\phi(x,y)|dxdy \tag{10}$$

where $\delta(\phi(x,y))$ will return non-zero values only for the pixels that are on the contour C.

2.3.3. Object Shape Prior—Term $J_3(\phi)$

This term has been introduced in [12] to reinforce an elliptical shape in heart MR images, but it can be changed by any other shape model depending on the specific object to be segmented. The addition of this prior will improve the performance of the general active contour implementation. For instance, if the target to segment has a circle-like shape, then the snake function can be constrained to satisfy an ellipse equation. In that case, the functional corresponding to this energy term can be defined as $J_3(\phi) = \int_C D^2(x,y)ds$ where $D(x,y)$ is the ellipse distance function defined as:

$$D(x,y) = ax^2 + bxy + cy^2 + dx + ey + f \tag{11}$$

The parameters $\theta = [a,b,c,d,e,f]$ are computed in such a way that the cloud of points around the contour C fits with this ellipse equation. This means that the parameters of θ must be computed for each contour C, and they will change the force direction in order to minimize this distance function. Finally, introducing the level set function ϕ, where the contour C is embedded, the shape prior is computed as in Equation (12), when integrating in all the space Ω.

$$J_3(\phi) = \int_\Omega D^2(x,y)\delta(\phi(x,y))|\nabla\phi(x,y)|dxdy \tag{12}$$

2.3.4. Contour Smoothing—Term $J_4(\phi)$

Finally, it is desirable that the generated contour is smooth. This can be achieved if the Euclidean arc length of the contour C is minimized. It follows that the contribution function for this prior is the one represented in Equation (13).

$$J_4(C) = \int_C ds \tag{13}$$

It is worth mentioning that if only this term is included in the functional, the shape of the contour will become a circle, and then it will start shrinking until it eventually disappears. Nonetheless, when all the terms are put together, this situation is avoided, and the effect is to smooth the curve. Again, adding the level set function where the contour is embedded, the final function for J_4 is defined in Equation (14).

$$J_4(\phi) = \int_\Omega \delta(\phi(x,y))|\nabla\phi(x,y)|dxdy \tag{14}$$

The following step is to combine all the functional together, and expand the minimization problem, in such a way the function $\phi(x,y)$, which contains the contour C as its level zero, evolves towards the edge of the object. The entire procedure is well explained in [12], and it consists of three tasks:

1. Define the statistical model constants, in such a way that they comply with the prior that the pixel distribution follows a Gaussian distribution.
2. Estimate the ellipse parameters to obtain the distance functional contribution.
3. Define the contour evolution equation. This can be done by applying the Euler-Lagrange (EL) equation to the functional of the four priors. Then, considering that ϕ is a function of time, the EL equation is equaled to the derivative of ϕ with respect to the time. The resulting function is given in Equation (15).

$$\frac{\partial \phi}{\partial t} = \left[\lambda_1(M_2 - M_1) - \nabla P \frac{\nabla \phi}{||\nabla \phi||} - P\kappa\right]\delta(\phi(x,y)) \tag{15}$$

where M_1, M_2 are the stochastic models of the object and the background, respectively, $\kappa = div\left(\frac{\nabla \phi}{||\nabla \phi||}\right)$ is the curvature of the contour, $\phi(x,y)$ is our level set function, and $P(x,y) = \lambda_2 Y(x,y) + \lambda_3 D^2(x,y) + \lambda_4$ is the potential function.

The different values of λ_1, λ_2, λ_3 and λ_4 will define the contribution of the corresponding energy term, from J_1 to J_4, and the one with the biggest value will enforce its properties over the others. In practice, the parameters setting is done empirically, and there is no rule that defines how to chose them. It depends on the quality and the properties of the input image. One solution is to make the weights to evolve at each iteration to obtain the best results. The general idea of this evolution is that at the beginning, the algorithm should minimize the energy functional trying to cover all the object, pushing the boundaries towards the edges (effect produced by λ_1 and λ_2), and when the algorithm is close to the end, the curve must enforce the shape of the contour and its smoothness (λ_3 and λ_4).

For the particular case of prostate segmentation, several objects with different shapes have to be considered. Therefore, the shape prior cannot be only an ellipse, as it happens in the case of the left ventricle of the heart. Thus for this implementation, the value of λ_3 has been set to zero.

Additionally, through several experiments, we concluded that the contribution produced by the smoothness prior is not noticeable. In fact, it produces small variations in the contour, and the result is that the algorithm takes more time to converge. This is the reason why the value of λ_4 has been set to zero too. Finally, the suggested evolution of the weights is shown in Figure 5.

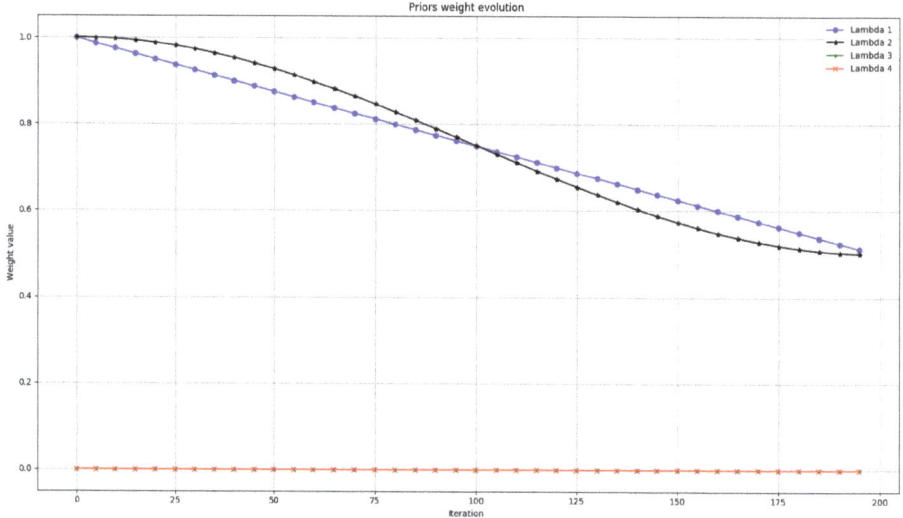

Figure 5. Evolution of λ_i weights for the energy functional.

2.4. Gradient Vector Flow Approach (GVF)

When dealing with snakes algorithms, there are two types of implementations: *Parametric Active Contours (PACs)* or *Geometric Active Contours (GACs)*. They differ in how they define the curve function, since equations formulated for the minimization problem stays almost the same. PACs are based on a parametric curve of a shape represented in Equation (16):

$$C(s) = \{[x(s), y(s)], s \in [0,1]\} \quad (16)$$

with the constraint that it should be closed, i.e., $C(0) = C(1)$. Geometric Active Contours, on the other hand, define the curve to be deformed as embedded in a level-set function, generally as its level zero. This last case is the one implemented and described in Section 2.3. GACs have advantages over PACs, since they are computationally more stable and they are able to change their topology as the function is deformed. Nonetheless, the implemented method is an edge-based method, since it uses the gradient as pushing force, and local intensity information to determine if a pixel belongs to the object or not. Due to this, several problems can appear, such as:

1. If the edges of the object are not well defined, a leaking problem occurs, leading the snake outside of the object's boundaries.
2. If the initial contour is not close to the limits of the object, the gradient will not be able to guide the snake to the edges of the object. If the image is just black and white with one object on it, an initial contour far away from the object will not evolve. On the other hand, if there are other objects around, the snake might be attracted to them, instead of the desired object.
3. Since the snake uses the local pixel information to determine the evolution of the curve, it is sensible to the image noise.

Additionally, the fact of using gradients only, brings another effect related to concavities, that is illustrated in Figure 6.

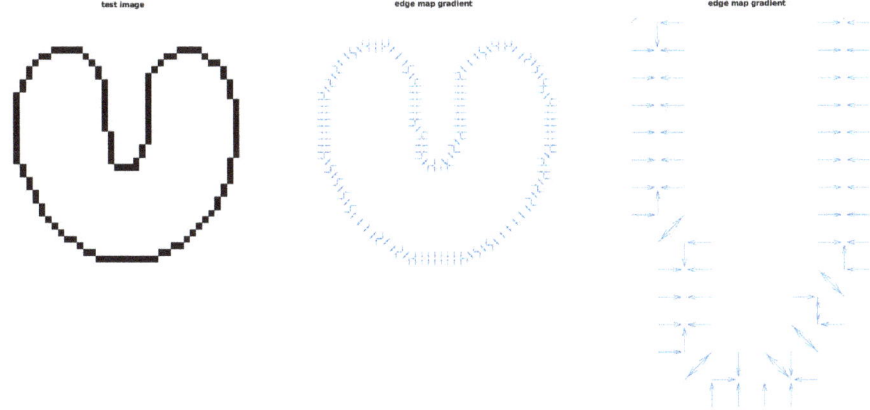

Figure 6. Example of Gradient vector field of a U shape object. (**Left**) Original image. (**Center**) Gradient of the object. (**Right**) Zoom of the vector field in the central concavity of the object.

In this case, a simple object with a narrow concavity, and its corresponding gradient vector field are shown. From it, it is easy to see that:

- In all the space where there the intensities are constant, the gradient is zero. There are gradient vectors only in the borders of the object. This is the main reason why (in an edge-based snake) an initial contour placed far away from the object might not converge to the real object boundaries.
- Narrow concavities start to have horizontal gradient vectors (as it can be seen in the right plot of the Figure 6). As a consequence, the snake will attach to the borders, but it will not address towards the interior of such concavity because the gradient does not have any downwards component.

These last two problems can be solved in the previously explained algorithm with an external force that, not only adds vectors where the gradient is zero, but that also adds a downwards component in the long concavities in such a way that the active contour will be pushed to the interior of this type of areas. This external force is called Gradient Vector Flow (GVF) [17]. Adding this component to the energy described in Section 2.3 will help to not only make the system more robust against initialization effects, but it will improve the outcome by attaching the resulting snake really close to the edges of the object.

The GVF is a dense vector field $\mathbf{v}(x,y) = [u(x,y), v(x,y)]$ derived from the original image, and it is the result of minimizing the energy term defined in Equation (17) [17].

$$\varepsilon = \iint \mu(u_x^2 + u_y^2 + v_x^2 + v_y^2) + |\nabla Y|^2 |\mathbf{v} - \nabla Y|^2 \, dxdy \qquad (17)$$

where u_x and v_x are the partial derivatives of u and v with respect to the variable x, respectively, u_y and v_y are the partial derivatives of u and v with respect to the variable y, respectively, and $Y(x,y)$ is the edge map of the original image. The parameter μ is a constant that serves as regularization: it adjusts the balance between the first and the second term of the integral, and it should be adjusted based on the noise. The higher the noise, the higher the value of μ. Interpreting the energy term presented in (17), it is possible to see that if the gradient of the edge map is too small, the energy term depends only on the partial derivatives of u and v. On the other hand, if this gradient is large, the integral is dominated by it, and the value of the GVF that minimizes the energy is $\mathbf{v} = Y$, i.e., the gradient vector flow is equal to the gradient of the edge map on those cases. It can be demonstrated that the vector field $\mathbf{v} = (u,v)$ that minimizes (17) is the result of the decoupled pair of differential Equations (18) and (19).

$$\mu \nabla^2 u - (u - Y_x)(Y_x^2 + Y_y^2) = 0 \qquad (18)$$
$$\mu \nabla^2 v - (v - Y_y)(Y_x^2 + Y_y^2) = 0 \qquad (19)$$

where ∇^2 is the Laplacian operator. Similarly as in Equation (17), it is possible to see that in the regions where the gradient of the edge map is small, the solution of the differential equations for the GVF are the solution of Laplace's equations. Furthermore, this solution is interpolated from the boundaries of the object, and that's the reason why the resulting field, even far away from the object, points to the edges of it. The gradient vector flow of the same image as in Figure 6, is shown in Figure 7. Now, the solution to the Equations (18) and (19) provides vectors in the areas where the gradient is zero, and the vectors in the concavity contains downwards components too.

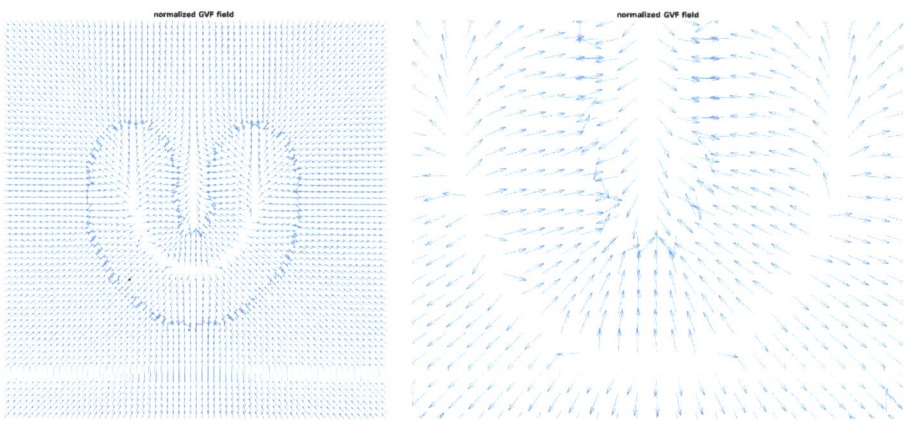

Figure 7. Example of normalized Gradient Vector Flow. (**Left**) GVF vector field for the same image used before. (**Right**) Zoom in the concavity.

Once the GVF has been computed, it is fixed for the entire the image, and what remains is the optimization equation that will guide the deformation of the active contour to the edges of the object, based on this new force. Several researchers have been working on adding gradient vector flow to the traditional snake equations. For the implementation made in Section 2.3, only GACs algorithms can be adapted to be added as an external force to the energy functional defined in the Equation (15), as it has been done in [18,19]. A simplified version of the GVF optimization equation from [19] is used, and defined as:

$$\gamma \frac{\partial \phi}{\partial t} = \left[\alpha \kappa - v . \frac{\nabla \phi}{|\nabla \phi|} \right] |\nabla \phi| \quad (20)$$

The parameter γ regularizes the step size, ϕ is the level-set function, $\kappa = div\left(\frac{\nabla \phi}{|\nabla \phi|}\right)$ is the curvature, v is the Gradient Vector Flow vector field, and the parameter α regulates the balance between the two forces. The right hand factor of (20) is added directly to Equation (15), giving Equation (21):

$$\frac{\partial \phi}{\partial t} = \left[\lambda_1(M_2 - M_1) - \nabla P \frac{\nabla \phi}{||\nabla \phi||} - P\kappa + \beta \left(\left[\alpha \kappa - v . \frac{\nabla \phi}{|\nabla \phi|} \right] |\nabla \phi| \right) \right] \delta(\phi(x,y)) \quad (21)$$

This new segmentation algorithm has been included in the list of options to segment the different prostate zones. After having implemented the *Basic ACS* in Python, the extension with a GVF component is trivial: all the components of this new force are already available in the code except for the vector field **v**. Since this vector field is fixed for a given image, a new class has been created that solves the optimization problem for the GVF. This new piece of code is executed before the main loop of the segmentation algorithm. Since there are no rule for setting both α and γ, we arbitrarily decided to set them to 1. In order to adjust the contribution of this new force, the β factor has been introduced. For the following experiments, this factor has been also set to 1. In the coming sections, the graphical user interface result of the integration of all the modules will be showed. Then, the described algorithms will be tested to show their performance.

3. Experimental Case of Use for Demonstration

In this section a case of use for demonstration is presented. Previously, the proposed GUI has been explained in Section 2.2. A detailed definition of this algorithm and the introduced improvements have been explained in Sections 2.3 and 2.4. The following study case demonstrates how an user can use the proposed tool to manage and segment a real prostate image.

First, the user must load an image in DICOM format. For this application, the snake initialization is required; an example of the initial contours for a study is shown in Figure 8. In the area of the GUI that corresponds to the initialization of the snake, the three first buttons are used for selecting the different zones of the prostate, whereas the fourth one gives the possibility of selecting a tumor.

Located below these buttons, there are two radio buttons, enabling to choose the shape of the initial contour, which can be circular or manual. The first option corresponds to an initial contour with a shape of a circle whose radius can be specified with the spin box located at the end of this area. The possible values are between 1 and 30 pixels. The manual input enables the user to enter a random polygon as initial contour. If selected, the user just has to make a click with the mouse in the vertices of the desired polygon. There are no limits for the amount of points, or the shape of the polygon.

The steps required to initialize the snake for any of the prostate areas are the following:

1. Select the type of contour to enter, circular or manual. In case of circular, enter also the radious.
2. Select an area: TZ, PZ, CZ or Tumour.
3. Create the initial contour for the snake in the left image. If it is a circle, the mouse cursor must be placed in the center of the area of interest, and click with the left button of the mouse. If manual contour has been chosen, the mouse must be placed in the point where the user wishes to start the contour and make click with the left button. Then move the cursor until the next point, make a left click and go to the next point. More than 2 points are required.
4. In manual mode, once the contour is finished, press the "Ok" button. If not, go to step 5.
5. A message box will appear informing if the contour has been correctly added or not.

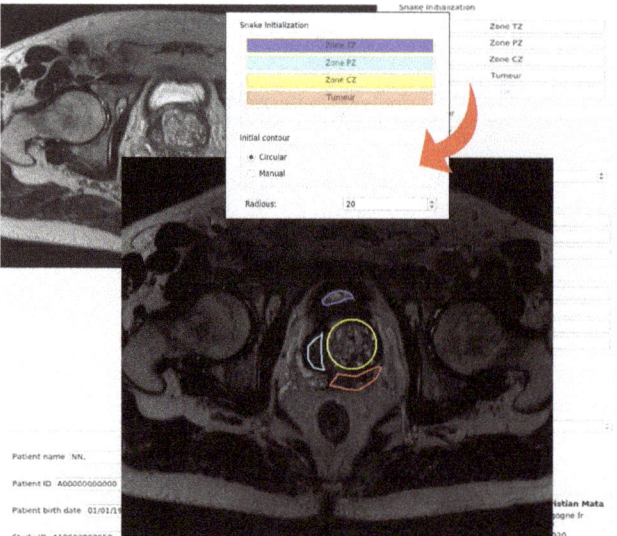

Figure 8. Example of snake initialization for the four zones.

The user can repeat the same procedure for all the zones, or just some of them. In order to differentiate the various selected areas, each initial contour will be drawn with a different color. There are no constraints about the type of contours to use. All the contours can be manual, all of them can be circles or they can be a combination of them.

The following area of the control panel is used for triggering the segmentation. This section is depicted in Figure 9. After an image has been loaded, at least one initial contour has been entered, then the segmentation process will start after pressing the *Run* button. The segmentation method will be triggered as many times as initial contours have been entered, and they will be executed sequentially. During this process, the user can cancel the segmentation at any moment, pressing the *Cancel* button. Once the algorithm had finished, the results will be shown in the right image. Additionally, the color code of the contours is the same for both, left and right images. For instance, the resulting contour of color blue in the right image has as initial contour the blue snake from the left image.

If some results have been produced, then a 3D representation of them can be visualized if the user presses the button *Show 3D model*. This representation consists only of the resulting contours, replicated several times along the Z axis. It is an extra option for users to visualize the main structure of the segmentation in a 3D model. In fact, this option should be improved using better visualization techniques, but it is out of scope of this work for the moment. The amount of repetitions has been set to 50. The axis are represented in real scale, in mm, if the DICOM file contains the information about slice thickness and spatial resolution. If they are not provided, a pop up message will appear reporting the situation, and the X and Y axis will be presented in pixels, and the Z axis will have a size of 10 units. An example of this 3D representation of a result is shown in Figure 10.

Regarding to file management tasks provided to this tool, users can open a DICOM formatted file or a folder that contains several DICOM formatted files. When the *Open file* button is pressed, a pop up window will appear, and it will only allow the user to select a file, not folders. If a file is not in DICOM format, then the program will reject it, and it will not do further actions. If the user wants to open a folder, it should click the *Open folder* button, navigate until the folder it wants, and go into that folder. Without touching any file, users should click the *Choose* button and the system will automatically search for files, and open only the DICOM formatted files. It is important to emphasize that the search system is not recursive. That means, if there are folders inside the selected one, and those folders contain DICOM files, the program will not open them. It will only open the files that are in the current directory.

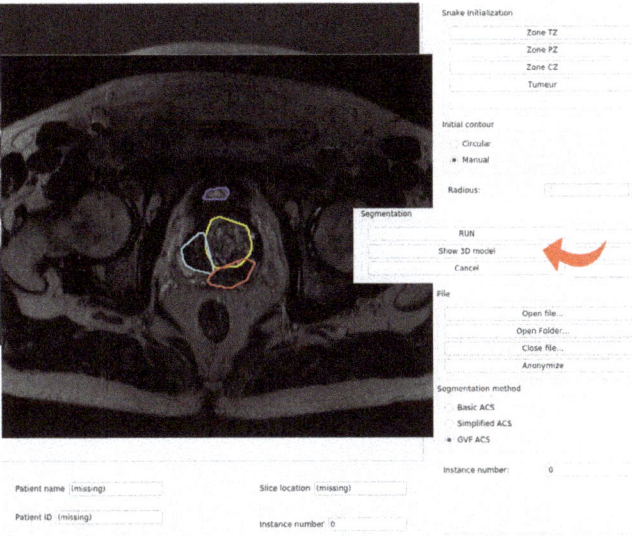

Figure 9. Example of snake results after the snake segmentation.

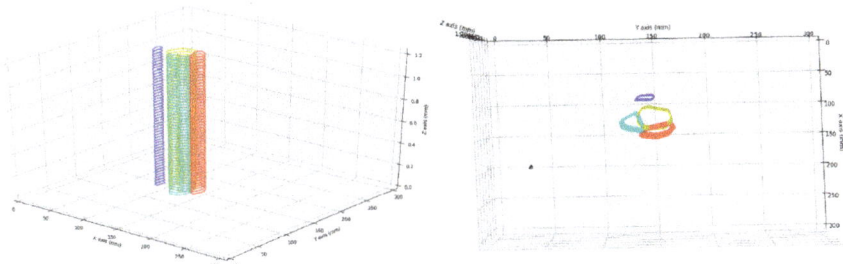

Figure 10. Example of 3D representation of the segmented prostate zones.

As it can be seen in the graphical user interface, there are three types of algorithms: *Basic ACS, Simplified ACS* and *GVF ACS*. The first and the second algorithms are based on [12], but the second one does not follow the mathematical approach described in this previous work. On the other hand, *Basic ACS* implements exactly what the paper states, as explained in Section 2.3. Both algorithms have been included so that there is an example in the code of how to add a new algorithm to this code-base. Additionally, the *Simplified ACS* performs a faster than *Basic ACS* but with less accuracy. Nonetheless, in order to produce improvements to the original paper, the *Basic ACS* was required.

Finally, considering that this application is focused on DICOM format and it can be used for radiologists and/or medical experts, it is important to maintain the private information of the patient. For this reason, an anonymization module is integrated in this tool. If the user wants to anonymize the opened file or files, it should click into the *Anonymize* button. If there is a file/files opened, a pop up window will be shown where the user must specify the destination folder of the anonymized files. The name of the output files will be the same as the source files, but the string *_anonymized* will be appended to it. For instance, if the original file is called *Image00001*, the output file will be called *Image00001_anonymized*. The fields that are anonymized are: *Patient Name*, *Patient ID* and the

Patient Date of Birth. Those fields are not cleared, but changed by some default data: *Patient Name* is changed by *NN*, *Patient ID* is transformed to *A00000000000*, and the date of birth is changed to 01/01/1970.

We believe that the proposed tool can be beneficial for the research community as it enables to integrate various image management tools thoroughly discussed in previous sections, as well as the capability to segment prostate cancer lesions and other areas as mentioned in the introduction. Even though the application includes the option of segmenting four zones only (CZ, TZ, PZ and Tumor), nothing stops the users of trying to segment other areas of their interest (additional buttons can be appended into the GUI in order to select more areas, or the already existing buttons can be used to segment those areas). These features, as well as the capability to integrate new segmentation models seamlessly make it very appealing for research and teaching purposes in clinical settings. In the former case, it can help in speeding up the creation of datasets for machine learning applications. However, in our experience, doctors are reluctant to use fully automated annotation tools and prefer to use interactive semi-automated tools that enable them to verify and contrast the results with other specialists. In order to test the performance of the proposed tool, we performed one experiment to assess the quality of the segmentation algorithm implemented in this work, which will be detailed in the following section.

4. Discussion of the Segmentation Method Results

In this section, we present a deep analysis of the results of a single segmentation experiment performed using the implemented algorithms, namely the *Basic ACS*, *Simplified ACS* and *GVF ACS* versions of the snake-based models. For all the cases, the initial contours used for all the zones are shown in Figure 11.

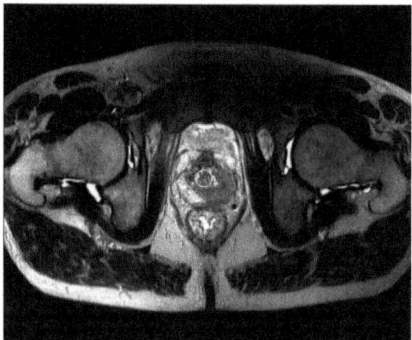

Figure 11. Initialization used for the testing of all the algorithms.

The results for all the algorithms and the ground truth for the selected image are shown in the Figure 12.

From this experiment, it is possible to confirm what it has been said in previous sections. The *Basic ACS* algorithm performs relatively well when there is some gradient information between different areas. In this image, the cyan and the blue contours (corresponding to the PZ and CZ, respectively) are practically attached to the borders; the contour corresponding to the TZ (yellow contour) is almost perfect. Nonetheless, the tumour area invades the TZ area, since the intensities contrast between them is not enough in order to define a good edge.

For the case of *Simplified ACS*, the results are not so satisfactory. This algorithm is uses simplifications of the formulas described in [12]. It has been tested for heart's left ventricle segmentation and it has a good performance in both, quality and speed, but for prostate segmentation, this is not true. Except for the TZ, all the results take part of the other zones, and only when the edge is too strong, the snake seems to be perfectly attached to it.

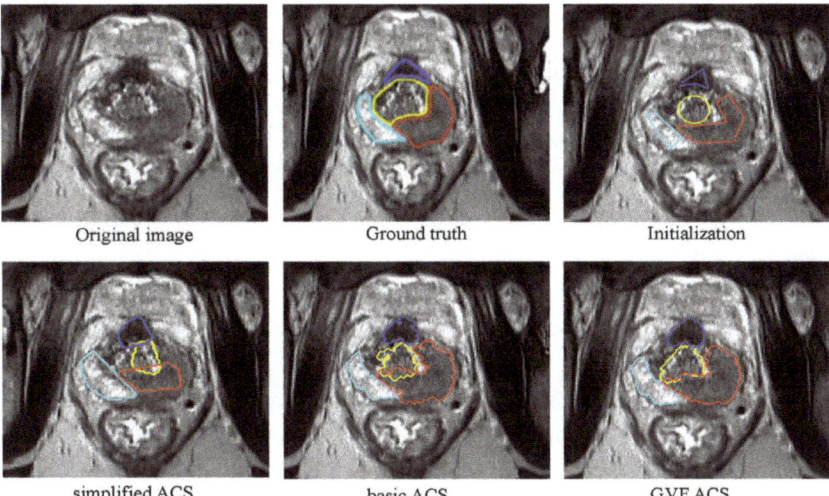

Figure 12. Segmentation results and ground truth for all the algorithms implemented.

Finally, as it is expected, the Gradient Vector Flow implementation overcomes all the problems, and the curves are strongly attached to the borders of each zone. There is only a little overlapping between the tumour and the TZ.

Another point to observe is the smoothness of the results from *Basic ACS* and *GVF ACS*. None of them include either a shape prior or the smoothing factor. This allows the snake to evolve in any shape, which is desired in this case, since there is not a single prior that work for all the prostate zones. Additionally, for the same reason, a generic post-processing that increases the smoothness of the curves is not trivial to implement. This problem is visible mainly in the result given by the *Basic ACS*, where all the contours do not present smooth borders. Nonetheless, the *GVF ACS* generates a result that even without these factors, the outcomes are not so jagged. Once again, the addition of the Gradient Vector Flow component surpasses the results given by the *Basic ACS*.

It is worth mentioning that the initialization (in all the cases) requires to be inside of the object to produce valid results. Since a lot of objects are present in an MR image, a larger contour than the object will produce poor segmentation results. In order to reduce this effect, the image to be segmented is cropped to an square of 150x150 pixels around the center of the initialization contour before starting the segmentation process. As a consequence, not only the influence of other objects over the snake is reduced, but also it reduces the execution time, since less operations are required at each iteration of the algorithm.

In order to measure quantitatively the efficiency of the three model implementations, a contour evaluation of this test was performed. For this evaluation, the Hausdorff distance (HD) and Dice index (DI) metrics for the various segmentation results were compared with a ground truth provided by a specialist. The Hausdorff distance between two finite set of points A and B is defined as follows:

$$HD(A, B) = max(h(A, B), h(B, A)) \tag{22}$$

where $h(A, B)$ is the directed Hausdorff distance defined by:

$$h(A, B) = \max_{a \in A} \min_{b \in B} \|a - b\| \tag{23}$$

where $\|.\|$ is the Euclidean distance and A and B are the resulting contours of the segmentation.

In computer vision and image processing applications, the largest segmentation errors quantified using the Hausdorff Distance can be a good measure of the usefulness of the segmentation for the intended task. Intuitively, *HD* is the longest distance one has to travel from a point in one of the two sets to its closest point in the other set. In image segmentation, this metric is computed between boundaries of the estimated and the ground-truth segmentation, which consist of curves in 2D. We computed the Hausdorff distance between the generated segmentation and the ground truth. The methods with the lowest distance are considered to have yielded the best segmentation results.

Another popular metric for image segmentation tasks is based on the Dice coefficient, which is essentially a measure of overlapping between two samples and it is equivalent to the F1 score. This measure ranges from 0 to 1, where a Dice coefficient of 1 denotes perfect and complete overlap. This metric is calculated as:

$$Dice(A, B) = \frac{2|A \cap B|}{|A \cup B|} \quad (24)$$

In Table 1, we summarize the results obtained from the performance analysis for the three segmentation methods, using the two above-mentioned metrics. This procedure has been done for each of the prostate's gland zones, which corresponds to the examples of the annotations depicted on Figure 12. The ground truth is used as a reference image to calculate all the measurements. First, according to the initialization image, a comparison of the results between *Simplified ACS*, *Basic ACS* and *GVF ACS* is performed. It can easily be inferred from the table that the *Basic ACS* yields more accurate segmentation results in all the prostate zones than the *Simplified ACS*. Moreover, it can be seen that the *GVF ACS* implementation improves the results in all the cases.

Table 1. Analyses of Hausdorff distance (in mm) and Dice index for the CZ, PZ, TZ and tumour area (TUM).

	Hausdorff Distance			Dice Index		
	Simplified ACS	Basic ACS	GVF ACS	Simplified ACS	Basic ACS	GVF ACS
CZ	11 ± 3	8 ± 1	7 ± 1	0.69 ± 0.20	0.79 ± 0.10	0.79 ± 0.10
PZ	4 ± 2	3 ± 2	2 ± 2	0.88 ± 0.10	0.93 ± 0.10	0.94 ± 0.10
TZ	9 ± 4	7 ± 3	6 ± 3	0.74 ± 0.20	0.73 ± 0.10	0.75 ± 0.10
TUM	5 ± 2	4 ± 2	3 ± 2	0.81 ± 0.10	0.92 ± 0.10	0.93 ± 0.10

The geometry of the *CZ* zone is considered the most difficult part of the prostate MR image because it is difficult sometimes to demarcate the edges of this area, given that it is surrounded by the other zones; for this reason, it is important to do a good initialization. The results for the *PZ* are good in all the cases, especially when GVF is used. Moreover, the results on the *TZ* area are good for all the algorithms considered in this study. Finally, the results for the tumor area indicate that the best segmentation is obtained using *GVF ACS* methods.

Finally, in order to assess the performance of the various studied segmentation methods, a time analysis has been performed. As in Table 1, the analysis has been divided by zones and by algorithm. Then, the execution time of the segmentation algorithm has been assessed for each zone, using the same initialization as in Figure 11. For this test, a computer with a microprocessor i7-8650U @ 1.90 GHz, 16 gb of RAM and running Linux 4.15.0-64 has been used. The execution times are depicted in Table 2. All the measurements has been done in milliseconds. Both *Simplified ACS* and *Basic ACS* run at maximum 200 iterations, and the *GVF ACS* runs at maximum 80 iterations. Both Tables 1 and 2 confirm what it has been said about the *Simplified ACS* algorithm. It is the least accurate, but it runs faster than the other ones. On the other hand, even though the *GVF ACS* runs less iterations than the *Basic ACS*, their running time are similar. This is due to the *GVF ACS* algorithm computes the same code, plus the additional ones in order to get the Gradient Vector Flow contribution. Nonetheless, for this work, this execution time could have been reduced if the equations related to the shape prior and the smoothness would have been removed. Only the weights have been set to zero for those priors. This code has not been erased so that other developers can prove other parameters values, and try to find other combination of weights to make this program work with either, other image modalities, or other organs to be studied.

Table 2. Execution time (in ms) for each segmentation algorithm, and for each prostate zone.

	CZ	PZ	TZ	TUM
Simplified ACS	605.79	231.69	317.19	616.93
Basic ACS	1054.97	574.30	819.18	1108.16
GVF ACS	641.66	644.95	725.72	1058.67

These results show that a good segmentation can be obtained in a reasonably time, which is important for both clinical and machine learning applications. As it is expected, one result is not representative of the quality of these algorithms. An analysis of a larger population must be done in order to have a real measure of quantitative error of our implementations. The work we introduced here is to present the tool, the algorithms implemented and how to use them. As future work, we plan to perform a more comprehensive study encompassing other methods known to have good results to contrast results as well as other regions of interest within the prostate. This will enable us to assess the validity of the proposed segmentation approach in other setting, and to get feedback from a larger pool of specialists. Other avenues of research pertain the validation of the proposed tool, as well as of the segmentation algorithm in a larger pool o prostate MRI images, as well as with a wider number of clinicians. We also plan to integrate other segmentation methods into the proposed GUI tool to carry out a more comprehensive quantitative comparison and to investigate its diagnostic differentiation with other prostate diseases such as BPH, chronic or acute prostatitis.

5. Conclusions

In this paper we described the implementation of a snake-based segmentation algorithm, based on an Active Contours Models (ACM), which has been integrated into a GUI based application. We focused our research in a method originally conceived for segmenting the shape of the heart's left ventricle. A modification of this specific prior has yielded very good results in the context of prostate cancer segmentation: the snake models tries to evolve and to adjust to the boundaries of the proposed zones. The problem with this implementation is that the performance of this previous model highly depends on the quality of the input image, as it uses the pixel intensities and the edges of the object in order to determine the correct curve evolution. As it can be expected, if the boundaries are not well defined, or if the intensities of different sections have similar values, then either the model will not be able to assess the difference, preventing the algorithm of evolving, or it will cause the snake to overlap with other elements in the image. This scenario can be observed in Figure 12, where the red contour overlaps with the area that corresponds to the TZ.

Furthermore, in order to get that segmentation, several shapes for the initial contours had been tested to obtain the best results, which might be very different from one run of the algorithm to another. This entails that the implemented snake-based algorithms are very sensitive to the initialization conditions. This type of problems have fostered researches in image analysis and computer vision to find novel ways of constraining the shape of the force that pushes the objects' boundaries in the right direction. Doing so, the segmentation algorithm becomes robust against to initialization conditions and less sensitive to the quality of the image.

Regarding the performance of both implementations, the *Simplified ACS* and *Basic ACS*, their behaviour are not the same. Since *Basic ACS* includes all the weights and all the functions described by the original document, the boundaries of the final segmentation tends to be closer to the real boundaries of the object to segment than in the case of *Simplified ACS*. Nonetheless, both of them fail in the task of finding the boundaries when the image intensities between two contiguous areas are not noticeably different, like in the case of the tumor and the central zone in Figure 12. This problem has been partially overcame when using the Gradient Vector Flow external force.

Further improvements to this algorithm will thus be directed towards implementing other types of Gradient Vector Flow energy optimization algorithms, or exploring how to include shape priors for each zone of the prostate separately. These modifications would help to create a segmentation that does not go too far from where the real object is. Additionally, no pre-processing nor post-processing functions have been included. Adding pre-processing operations might help to remove the noise that addresses the snake towards the wrong directions, and post-processing of the resulting contour will help to make it smoother, and closer to the real boundaries of the object.

Moreover, since the DICOM files can contain different image modalities, and each modality has its particularities, a profiles section can be added to the program. Each profile will contain a set of parameters (priors weights, GVF weight, regularization constants, and iterations) specific for each algorithm. These profiles will be chosen in a way that they will produce the best segmentation results for the selected image modality, increasing the scope of application of the program.

Other avenues of research pertain the validation of the proposed tool, as well as of the segmentation algorithm in a larger pool o prostate MRI images, as well as with a wider number of clinicians. We also plan to integrate other segmentation methods into the proposed GUI tool to carry out a more comprehensive quantitative comparison and to investigate its diagnostic differentiation with other prostate diseases such as BPH, chronic or acute prostatitis

Author Contributions: Conceptualization, C.M. and J.R.; methodology, all authors.; software, J.R.; validation, C.M., G.O.-R.; resources , C.M and G.O.-R.; data curation, C.M.; writing—original draft preparation, J.R. and C.M.; writing—review and editing, all authors; visualization, all authors; supervision, C.M., G.O.-R. All authors have read and agreed to the published version of the manuscript.

Funding: This work was partially funded by the Spanish R+D+I grant n. TIN2012-37171-C02-01, by UdG grant MPCUdG2016/022. The Regional Council of Burgundy under the PARI 1 scheme also sponsored this work. C. Mata held a Mediterranean Office for Youth mobility grant.

Conflicts of Interest: The authors declare that they have no known competing financial interests or personal relationships that could have appeared to influence the work reported in this paper.

Abbreviations

The following abbreviations are used in this manuscript:

PCa	Prostate Cancer
ICD-O	International Classification of Diseases for Oncology
ICCC	International Classification of Childhood Cancer
EU	European Union
MRI	Magnetic Resonance Imaging
ROI	Region of Interest
T2WI	T2-Weighted Imaging
DWI	Diffusion Weighted Imaging
DCE	Perfusion based on the Dynamic Contrast Enhancement
MRS	Magnetic Resonance Spectroscopy
PI-RADS	Prostate Imaging-Reporting and Data System
CZ	Central Zone
PZ	Peripheral Zone
TZ	Transition Zone
AFT	Anterior Fibromuscular Tissue
Tum	Tumor lession
ACM	Active Contour Models
GVF	Gradient Vector Flow
DICOM	Digital Imaging and Communication On Medicine
HD	Hausdorff distance
DI	Dice Index

References

1. Siegel, R.L.; Miller, K.D.; Jemal, A. An Enhanced Contextual Fire Detection Algorithm for MODIS. *CA Cancer J. Clin.* **2020**, *70*, 7–30. [CrossRef] [PubMed]
2. Carioli, G.; Bertuccio, P.; Boffetta, P.; Levi, F.; La Vecchia, C.; Negri, E.; Malvezzi, M. European cancer mortality predictions for the year 2020 with a focus on prostate cancer. *Ann. Oncol.* **2020**, *31*, 650–658. [CrossRef] [PubMed]
3. Shah, V.; Turkbey, B.; Mani, H.; Pang, Y.; Pohida, T.; Merino, M.J.; Pinto, P.A.; Choyke, P.L.; Bernardo, M. Decision support system for localizing prostate cancer based on multiparametric magnetic resonance imaging. *Med. Phys.* **2012**, *39*, 4093–4103. [CrossRef] [PubMed]
4. Dickinson, L.; Ahmed, H.U.; Allen, C.; Barentsz, J.O.; Carey, B.; Futterer, J.J.; Heijmink, S.W.; Hoskin, P.J.; Kirkham, A.; Padhani, A.R.; et al. Magnetic resonance imaging for the detection, localisation, and characterisation of prostate cancer: Recommendations from a European consensus meeting. *Eur. J. Neurol.* **2011**, *59*, 477–494. [CrossRef] [PubMed]
5. Fradet, V.; Kurhanewicz, J.; Cowan, J.E.; Karl, A.; Coakley, F.V.; Shinohara, K.; Carroll, P.R. Prostate cancer managed with active surveillance: Role of anatomic MR imaging and MR spectroscopic imaging. *Radiographics* **2010**, *256*, 176–183. [CrossRef] [PubMed]
6. Ghose, S.; Oliver, A.; Mitra, J.; Martí, R.; Lladó, X.; Freixenet, J.; Meriaudeau, F.; Sidibé, D.; Vilanova, J.C.; Comet, J. A supervised learning framework of statistical shape and probability priors for automatic prostate segmentation in ultrasound images. *Med. Image Anal.* **2013**, *17*, 587–600. [CrossRef] [PubMed]
7. Ghose, S.; Oliver, O.; Martí, J.; Lladó, X.; Vilanova, J.; Freixenet, J. A survey of prostate segmentation methodologies in ultrasound, magnetic resonance and computed tomography images. *Comput. Methods Programs Biomed.* **2012**, *108*, 262–287. [CrossRef] [PubMed]
8. Vos, P.C.; Hambrock, T.; Barenstz, J.O.; Huisman, H.J. Computer-assisted analysis of peripheral zone prostate lesions using T2-weighted and dynamic contrast enhanced T1-weighted MRI. *Phys. Med. Biol.* **2010**, *55*, 1719–1734. [CrossRef] [PubMed]
9. Chen, M.; Dang, H.; Wang, J.; Zhou, C.; Li, S.; Wang, W. Prostate cancer detection: Comparison of t2-weighted imaging, diffusion-weighted imaging, proton magnetic resonance spectroscopic imaging, and the three techniques combined. *Acta Radiol.* **2008**, *49*, 602–610. [CrossRef] [PubMed]
10. Brancato, V.; Di Costanzo, G.; Basso, L.; Tramontano, L.; Puglia, M.; Ragozzino, A.; Cavaliere, C. Assessment of DCE Utility for PCa Diagnosis Using PI-RADS v2.1: Effects on Diagnostic Accuracy and Reproducibility. *Diagnostics* **2020**, *10*, 164. [CrossRef] [PubMed]
11. Mata, C.; Walker, P.; Oliver, A.; Brunotte, F.; Martí, J.; Lalande, A. Prostateanalyzer: Web-based medical application for the management of prostate cancer using multiparametric mr images. *Inform. Health Soc. Care* **2015**, *87*, 1–21. [CrossRef] [PubMed]
12. Pluempitiwiriyawej, C.; Moura, J.M.; Wu, Y.J.L.; Ho, C. STACS: New active contour scheme for cardiac MR image segmentation. *IEEE Trans. Med. Imaging* **2005**, *24*, 593–603. [CrossRef] [PubMed]
13. De Marzo, A.; Platz, E.; Sutcliffe, S.; Xu, J.; Grönberg, H.; Drake, C.; Nakay, Y. Inflammation in prostate carcinogenesis. *Nat. Rev. Cancer* **2007**, *7*, 256–269. [CrossRef] [PubMed]
14. Verma, S.; Rajesh, A. A clinically relevant approach to imaging prostate cancer: Review. *Am. J. Roentgenol.* **2011**, *196*, S1–S10. [CrossRef] [PubMed]
15. Rodríguez, J.; Ochoa-Ruíz, G.; Mata, C. Prostate-MRI-segmentation-App. GitHub Repos. 2020. Available online: https://github.com/joako1991/Prostate-MRI-segmentation-App (accessed on 2 September 2020).
16. Chan, T.F.; Vese, L.A. Active contours without edges. *IEEE Trans. Image Process.* **2001**, *10*, 266–277. [CrossRef] [PubMed]
17. Xu, C.; Prince, J.L. Snakes, shapes, and gradient vector flow. *IEEE Trans. Image Process.* **1998**, *7*, 359–369. [CrossRef] [PubMed]

18. Paragios, N.; Mellina-Gottardo, O.; Ramesh, V. Gradient vector flow fast geometric active contours. *IEEE Trans. Pattern Anal. Mach. Intell.* **2004**, *26*, 402–407. [CrossRef] [PubMed]
19. Xu, C.; Yezzi, A.; Prince, J.L. On the relationship between parametric and geometric active contours. In Proceedings of the Conference Record of the Thirty-Fourth Asilomar Conference on Signals, Systems and Computers (Cat. No.00CH37154), Pacific Grove, CA, USA, 29 October–1 November 2000; Volume 1, pp. 483–489. [CrossRef]

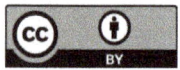

© 2020 by the authors. Licensee MDPI, Basel, Switzerland. This article is an open access article distributed under the terms and conditions of the Creative Commons Attribution (CC BY) license (http://creativecommons.org/licenses/by/4.0/).

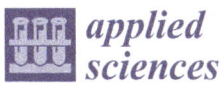

Article

Medical Assistant Mobile Application for Diabetes Control by Simulating a Compartmental Model

Martín Hernández-Ordoñez [1,*], Marco Aurelio Nuño-Maganda [2], Carlos Adrián Calles-Arriaga [2], Abelardo Rodríguez-León [3,*], Guillermo Efren Ovando-Chacon [1,*], Rolando Salazar-Hernández [4], Omar Montaño-Rivas [5] and José Margarito Canseco-Cortinas [2]

1. Department of Metal-Mechanics, México National Technological/I.T. Campus, Veracruz 91860, Mexico
2. Intelligent Systems Department, Polytechnic University of Victoria, Tamaulipas 87138, Mexico; mnunom@upv.edu.mx (M.A.N.-M.); ccallesa@upv.edu.mx (C.A.C.-A.); 1229002@upv.edu.mx (J.M.C.-C.)
3. Department of Systems and Computing, México National Technological/I.T. Campus, Veracruz 91860, Mexico
4. Facultad de Comercio, Administración y Ciencias Sociales, Universidad Autónoma de Tamaulipas, Tamaulipas 87000, Mexico; rsalazar@uat.edu.mx
5. Academy of Information Technologies, Polytechnic University of San Luis Potosí, San Luis 78369, Mexico; omar.montano@upslp.edu.mx
* Correspondence: martin.ho@veracruz.tecnm.mx (M.H.-O.); abelardo.rl@veracruz.tecnm.mx (A.R.-L.); guillermo.oc@veracruz.tecnm.mx (G.E.O.-C.)

Received: 29 July 2020; Accepted: 25 September 2020; Published: 29 September 2020

Featured Application: Mobile application for iterative simulation of a diabetic model.

Abstract: This paper presents an educational mobile assistant application for type 1 diabetes patients. The proposed application is based on four mathematical models that describe the glucose-insulin-glucagon dynamics using a compartmental model, with additional equations to reproduce aerobic exercise, gastric glucose absorption by the gut, and subcutaneous insulin absorption. The medical assistant was implemented in Java and deployed and validated on several smartphones with Android OS. Multiple daily doses can be simulated to perform intensive insulin therapy. As a result, the proposed application shows the influence of exercise periods, food intakes, and insulin treatments on the glucose concentrations. Four parameter variations are studied, and their corresponding glucose concentration plots are obtained, which show agreement with simulators of the state of the art. The developed application is focused on type-1 diabetes, but this can be extended to consider type-2 diabetes by modifying the current mathematical models.

Keywords: mathematical models; Iterative simulation; compartmental model; diabetes control; mobile assistant

1. Introduction

In recent years, obesity and overweight have become a severe problem for human health. In 2014 more than 1.9 billion adults aged 18 and older were overweight globally, from which over 600 million were obese. The data indicated that 39% of these adults were overweight and 13% were obese [1]. Body mass index (BMI) provides the most useful population-level measure of overweight and obesity as it is the same for both sexes and all ages of adults. Patients with higher BMI are at greater risk for having diabetes. In 2014, more than 422 million people had diabetes in the world, with a global prevalence of 8.5% among adults over 18 years old. Diabetes is a leading cause of blindness, kidney failure, heart attacks, stroke and lower limb amputation. In 2012, an estimated 1.5 million deaths were directly caused by diabetes, and another 2.2 million deaths were attributable to high blood glucose [2]. Diabetes was promoted from 21st place in 1990 to the 14th in 2010 in the list of death causes worldwide [3], and recently, to the 6th place in 2016 [4].

In Mexico, about 72.5% of adults from 18 years and over, 36.3% of teenagers, and 33.2% of children were overweight or obese in 2016. Diabetes statistics are not too optimistic; Mexico is in sixth place in countries with more diabetes, just behind China, India, US, Brazil and Russia [5]. Recent statistics show that 9.17% of adults from 18 years (about 6.4 million people) have diabetes [6]. Type 2 diabetes has become the leading cause of death in Mexico. The disease claims nearly 80,000 lives each year, and forecasters say the health problem is expected to get worse in the decades to come [7].

On the other hand, smartphones have been accessible to more people due to the high worldwide market growth rate. In 2016, around 1.5 billion smartphones were sold worldwide [8]; by the end of 2016, more than 3.2 billion individuals worldwide used the Internet regularly, accounting for nearly 45% of the world's population; about 2.5 billion people access the web via mobile phone [9], which represents novel opportunities for designing applications running on smartphones, accessible to large population groups. Specifically, healthcare and disease management have benefited with applications such as fitness tracking, drug dose calculators, information apps, tutorials, surveys, diaries, and other tools created to help empower users to put more emphasis on their health care. Some benefits of using smartphones with Internet connectivity consists of the possibility of sharing data with family, friends, classmates, colleges, collaborators but especially with professionals who can guide the user and give feedback regarding treatment to be followed.

This paper is structured as follows. In Section 2, a concise review of the state of the art is given. A description of the models used in the developed application is provided in Section 3. In Section 4, the results and discussion are described. Finally, in Section 5, the conclusion is presented where final recalls are established, and future work is outlined.

2. State of the Art

2.1. PC or Web Simulators for Glucose Concentration Levels

In recent years, an effort to implement glucose levels simulators has been made. One standard option for implementing simulators are PCs or Laptops. PCs have as their main advantage the inherent high computational power for performing simulations. In addition, there has been a trend to replace PCs with much more compact devices, such as smartphones, but most simulators for glucose concentration are PC-based. Another implementation option consists of Web systems, allowing for a broad range of devices to access such simulation systems. Web-based simulators have an advantage: many platforms can access the simulator compared to a particular PC implementation. Web-based simulators have as main disadvantage the requirement of Internet connectivity, making the simulator difficult to access in places with connectivity problems.

In [10], the AIDA diabetes simulator is presented, and extensive evaluation about this simulator has been reported in [11]. Recently, new types of rapid-acting insulins have been added to the AIDA diabetes simulator [12]. AIDA's mathematical model was created to simulate glucose tolerance; however, its use is not based on daily periods.

In [13], the REACTION project is presented. This project consists of a set of healthcare services oriented to diabetic patients and caregivers through a cloud-based application focusing on management and therapy services. The REACTION project is a management system created for the implementation of logistics related to medical personnel. The dosage management algorithm is based on basic rules, and it is not a pharmacological-dynamic behavioral study of insulin. In other words, it is a mathematical model with experimental parameters.

In [14], GLUCOSIM is proposed as a desktop application designed to do virtual experiments to show the effects of food intake changes and insulin therapy on glucose levels. A more detailed version of this system is reported in [15], where a Web-based solution was included. It is important to mention that GLUCOSIM is a tool designed to study, train and analyze the external effects that modify glucose concentration. It uses three mathematical models to consider all the mentioned effects; however, it does not describe periods of exercise or other modeled effects.

In [16], a system is proposed based on the combination of Compartmental Models (CMs) and artificial Neural Networks (NNs). Data from a Type 1 diabetes patient, which contains information about measured blood glucose levels, insulin intake, and food intake description, along with the corresponding time, were used as input to the model. The proposed strategy was not adequately validated. Furthermore, no performance criteria were mentioned to assess the results objectively.

The literature review indicates that early studies of compartmental modelling of glucose/insulin interactions were proposed since the 1980s in [17–19]. On the other hand, recently, different research groups have reported important works related with the implementations of compartmental models to develop glucose level simulators, for example, in [20,21] are presented a glucose forecasting algorithm based on a compartmental composite model of glucose-insulin dynamics. In [22] is developed a dynamic model for type 1 diabetic patient that focuses on blood glucose regulation. A first model for insulin adsorption in infusion sets using a minimal lumped two-compartment modelling approach is reported in [23]. A review of the key role of the UVA/Padova simulator is presented in [24], which has tested the use of new molecules for better glucose control.

2.2. Mobile Applications for Diabetes Management

The universe of mobile applications for diabetes care is enormous. A first step consists in determining the utility of apps. One standard classification includes exercise and fitness apps, med adherence, weight management, blood glucose trackers, support, healthcare professional apps, and educational simulators. There is extensive availability of applications related to any of the previously mentioned apps, but few efforts are related to educational simulators for smartphones.

One interesting branch of smartphone applications for health care is the simulators. In this paper, we are specifically interested in creating a smartphone-based simulator of glucose-insulin metabolism. In recent years, there have been advances in creating models that can replicate the behavior of parts (or entire) of human organisms and their corresponding implementation as a computer simulation. A smartphone-based simulation can be useful for patients with recently diagnosed diabetes to help them estimate the insulin doses and food intake, but also for patients at risk of developing diabetes or without diabetes, for contributing to raising awareness of the benefits of changing their food consumption and exercise habits. In [25], a review of several diabetes simulators is presented, but the applications reported in that paper is out of the scope of this work, since there is an interest in providing a realistic simulation of blood glucose levels.

There are several reviews of applications for diabetes management. In [26], a set of critical factors to be considered when designing diabetes management applications are explored. These factors come from patient demographics, technology costs, platform varieties, and ease of use. They also categorize the applications in the following classes: blood glucose logging, nutrition databases, carbohydrate tracking, tracking physical activity and weight, data-sharing and social support, and short messages and reminders. An important point to consider is that the FDA does not approve most applications. In [27], several commercial applications for diabetes management available on the Apple App Store and articles published in relevant databases are reviewed. The reviewed applications support self-management tasks such as physical exercise, insulin dosage or medication, blood glucose testing, and diet. Other support tasks considered include decision support, notification/alert, tagging of input data, and social media integration. Analysis indicates that application usage is associated with improved attitudes favorable to diabetes self-management. Limitations of the applications include lack of personalized feedback; usability issues, particularly the ease of data entry; and integration with patients and electronic health records. In much more detail, in [28], it is concluded that a critical feature strongly recommended by clinical guidelines—namely, personalized education is not assimilated in current diabetes applications. In [29] a critical assessment was reported of several smartphone apps for calculating insulin dose. The conclusion was that popular apps offering insulin dose calculations carry a risk of incorrect dose recommendations ranging from those that might lead to suboptimal disease control to those with potentially life-threatening consequences. In [30], an analysis of the benefits of smartphone apps for type 2 diabetes mellitus (T2DM) self-management was presented. It can be concluded that more research with valid study designs and longer follow-up is needed to evaluate the impact of health apps for diabetes care and self-management, specifically for T2DM. In [31], both Heuristic and keystroke level modeling (KLM) are used to measure efficiency for each analyzed mobile diabetes management application for patients with Type-1 Diabetes Mellitus.

With recent advances in connectivity technologies, there are some efforts to build tools based on cloud computing [32] or social network support [33,34]. One disadvantage of these tools is that they always require Internet connectivity at all times, which makes them useless in places with connectivity problems. Some applications are targeted to a particular segment of the population, such as pregnant women; one of these applications is reported in [35,36], where a tool to follow patients with gestational diabetes is described. In [37], an application for insulin dose calculation is reported. The authors establish that this application's innovation consists of the incorporation of exercise and alcohol intake to the calculator in addition to carbohydrates intake. In [38], an application created explicitly for controlling an insulin pump taking as real-time input data from a continuous glucose monitor is reported. A closed-loop control system used to automatically manage insulin infusion to maintain the desire range´s glucose level is proposed. To summarize, there is a strong interest from the scientific community in developing applications around the problems associated with diabetes. This article adds to this trend with an emphasis on the exercise model.

3. Models

The idea of creating an artificial model for a glucose-insulin system for several purposes has been widely explored. In [39], a minimal glucose-insulin system is proposed; the model starts with the Bergman model [17] and presents modifications to improve, considering the glucose level´s description in the subcutaneous layer and a meal disturbance term. The developed application uses four mathematical models related to them, following the different dynamics that they describe:

1. Glucose-Insulin Model: Sorensen in [40] proposed it. This model comprises 19 nonlinear differential equations, which include significant metabolic effects related to glucose regulation. The model was obtained through a compartmental technique, where the pancreas compartment is omitted to consider a type 1 diabetic patient. Recently, this glucose-insulin model was extended to consider exercise periods [41].
2. Subcutaneous Insulin model: Berger and Rodbard [42] obtained it. This model describes the subcutaneous insulin uptake pattern after an insulin injection. The model considers interactions between components after subcutaneous injections such as insulin absorption and elimination in plasma insulin, active insulin, glucose utilization, plasma glucose, and glucose input. The model is based on a set of differential equations. Variations in plasma insulin concentration (I) can be estimated by Equation (1).

$$\frac{dI}{dt} = \frac{I_{abs}}{V_i} - k_e I \tag{1}$$

where I_{abs} represents the rate of insulin absorption, V_i is the volume of insulin distribution, and k_e is the first-order rate constant of insulin elimination. The absorption of insulin can be calculated as follows:

$$I_{abs} = \frac{st^2 T_{50}^s D}{t\left(T_{50}^s + t^s\right)^2} \tag{2}$$

where s is a parameter associated with the insulin absorption pattern, t represents the time of the injection, T_{50} is when the dose (D) is absorbed in an amount of 50%.

3. To estimate steady-state conditions, insulin profile (I_{ss}) using the superposition principle is computed assuming three days as follows:

$$I_{ss}(t) = I(t) + I(t+24) + I(t+48) \tag{3}$$

$$I_{a,ss}(t) = I_a(t) + I_a(t+24) + I_a(t+48) \tag{4}$$

where I_a is the build-up and the deactivation of the insulin pump.

4. Meal Intake model: this model was proposed in 1992 by Lehmann and Deutsch [43]. It describes the gastric glucose absorption into the bloodstream by a meal intake represented by its carbohydrates content. According to this model, glucose utilization G_{out} (G) at plasma insulin concentration is:

$$G_{out}(G) = \frac{V_{max} G}{K_m + G} \tag{5}$$

G represents the glucose concentration, V_{max} maximal glucose utilization for reference insulin concentration, and K_m is glucose concentration for the half-maximal response. V_{max} depends on insulin; mathematically, this is

$$V_{max}(I_{ss}) = \frac{G_{out}(I_{ss})(K_m + G_x)}{G_x} \tag{6}$$

where I_{ss} is plasma insulin concentration equivalent to steady-state insulin, and G_x is the reference glucose value. Glucose utilization for any combination of plasma glucose and insulin levels is given by

$$G_{out}(G, I_{ss}) = \frac{G(c \cdot I_{ss} + d)(K_m + G_x)}{G_x(K_m + G)} \tag{7}$$

where c is insulin sensitivity, and d represents insulin-independent glucose utilization. The insulin absorption dynamics for regular, NPH, lente, ultralente formulations were characterized in [42] just by changing some specific parameters in the general model. Recently, in [44], the Lispro insulin formulation was also characterized by the model in [42].

5. The exercise model was considered from [41]. The liver's glycogen reservoir (GLY) can be calculated as shown in Equation (8).

$$\frac{dGLY(t)}{dt} = -\varnothing(PVO_2^{max}(t), GLY(t)) + \Psi(G_{abs}(t) + GLY(t)) \tag{8}$$

$$\varnothing(PVO_2^{max}, GLY) = \begin{cases} \zeta(PVO_2^{max}) & \text{if } 0 < GLY \le GLY_{max} \\ 0 & \text{if } GLY \ge 0 \end{cases} \tag{9}$$

$$\Psi(G_{abs}, GLY) = \begin{cases} G_{abs} & \text{if } GLY < GLY_{max} \\ 0 & \text{if } GLY > GLY_{max} \end{cases} \tag{10}$$

$$\zeta(PVO_2^{max}) = 0.006(PVO_2^{max})^2 + 1.226 PVO_2^{max} - 10.1958 \text{ mg/min} \tag{11}$$

where φ is the net glycogenolysis rate, Ψ represents the absorptive period, ζ is the glucose uptake due to exercise intensity, and PVO_2^{max} is the percentage of the maximum oxygen consumption rate.

In Figure 1, the block diagram of the diabetic patient utilized in this work is shown. There are four subsystems, each one corresponds to a previously described model, and their interactions are shown as solid arrows. The dotted lines delimit the mathematical models proposed in the literature, which describe different but comparable physiological phenomena because they have the same scale.

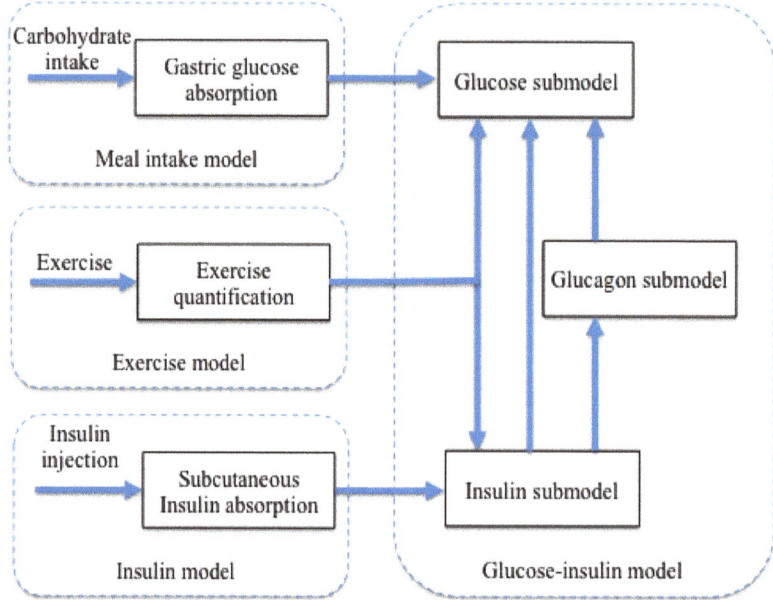

Figure 1. The diabetic patient model utilized for the implementation of simulations reported in this work.

4. Results and Discussion

4.1. Mobile Application for Educational Similar

4.1.1. Hardware and Software Tools

The proposed education simulator was developed based on the models described in the last section. The models were implemented in Java using Android Studio IDE with Android Studio SDK and Java SE Development Kit; besides, Android MPChart Library is used for showing results of the glucose level simulation in a plot [45].

The proposed application was validated on devices with several versions of Android. Table 1, shows the list of devices and its specifications used for testing the proposed application.

Table 1. Devices utilized for testing the proposed application.

Device	Processor	RAM	Android Version
Galaxy S2	Dual-core 1.2 GHz Cortex-A9	1 GB	4.1
Galaxy S4	Dual-core 1.7 GHz Krait 300	1.5 GB	5.0.1
Polaroid Tab	Dual-core 1.0 GHz Broadcom 21663	1 GB	4.2.2
Galaxy Tab 10.1	Quad-core 2.3 GHz Krait 400	3 GB	5.1.1
LG G3 Stylus	Quad-core 1.3 GHz Cortex-A7	1 GB	5.0.2

4.1.2. System Architecture

In Figure 2, the architecture of the proposed application is shown. The architecture takes as an input the following data:

1. Meal parameters: these parameters are related to carbohydrate intake (in grams) and the day's carbohydrate intake schedule.

2. Insulin dose parameters: these parameters are related to the type (fast or slow actions) and the dose of insulin (in units).
3. Exercise parameters: these parameters are related to the quantity and intensity of exercise.
4. Simulation configuration: these parameters are related to the simulation's duration and the type of plot to be generated.
5. The architecture contains the following blocks:
6. Simulation variables container: this block stores data required to be accessed and shared by all model blocks. It contains three profiles: meal dosing, insulin dosing, and exercise quantification.
7. Meal model block: this block takes as input the meal profile and generates as output the glucose obtained according to the carbohydrate intake grams.
8. Insulin model block: this block takes as input the insulin dosing profile and generates as output the quantity and duration of insulin in the blood flow.
9. Exercise model block: this block takes as input the exercise dosing profile and generates as output the blood redistribution volume according to the quantity of exercise.
10. Simulation loop block: this block updates each model block with required data from others and controls the simulation's start and end.
11. Plot generation module: this block generates data from the simulation to be used for generating a plot.
12. Plot visualization module: this block takes as input the vector generated by the plot generation module and displays the plot.

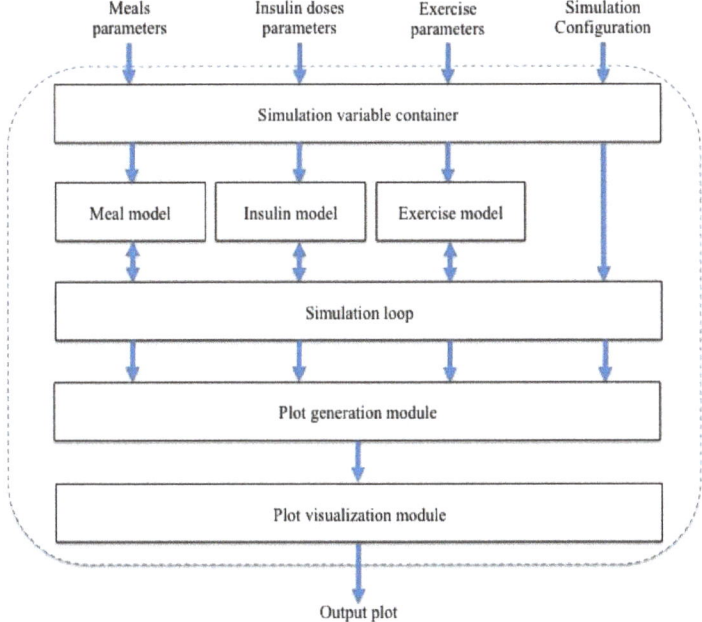

Figure 2. The system architecture.

Finally, the architecture generates as the output the plot with the information according to the user's input.

4.1.3. User Interface

In Figure 3a, a welcome screen of the proposed application is shown. The proposed application's main objective is the generation of a plot of the blood glucose concentration based on the parameters defined in the previous section. For user commodity and better distribution application's controls, a tabbed document interface (TDI) was conceived as the main container for hosting all the needed user controls required to set the simulation parameters and show the results. Specifically, for the Android SDK environment, a tab host container was utilized. This control enables the integration of plenty of components in a single form. The proposed application contains four tabs: the first three tabs allow the user to define the parameters of meal, insulin, and exercise models, and the last one is designed to generate simulation data and show the blood glucose concentration in a plot.

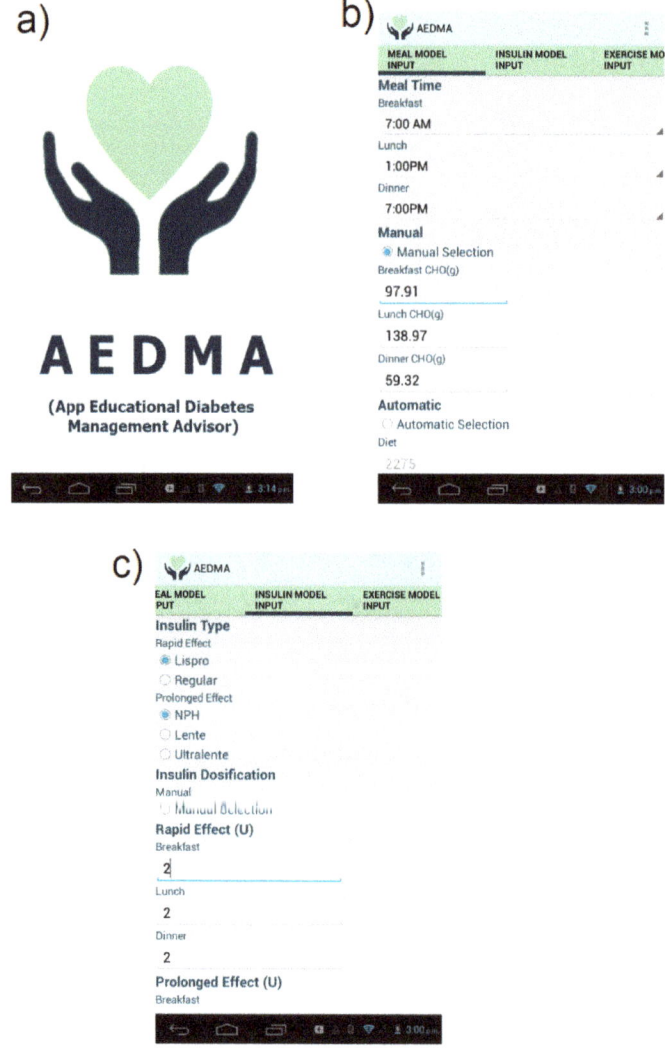

Figure 3. Screens of the proposed AEDMA app. (**a**) Main screen of the proposed applications. (**b**) Components of the meal model input Table. (**c**) Components of the insulin model tab.

In Figure 3b, the tab for the meal model parameters is shown. This tab contains interface controls where users can define each meal's time and its estimated carbohydrate contents (in grams). The estimated carbohydrate contents also can be automatically calculated based on a default estimation of calories for a day, or user can input the total calories, and the application estimates the carbohydrate content in grams based on the given calories.

In Figure 3c, the tab for the insulin model is shown. This tab contains interface controls that define the type of insulin and the unit to be dosed in each meal, for both the rapid and prolonged effect.

In Figure 4a, the tab for the exercise model is shown. This tab contains interface controls where the user defines the intensity, duration, start time, and exercise routine.

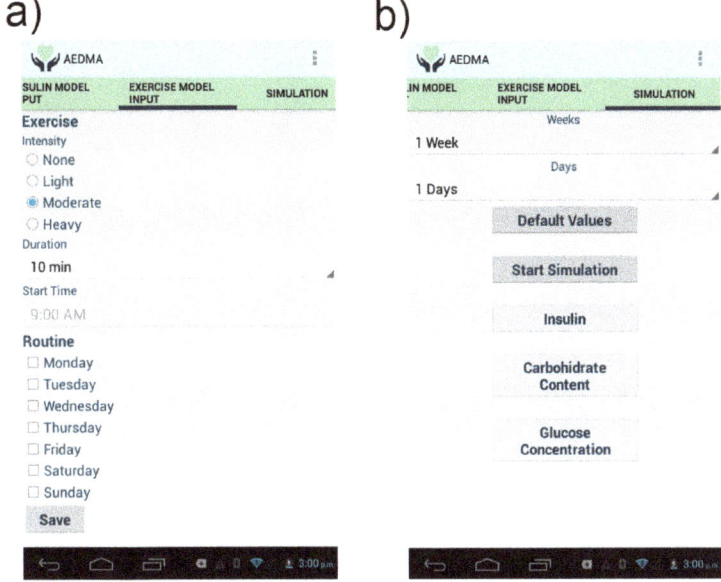

Figure 4. The last two configuration screens. (a) Components of the exercise model Table. (b) Components of the simulations tab.

In Figure 4b, the tab for simulation is shown. In this tab, the user defines the time of the simulation in weeks and days. It is also possible to set all variables to their default values, start simulation, shown insulin, carbohydrate, or glucose concentration plots.

In Table 2, the application's default values are listed, but the user can syntonize this to get a better understanding of the model behavior.

Table 2. Default parameter values for the proposed application.

Meal Model	
Breakfast time	7:00 AM
Lunch time	1:00 PM
Dinner time	7:00 PM
Breakfast CHO (g)	97.91
Lunch CHO (g)	138.97
Dinner CHO (g)	59.32

Table 2. Cont.

Insulin Model	
Rapid effect insulin type	Lispro
Prolonged effect insulin Type	NPH
Rapid effect insulin units at breakfast	2
Rapid effect insulin units at lunch	2
Rapid effect insulin units at dinner	2
Prolonged effect insulin units at breakfast	3
Prolonged effect insulin units at dinner	3
Exercise Model	
Intensity	Light
Duration	10 min
Start time	9:00 AM
Routine	Monday checked

4.2. Reported Experiments

In Table 3, the parameters utilized for validating the meal and insulin models are shown. The abbreviations in the column names are experiment number (Exp), carbohydrate grams in breakfast

Table 3. Selected parameters set of four experiments.

Exp	Meal									Insulin Dossification
	Carbohydrate Grams Intake			Rapid Effect				Prolongated Effect		
	B-CHO	L-CHO	D-CHO	Type	B-u	L-u	D-u	Type	B-u	D-u
1	97.91	138.97	59.32	Lispro	2	2	2	NPH	3	3
2	49.85	69.48	29.66	Lispro	2	2	2	NPH	3	3
3	97.91	138.97	59.32	Lispro	4	4	4	NPH	6	6
4	49.85	69.48	29.66	Lispro	4	4	4	NPH	6	6

(B-CHO), carbohydrate grams in lunch (L-CHO), carbohydrate grams in dinner (D-CHO), insulin units at breakfast (B-u), insulin units at lunch (L-u), insulin units at dinner (D-u). In the first experiment, the default values for carbohydrate and insulin units are used. In the second experiment, carbohydrate grams are reduced to half, but the insulin units are left at their default values. In the third experiment, default values for carbohydrate grams are used, but the insulin dose is doubled, and in the last experiment, carbohydrate grams are reduced to half, and the insulin dose is doubled.

Figure 5 shows a glucose concentration plot for a 5-day simulation for each experiment reported in Table 3. In Figure 5a, the maximum glucose peak is close to 195 mg/dL every day of the reported simulation. In contrast, in Figure 5b, the maximum glucose peak surpasses 175 mg/dL due to the reduction of carbohydrate intake. In Figure 5c, the same carbohydrate intake is used, but both prolonged and rapid insulin doses are doubled. It can be shown that glucose levels are lower when compared with the plot of experiment 1, and in Figure 5d, also the carbohydrate intake is reduced to half to validate both meal and insulin models. In both experiments (3 and 4), it can be shown for its corresponding plots that even a risk of hyperglycemia is present due to the high insulin dose.

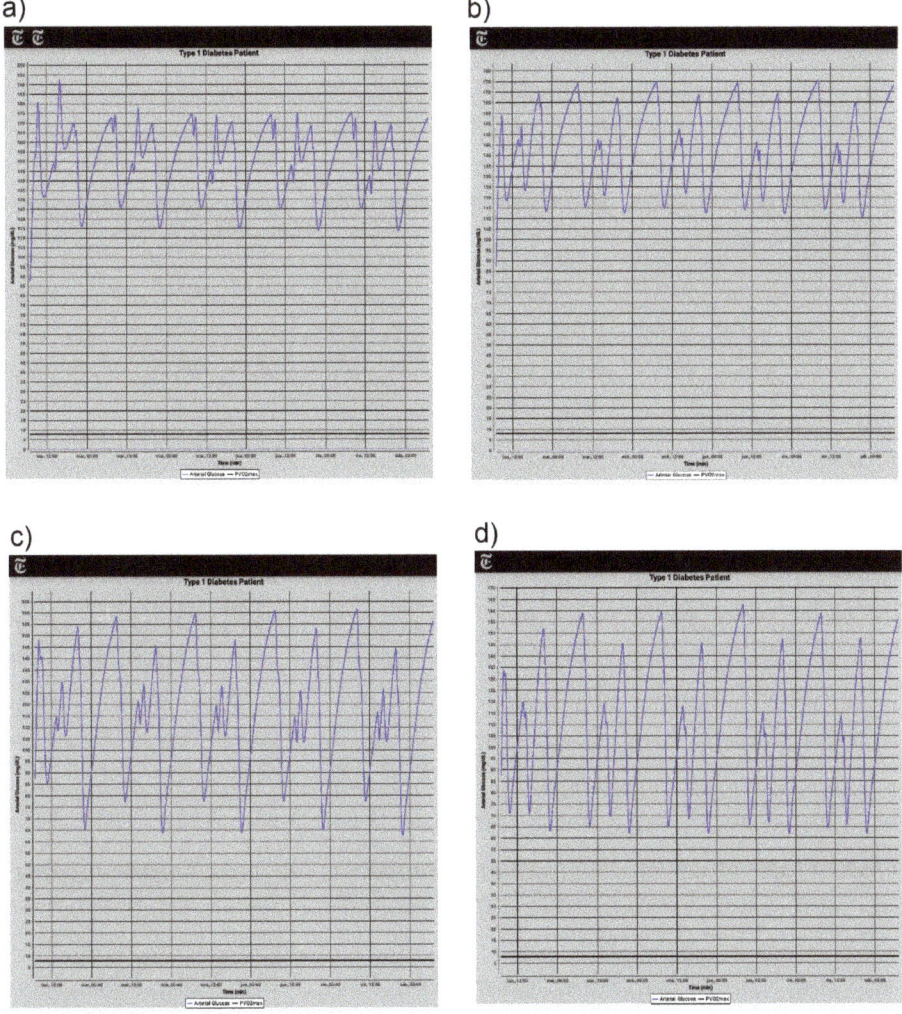

Figure 5. Comparison of blood glucose plots generated by AEDMA application for several values of carbohydrate grams and insulin units. (**a**) Experiment 1. (**b**) Experiment 2. (**c**) Experiment 3. (**d**) Experiment 4.

In Figure 6, a validation of the exercise models through the corresponding simulation plots are shown. In order to obtain the reported plots, the used exercise intensities are light, moderate, and heavy, and the exercise durations are 10, 30, and 90 min. The default values for grams of carbohydrate intake and insulin doses are used. In Figure 6a, the simulation using 10 min of light exercise is shown. The value of the glucose peaks after exercise (at 9:00 AM) is close to 185 mg/dL, but using 30 min of light exercise, this is under 180 mg/dL (Figure 6b), and when using 90 min of light exercise, the glucose peaks is close to 175 mg/dL (Figure 6c). Similar behavior is shown when using the same duration but with moderate exercise (Figure 6d–f). The value of the glucose peaks after exercise (at 9:00 AM) is close to 175 mg/dL, and it is low when compared with the same peak obtained when using light exercise (180 mg/dL). Finally, this behavior remains when using heavy exercise (Figure 6g–i). For comparing exercise intensities, it can be shown from plots that the glucose peaks after 10 min exercise are: close to

185 mg/dL for light exercise, over 175 mg/dL for moderate exercise, and below 170 mg/dL for heavy exercise. Similar results are obtained for 30 and 90 min of exercise duration. In general, there are many applications, however, long-term prediction of glucose still remains a challenge [20]. In this work, an app has been developed capable of predicting the behavior of glucose levels for several days (see Figure 5) or during a day with different exercise regimes (see Figure 6).

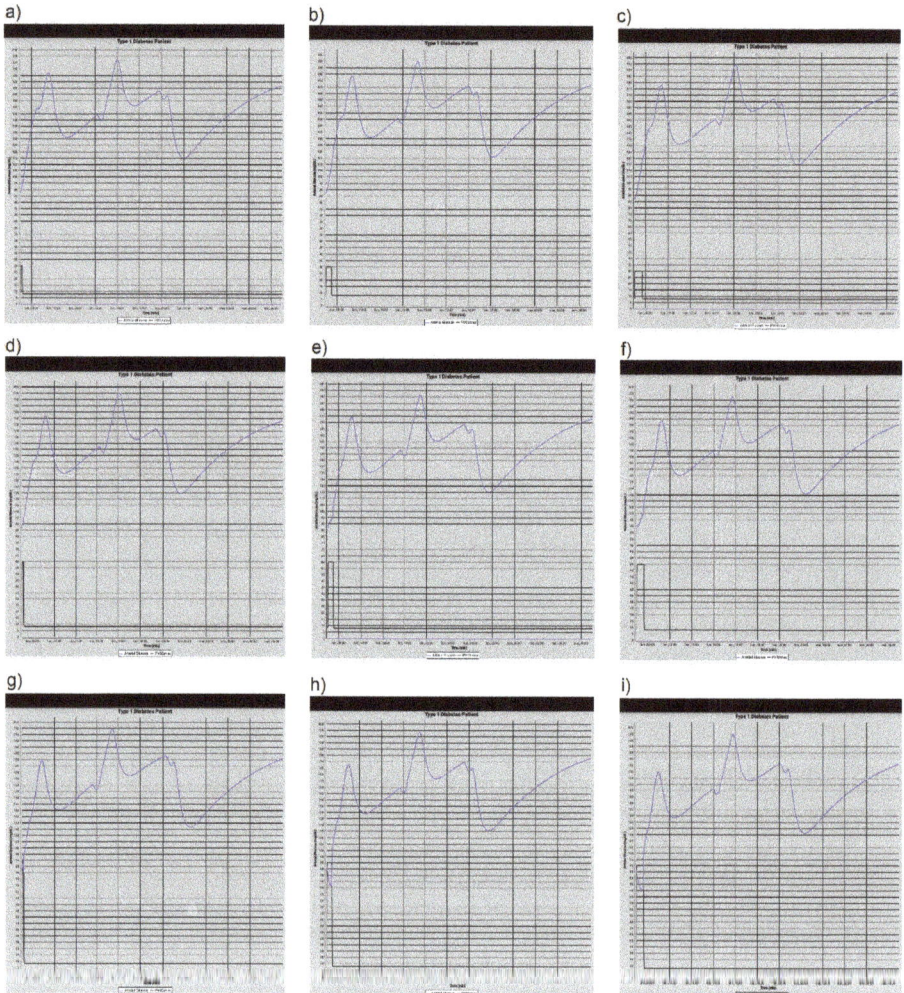

Figure 6. Comparison of blood glucose plots generated by AEDMA application for several exercise intensities using experiment 1 settings. (**a**) Light exercise—10 min. (**b**) Light exercise—30 min. (**c**) Light exercise—90 min. (**d**) Moderate exercise—10 min. (**e**) Moderate exercise—30 min. (**f**) Moderate exercise—90 min. (**g**) Heavy exercise—10 min. (**h**) Heavy exercise—30 min. (**i**) Heavy exercise—90 min.

Until now, the complete software of the presented application has not been compared with other applications since our priority is to focus on the diet and physical activity of the Mexican population with diabetes. There are many applications, but with European or United States standards. However, each submodel has been compared and validated separately by its respective authors. It is important to point out that the current version of the application presented in this work is an extension of a previous compartmental model that takes into account exercise periods. This model was developed by the main author, who validated and compared its results with experimental data [41]. So far, we have performed a prototype test on 26 young adults and execution times comparison for different devices.

4.3. Qualitative Study

For validating the AEDMA, we perform a prototype test using a questionnaire to evaluate the main points of the proposed system. We applied a questionnaire to 26 young adults (age 15–25). This application is focused mainly on this user group, which is highly familiar with tablet or smartphone devices, and they are regular users of mobile apps. We restrict the participants of the prototype test to have an android device because we designed AEDMA specifically for this mobile OS. In Table 4, relevant information about the distribution of the testing subjects is shown.

Table 4. Relevant data of testing subjects.

Gender		Age		Previous Knowledge of Mobiles Apps for Diabetes Treatment	
Male	Female	15–19	20–25	Yes	No
76.9%	23.1%	38.5%	61.5%	15.4%	84.6%

After testing the ADEMA by at least 1 h in the participant's device, they were asked to answer a questionnaire that contains 10 questions related to the key aspects of the AEDMA. Each question has 5 options, rated from NO, Rather NO, Do not know, Rather YES, and YES. The questions and the percentage of responses for each option are summarized in Table 5. From the obtained responses, we can summarize the following remarks:

1. From questions 1, 3, 4, and 5, a preliminary conclusion about important points to be improved to the AEDMA can be guessed. These points are related to improving the user interface, the clarity, and legibility of presented glucose level graphs, and the ease of use of the app. Question 8 gives a general panorama showing that the mobile app in its current state can be improved. From question 9, the variability of glucose levels is adequate from the user's perspective.
2. In general, from questions 2 and 7, we can conclude that the AEDMA is useful and to give an appropriate impression to the test user, to reuse the application if a next version is released. Question 10 allows highlighting the importance of giving users an important role to involve them in the design of these types of apps.

Table 5. Results of the questionnaire for the test group.

Question	1 (No)%	2 (Rather No)%	3 (Do Not Know)%	4 (Rather Yes)%	5 (Yes)%
(1) Are the user interface controls adequate to the type of data required by the app?	15.4%	15.4%	15.4%	38.5%	15.4%
(2) Is the application useful?	23.1%	0%	0%	0%	76.9%
(3) Are the generated graphs easy to understand?	7.7%	0%	23.1%	46.2%	23.1%
(4) Do the application's user interface controls allow to manage the application in an ease way?	0%	7.7%	7.7%	46.2%	38.5%
(5) How difficult has been the use of the app?	15.4%	38.5%	30.8%	15.4%	0%
(6) Does the application motivate to study more in depth the phenomena?	0%	0%	15.4%	46.2%	38.5%
(7) Will you reuse the app?	0%	7.7%	7.7%	15.4%	69.2%
(8) Do you consider that current app can be improved?	7.7%	0%	0%	23.1%	69.2%
(9) Do you consider appropriate the functionality of the application for learning the glucose levels variability?	0%	0%	7.7%	38.5%	53.8%
(10) Do you consider the mobile application are sufficient to assess whether in the future you would like to participate in similar experiences with mobile apps?	0%	0%	23.1%	38.5%	38.5%

4.4. Execution Time Comparison

We obtain a measurement of the time required to conclude the simulation using several parameters for each application's deployment device. Table 6 shows the obtained measurements for each device. We compute each measurement using only one thread environment because a multithread environment was not conceived in the original application. We choose the following simulation times: 4 days, one week, two weeks, and three weeks. A Polaroid tablet device obtained the biggest execution time, while a Galaxy Tab 10.1 device obtained the shortest one. The rows in Table 6 start from the slower to the higher simulation time. The mobile devices used for the application's deployment were not recent models, because even when some of them were featured as high-end devices when released, they are old devices and, with recent advances in mobile technology, many of them can be featured as low or middle-end devices when compared with the existing technology available at the time of writing this paper.

Table 6. Time to complete computation of glucose concentration plots (in seconds) using several simulation time durations.

Device	Simulation Time Duration			
	4 Days	1 Week	2 Weeks	3 Weeks
Polaroid Tab	12.30	13.53	16.24	21.11
Galaxy S2	9.53	10.97	13.16	18.16
Galaxy S4	6.53	7.64	9.17	12.84
LG G3 Stylus	5.53	6.59	7.90	11.30
Galaxy Tab 10.1	5.53	6.70	8.04	11.73

5. Conclusions

In this paper, an application for diabetes education is proposed. The proposed application was designed to provide a software tool to help support therapy in patients with diabetes, seeking to improve the quality of life. The simulation is fixed, but an interactive simulation functionality can be added to provide a richer user experience. The software is based on four mathematical models originally designed as a desktop computer program. An exercise option in the interface helps patients to schedule their routines and to estimate in advance its impact on blood glucose. This app could also be developed for Apples' iOS products. Besides, this app could potentially be implemented as a smartwatch app. The most important conclusions are:

1. The App includes glucose regulation associated with metabolism and the application of an insulin injection.
2. The App is capable of taking into account the effects of food intake and physical activity.
3. The developed application can simulate the behavior of glucose levels for long periods.
4. The App is capable of considering three types of physical activity: light, moderate and heavy.
5. The developed application is focused on type-1 diabetes, but this can be extended to consider type-2 diabetes.
6. As a future improvement, the application should be modified to split the simulation processing into smaller operations running on multiple threads. This could be beneficial in devices with more than one core.

Author Contributions: Conceptualization, M.H.-O., M.A.N.-M.; Formal Analysis, C.A.C.-A., A.R.-L.; Investigation, M.A.N.-M., G.E.O.-C., J.M.C.-C.; Methodology, M.H.-O., C.A.C.-A., G.E.O.-C., R.S.-H., O.M.-R.; Project Administration, M.H.-O., R.S.-H.; Software, M.H.-O., G.E.O.-C., J.M.C.-C., O.M.-R.; Supervision, M.H.-O., M.A.N.-M., A.R.-L., O.M.-R.; Validation, A.R.-L., R.S.-H., J.M.C.-C.; Visualization, A.R.-L., J.M.C.-C., O.M.-R.; Writing Original Draft, M.H.-O., M.A.N.-M., C.A.C.-A., G.E.O.-C.; Writing Review and Editing, M.A.N.-M., C.A.C.-A., R.S.-H. All authors have read and agreed to the published version of the manuscript.

Funding: This research received no external funding.

Acknowledgments: The present project was partially funded by the National Council of Science and Technology of México (CONACYT) through a scholarship (no. 337087) granted to José Margarito Canseco-Cortinas. The authors are grateful for the support provided by TNM-ITV, CONACYT and PRODEP.

Conflicts of Interest: The authors declare no conflict of interest.

References

1. World Health Organization. *Obesity and Overweight Fact Sheet*; WHO: Geneva, Switzerland, 2016.
2. World Health Organization. *Diabetes Fact Sheet*; WHO: Geneva, Switzerland, 2016.
3. Institute for Health Metrics and Evaluation. *The Global Burden of Disease: Generating Evidence, Guiding Policy*; IHME: Washington, DC, USA, 2013.
4. World Health Organization. *The Top 10 Causes of Death*; WHO: Geneva, Switzerland, 2017.
5. International Diabetes Federation. *IDF Diabetes Atlas*, 7th ed.; International Diabetes Federation: Brussels, Belgium, 2015.
6. Levy, T.S.; Nasu, L.C.; Dommarco, J.R.; Ávila, M.H. *Informe Final de Resultados, Encuesta Nacional de Salud y Nutrición de Medio Camino 2016*; Instituto Nacional de Salud Pública INSP: Mexico City, Mexico, 2016.
7. Institute for Health Metrics and Evaluation (IHME). Country Profile Mexico. Mexico, 2017. Available online: http://www.healthdata.org/ (accessed on 7 October 2018).
8. Statista Inc. Global Smartphone Sales to End Users 2007–2016. Available online: https://www.statista.com/statistics/263437/global-smartphone-sales-to-end-users-since-2007/ (accessed on 12 October 2018).
9. eMarketer. Worldwide Internet and Mobile Users: eMarketer's Updated Estimates and Forecast for 2015–2020. 2016. Available online: https://www.emarketer.com/Report/Worldwide-Internet-Mobile-Users-eMarketersUpdated-Estimates-Forecast-20152020/2001897#moreReport (accessed on 25 September 2018).
10. Lehmann, E. Preliminary experience with the Internet release of AIDA—An interactive educational diabetes simulator. *Comput. Methods Programs Biomed.* **1998**, *56*, 109–132. [CrossRef]
11. Hernandez-Ordonez, M.; Montano, O.; Campos-Delgado, D.U.; Palacios, E. Development of an Educational Simulator and Graphical User Interface for Diabetic Patients. In Proceedings of the 2007 4th International Conference on Electrical and Electronics Engineering, Mexico City, Mexico, 5–7 September 2007; pp. 82–85. [CrossRef]
12. Lehmann, E.D.; Tarín, C.; Bondia, J.; Teufel, E.; Deutsch, T. Development of AIDA v4.3b Diabetes Simulator: Technical Upgrade to Support Incorporation of Lispro, Aspart, and Glargine Insulin Analogues. *J. Electr. Comput. Eng.* **2011**, *2011*, 427196. [CrossRef]
13. Thestrup, J.; Gergely, T.; Beck, P. Exploring new care models in diabetes management and therapy with a wireless mobile eHealth platform. In *Wireless Mobile Communication and Healthcare: Second International ICST Conference, MobiHealth 2011, Kos Island, Greece, 5–7 October 2011*; Revised Selected Papers; Nikita, K.S., Lin, J.C., Fotiadis, D.I., Arredondo Waldmeyer, M.T., Eds.; Springer: Berlin/Heidelberg, Germany, 2012; pp. 203–210.
14. Erzen, F.C.; Birol, G.; Cinar, A. Glucosim: A simulator for education on the dynamics of diabetes mellitus. In Proceedings of the 23rd Annual International Conference of the IEEE Engineering in Medicine and Biology Society, Istambul, Turkey, 25–28 October 2001; Volume 4, pp. 3163–3166. [CrossRef]
15. Agar, B.U.; Eren, M.; Cinar, A. Glucosim: Educational software for virtual experiments with patients with type 1 diabetes. In Proceedings of the 2005 IEEE Engineering in Medicine and Biology 27th Annual Conference, Shanghai, China, 17–18 January 2006; pp. 845–848. [CrossRef]
16. Mougiakakou, S.G.; Prountzou, K.; Nikita, K.S. A Real Time Simulation Model of Glucose-Insulin Metabolism for Type 1 Diabetes Patients. In Proceedings of the 2005 IEEE Engineering in Medicine and Biology 27th Annual Conference, Shanghai, China, 17–18 January 2005; pp. 298–301. [CrossRef]
17. Bergman, R.N.; Phillips, L.S.; Cobelli, C. Physiologic evaluation of factors controlling glucose tolerance in man: Measurement of insulin sensitivity and beta-cell glucose sensitivity from the response to intravenous glucose. *J. Clin. Investig.* **1981**, *68*, 1456–1467. [CrossRef] [PubMed]
18. Cobelli, C.; Caumo, A.; Omenetto, M.; Sacca, L. Minimal model SG overestimation and SI underestimation: Improved accuracy by a Bayesian two-compartment model. *Am. J. Physiol.* **1999**, *277*, E481–E488.

19. Hovorka, R.; Shojaee-Moradie, F.; Carroll, P.V.; Chassin, L.J.; Gowrie, I.J.; Jackson, N.C.; Tudor, R.S.; Umpleby, A.M.; Jones, R.H. Partitioning glucose distribution/trans-port, disposal, and endogenous production during IVGTT. *Am. J. Physiol.* **2002**, *282*, E992–E1007.
20. Liu, C.; Vehí, J.; Avari, P.; Reddy, M.; Oliver, N.; Georgiou, P.; Herrero, P. Long-Term Glucose Forecasting Using a Physiological Model and Deconvolution of the Continuous Glucose Monitoring Signal. *Sensors* **2019**, *19*, 4338. [CrossRef]
21. Liu, C.; Avari, P.; Leal, Y.; Wos, M.; Sivasithamparam, K.; Georgiou, P.; Reddy, M.; Fernández-Real, J.M.; Martin, C.; Fernández-Balsells, M.; et al. A Modular Safety System for an Insulin Dose Recommender: A Feasibility Study. *J. Diabetes Sci. Technol.* **2019**, *14*, 87–96. [CrossRef]
22. Sangeetha, S.; Sreepradha, C.; Sobana, S.; Bidisha, P.; Panda, R.C. Modeling and Control of the Glucose-Insulin-Glucagon System in Type I Diabetis Mellitus. *ChemBioEng Rev.* **2020**, *3*, 89–100. [CrossRef]
23. Knopp, J.L.; Hardy, A.R.; Vergeer, S.; Chase, J.G. Modelling insulin adsorption in intravenous infusion sets in the intensive care unit. *IFAC J. Syst. Control* **2019**, *8*, 100042. [CrossRef]
24. Visentin, R.; Schiavon, M.; Basu, R.; Basu, A.; Man, C.D.; Cobelli, C. Physiological models for artificial pancreas development. In *The Artificial Pancreas: Current Situation and Future Directions*, 1st ed.; Sánchez-Peña, R.S., Cherñavvsky, D.R., Eds.; Academic Press: Cambridge, MA, USA, 2019; Volume 1, pp. 123–152.
25. Maas, A.H.; van der Molen, P.; van de Vijver, R.; Chen, W.; van Pul, C.; Cottaar, E.J.; van Riel, N.A.; Hilbers, P.A.; Haak, H.R. Concept Development of the Eindhoven Diabetes Education Simulator Project. *Games Health J.* **2016**, *5*, 120–127. [CrossRef]
26. Ristau, R.A.; Yang, J.; White, J.R. Evaluation and Evolution of Diabetes Mobile Applications: Key Factors for Health Care Professionals Seeking to Guide Patients. *Diabetes Spectr.* **2013**, *26*, 211–215. Available online: http://spectrum.diabetesjournals.org/content/26/4/211.full.pdf (accessed on 17 September 2018). [CrossRef]
27. El-Gayar, O.; Timsina, P.; Nawar, N.; Eid, W. Mobile Applications for Diabetes Self-Management: Status and Potential. *J. Diabetes Sci. Technol.* **2013**, *7*, 247–262. [CrossRef] [PubMed]
28. Chomutare, T.; Fernandez-Luque, L.; Arsand, E.; Hartvigsen, G. Features of mobile diabetes applications: Review of the literature and analysis of current applications compared against evidence-based guidelines. *J. Med Internet Res.* **2011**, *13*, e65. [CrossRef] [PubMed]
29. Huckvale, K.; Adomaviciute, S.; Prieto, J.T.; Leow, M.K.S.; Car, J. Smartphone apps for calculating insulin dose: A systematic assessment. *BMC Med.* **2015**, *13*, 106. [CrossRef] [PubMed]
30. Cui, M.; Wu, X.; Mao, J.; Wang, X.; Nie, M. T2DM Self-Management via Smartphone Applications: A Systematic Review and Meta-Analysis. *PLoS ONE* **2016**, *11*, e0166718. [CrossRef] [PubMed]
31. Garcia, E.; Martin, C.; Garcia, A.; Harrison, R.; Flood, D. Systematic Analysis of Mobile Diabetes Management Applications on Different Platforms. In Proceedings of the 7th Conference on Workgroup Human-Computer Interaction and Usability Engineering of the Austrian Computer Society: Information Quality in e-Health, Graz, Austria, 25–26 November 2011; Springer: Berlin/Heidelberg, Germany, 2011. USAB'11. pp. 379–396.
32. Baskaran, V.; Prescod, F.; Dong, L. A Smartphone-Based Cloud Computing Tool for Managing Type 1 Diabetes in Ontarians. *Can. J. Diabetes* **2015**, *39*, 200–203. [CrossRef]
33. Chomutare, T.; Tatara, N.; Arsand, E.; Hartvigsen, G. Designing a diabetes mobile application with social network support. In *Studies in Health Technology and Informatics*; IOS Press: Clifton, NJ, USA, 2013.
34. Nguyen, H.D.; Jiang, X.; Poo, D.C.C. Designing a Social Mobile Platform for Diabetes Self-management: A Theory-Driven Perspective. In *Social Computing and Social Media: 7th International Conference, SCSM 2015, Held as Part of HCI International 2015, Los Angeles, CA, USA, 2–7 August 2015, Proceedings*; Meiselwitz, G., Ed.; Springer International Publishing: Cham, Switzerland, 2015; pp. 67–77.
35. Garnweidner-Holme, L.M.; Borgen, I.; Garitano, I.; Noll, J.; Lukasse, M. Designing and Developing a Mobile Smartphone Application for Women with Gestational Diabetes Mellitus Followed-Up at Diabetes Outpatient Clinics in Norway. *Healthcare* **2015**, *3*, 310–323. [CrossRef]
36. Borgen, I.; Garnweidner-Holme, L.M.; Jacobsen, A.F.; Bjerkan, K.; Fayyad, S.; Joranger, P.; Lilleengen, A.M.; Mosdøl, A.; Noll, J.; Småstuen, M.C.; et al. Smartphone application for women with gestational diabetes mellitus: A study protocol for a multicentre randomised controlled trial. *BMJ Open* **2017**, *7*, e013117. Available online: http://bmjopen.bmj.com/content/7/3/e013117.full.pdf (accessed on 12 December 2018). [CrossRef]
37. Lloyd, B.; Groat, D.; Cook, C.; Kaufman, D.; Grando, A. IDECIDE: A mobile application for insulin dosing using an evidence based equation to account for patient preferences. In *Studies in Health Technology and Informatics*; IOS Press: Clifton, NJ, USA, 2015; Volume 216, pp. 93–97. [CrossRef]

38. Keith-Hynes, P.; Mize, B.; Robert, A.; Place, J. The Diabetes Assistant: A Smartphone-Based System for Real-Time Control of Blood Glucose. *Electronics* **2014**, *3*, 609–623. [CrossRef]
39. González, A.A.; Voos, H.; Darouach, M. Glucose-Insulin System Based on Minimal Model: A Realistic Approach. In Proceedings of the 2015 17th UKSIM-AMSS International Conference on Modelling and Simulation, Cambridge, UK, 25–27 March 2015; IEEE Computer Society: Washington, DC, USA, 2015. UKSIM '15. pp. 55–60. [CrossRef]
40. Sorensen, J.T. A Physiologic Model of Glucose Metabolism in Man and Its Use to Design and Assess Improved Insulin Therapies for Diabetes. Ph.D. Thesis, Massachusetts Institute of Technology. Dept. of Chemical Engineering, Berkeley, CA, USA, 1985.
41. Hernández-Ordoñez, M.; Campos-Delgado, D. An extension to the compartmental model of type 1 diabetic patients to reproduce exercise periods with glycogen depletion and replenishment. *J. Biomech.* **2008**, *41*, 744–752. [CrossRef]
42. Berger, M.; Rodbard, D. Computer simulation of plasma insulin and glucose dynamics after subcutaneous insulin injection. *Diabetes Care* **1989**, *12*, 725–736. [CrossRef] [PubMed]
43. Lehmann, E.; Deutsch, T. A physiological model of glucose-insulin interaction in type 1 diabetes mellitus. *J. Biomed. Eng.* **1992**, *14*, 235–242. [CrossRef]
44. Wilinska, M.E.; Chassin, L.J.; Schaller, H.C.; Schaupp, L.; Pieber, T.R.; Hovorka, R. Insulin kinetics in type-1 diabetes: Continuous and bolus delivery of rapid acting insulin. *IEEE Trans. Biomed. Eng.* **2005**, *52*, 3–12. [CrossRef] [PubMed]
45. Jahoda, P. MPAndroidChart. 2016. Available online: https://github.com/PhilJay/MPAndroidChart (accessed on 15 November 2018).

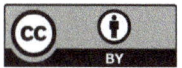

© 2020 by the authors. Licensee MDPI, Basel, Switzerland. This article is an open access article distributed under the terms and conditions of the Creative Commons Attribution (CC BY) license (http://creativecommons.org/licenses/by/4.0/).

MDPI\
St. Alban-Anlage 66\
4052 Basel\
Switzerland\
Tel. +41 61 683 77 34\
Fax +41 61 302 89 18\
www.mdpi.com

Applied Sciences Editorial Office\
E-mail: applsci@mdpi.com\
www.mdpi.com/journal/applsci

www.ingramcontent.com/pod-product-compliance
Lightning Source LLC
LaVergne TN
LVHW070440100526
838202LV00014B/1639